MANAGEMENT OF UPPER GASTROINTESTINAL CANCER

Commissioning Editor: **Rachael Stock**
Development Editor: **Tim Kimber**
Project Supervisor: **Mark Sanderson**
Cover Design: **Pete Wilder**

MANAGEMENT OF UPPER GASTROINTESTINAL CANCER

Edited by

JOHN M. DALY MD
PROFESSOR OF SURGERY,
WEILL MEDICAL COLLEGE OF CORNELL UNIVERSITY,
NEW YORK PRESBYTERIAN HOSPITAL,
NEW YORK, USA

THOMAS P. J. HENNESSY MD, FRCS, FRCSI
REGIUS PROFESSOR OF SURGERY,
ST JAMES' HOSPITAL,
DUBLIN, IRELAND

JOHN V. REYNOLDS MD, FRCSI
DEPARTMENT OF CLINICAL SURGERY,
ST JAMES' HOSPITAL,
DUBLIN, IRELAND

 W. B. SAUNDERS COMPANY LTD

London · Edinburgh · New York · Philadelphia · Toronto · Sydney · Tokyo

WB SAUNDERS
An imprint of Harcourt Brace and Company Limited

© Harcourt Brace and Company 1999

 is a registered trademark of Harcourt Brace and Company Limited

The right of J M Daly, T P J Hennessy and J V Reynolds to be identified as editors of this work has been asserted by them in accordance with the Copyright, Designs and Patents Act 1988

ISBN 0 7020 2147 4

British Library Cataloguing in Publication Data
A catalogue record for this book is available from the British Library

Library of Congress Cataloging in Publication Data
A catalog record for this book is available from the Library of Congress

Note
Medical knowledge is constantly changing. As new information becomes available, changes in treatment, procedures, equipment and the use of drugs become necessary. The editors, contributors, and the publishers have, as far as it is possible, taken care to ensure that the information given in this text is accurate and up-to-date. However, readers are strongly advised to confirm that the information, especially with regard to drug usage, complies with the latest legislation and standards of practice.

The publishers have made every effort to trace the copyright holders for borrowed material. If they have inadvertently overlooked any, they will be pleased to make the necessary arrangements at the first opportunity.

The
Publisher's
policy is to use
**paper manufactured
from sustainable forests**

Typeset by Keyword Publishing Services, Barking, Essex, UK
Printed in China

CONTENTS

PREFACE

The remarkable renewal of interest in all aspects of upper gastrointestinal cancer in recent years can be attributed to the great expansion of technological advances in investigative techniques, management strategies and treatment modalities. We felt that it would be appropriate to collate this accumulated knowledge in a single volume, and consider ourselves fortunate to have successfully recruited a team of leading authors, who have made substantial contributions to the clinical and technological advances that have occurred.

The book has been divided into four parts. The first, *General Management*, deals with the important subject of staging techniques, so vital for modern management and audit. Barrett's Esophagus and its significance in the development of adenocarcinoma is also considered in this section. Part 1 concludes with a detailed discussion of quality of life issues.

In Part 2, *Gastric Cancer*, the contributors have separately looked at the Western Experience, the Japanese Experience, Early Gastric Cancer and Gastric Lymphoma. The authors of the chapters on the Western Experience have been careful to point out that adherence to Japanese treatment principles has enabled many specialized centres in the US and Europe to achieve outcomes more akin to those of the Japanese Experience.

The four chapters in Part 3 are devoted to *Esophageal Cancer*. These contributions consider both the Western Experience and Japanese Experience and, once again, while acknowledging such differences as a consequence of differing histological types, the point is made that outcome differences probably depend on treatment techniques and the stage at which the disease is treated. There is also a chapter on Combined Modality Therapy and a comprehensive chapter on Complications.

The final two chapters which make up Part 4 of the book look at *Palliation* from the point of view of radiotherapy and other modalities. It is hardly necessary to emphasize the importance of palliation in a disease which so frequently presents at a late stage and with a poor prognosis.

The aim of this book is to provide a comprehensive and balanced account of current approaches to the diagnosis and management of upper gastrointestinal cancer and it is our hope that this aim has been achieved.

John M. Daly
Thomas P. J. Hennessy
John V. Reynolds

CONTRIBUTORS

Hiroshi Akiyama   Department of Surgery, Toranomon Hospital, Tokyo, Japan

Derek Alderson   Bristol Royal Infirmary, University Department of Surgery, Bristol, UK

Stephen Attwood   Hope Hospital, Division of Oesophageal and Gastric Surgery, Salford, UK

Jane M. Blazeby   Bristol Royal Infirmary, University Department of Surgery, Bristol, UK

Knut Böttcher   Technischen Universität, Klinikum rechts der Isar, Munich, Germany

Murray F. Brennan   Memorial Sloan-Kettering Cancer Center, Department of Surgery, New York, New York, USA

Linda S. Callans   University of Pennsylvania School of Medicine, Department of Surgery, Pennsylvania, USA

Lawrence R. Coia   Community Medical Center, Department of Radiation Oncology, Toms River, New Jersey, USA

John M. Daly   Weill Medical College of Cornell University, Department of Surgery, New York Presbyterian Hospital, New York, New York, USA

Thomas P. J. Hennessy   St James' Hospital, Department of Clinical Surgery, Dublin, Ireland

Robert Ivker   Department of Radiation Oncology, Community Medical Center, Tomes River, New Jersey, USA

Glyn G. Jamieson   Department of Surgery, Royal Adelaide Hospital, Adelaide, Australia

Martin S. Karpeh   Memorial Sloan-Kettering Cancer Center, Department of Surgery, New York, New York, USA

David Kelsen   Memorial Sloan-Kettering Cancer Center, Department of Medicine, New York, New York, USA

Simon Y. K. Law   Queen Mary Hospital, Department of Surgery, University of Hong Kong Medical Centre, Hong Kong

Iain G. Martin   Division of Surgery, Leeds General Infirmary, Leeds, UK

George Mathew   Department of Surgery, Royal Adelaide Hospital, Adelaide, Australia

Alexander A. Parikh   University of Cincinnati College of Medicine, Department of Surgery, Cincinnati, USA

John V. Reynolds   St James' Hospital, Department of Clinical Surgery, Dublin, Ireland

Mitsuru Sasako   Department of Surgical Oncology, National Cancer Center Hospital, Tokyo, Japan

Roderich E. Schwarz   City of Hope Medical Center, Department of Oncologic Surgery, California, USA

Andreas Sendler   Technische Universität, Department of Surgery, Klinikum rechts der Isar, Munich, Germany

J. Rüdiger Siewert   Technische Universität, Department of Surgery, Klinikum rechts der Isar, Munich, Germany

Harushi Udagawa   Department of Surgery, Toranomon Hospital, Tokyo, Japan

John Wong   Queen Mary Hospital, Department of Surgery, University of Hong Kong Medical Centre, Hong Kong

PART
1

General

1

STAGING OF ESOPHAGEAL AND GASTRIC CARCINOMA

IAIN G. MARTIN

INTRODUCTION

The "staging" process is the sequential acquisition of information designed to give the clinician accurate and comparative prognostic information. Accurate staging of upper gastrointestinal malignancies is central to good clinical practice, research, and audit. Information obtained from staging investigations enters every decision made in the treatment of patients with esophageal or gastric carcinoma. It is important that the patient with early disease does not receive inappropriately aggressive treatment, that the patient with very advanced disease is not subjected to treatments with no hope of success, and that the patient with significant chance of recurrence after single modality therapy receives appropriate adjuvant therapy. Without reliable staging information, each of these possibilities are much more likely.

The methodologies available for staging these cancers have increased considerably over the past 10 years. While these technologies have undoubtedly produced more accurate information, the optimal staging methods remain controversial. With current trends towards multi-modality therapy for upper gastrointestinal cancers, and neoadjuvant therapy in particular, accurate staging is becoming increasingly important.

All staging information obtained requires that a framework or system is devised to enable the accurate and consistent recording of the findings from the patient. Not only should such a system be unambiguous and easily understood, but it should convey to the clinician information of prognostic and therapeutic importance. The aim of this chapter is to describe currently utilized staging systems for both esophageal and gastric malignancy, the methods for obtaining such staging data points, and the therapeutic and prognostic importance of the information acquired.

The process of acquiring staging information is a continuum from the initial clinical assessment of the patient, through preoperative investigations, the findings at operation and the final histopathologic examination of any resected specimen. An important area for the future will be the molecular classification of tumors from which much important prognostic information will be derived. Developments are already being made in this area and in years to come, molecular staging will I am sure be a very important tool in the classification and treatment of patients with upper gastrointestinal cancer. This area cannot be included within the confines of this chapter given its great complexity and very rapid evolution.

An individual patient may therefore have staging information derived from any one, or indeed, all of these processes. The summation of these data points gives a final definitive, "stage". This chapter will describe this process for both esophageal and gastric cancer, highlighting difficulties, controversies, and current "best practice".

ESOPHAGEAL CANCER

Staging systems

There is no doubt that a system for the accurate classification and recording of staging information is crucial to both clinical and research oncology. However, to date, no entirely satisfactory system has been devised for cancer of the esophagus. Although the past decade has seen much progress towards the development of such a system, many of the more detailed points remain to be clarified. In particular, and in contrast to several other gastrointestinal malignancies, an internationally recognized method for the mapping of lymph node stations is not available. Despite these difficulties, it is the TNM system of the UICC (Union Internationale Contre le Cancer) that forms the mainstay of current clinical and pathological staging systems.

TNM classification

The UICC TNM classification for esophageal cancers first appeared in the 1st edition of the TNM manual in 1968.[1] This system was revised in 1974 and 1978.[2,3] Despite these frequent revisions, the TNM system had several shortcomings, notably its poor ability to predict survival. Following suggestions from the Japanese Committee for Registration of Esophageal Carcinoma in 1985, a fourth fully revised system was proposed in 1987.[4] It is the 1987 system which is currently in use, and which internationally remains the accepted method for staging esophageal carcinomas. There still remain however a number of difficulties with the 1987 TNM classification, in particular the classification of involved lymph nodes. These are discussed in more detail in the paragraphs following the description of the Japanese staging system.

As with any tumor, the TNM system aims to describe the extent of disease in terms of the local tumor (T), lymph node metastases (N) and distant metastases (M). The TNM system also provides for a stage classification (I–IV) based upon tumor groups with a similar prognosis.

T classification
- T1 – tumor localized to the mucosa or submucosa
- T2 – tumor invading the muscularis propria
- T3 – tumor invading the adventitia
- T4 – tumor invading other structures

As distinct from the stomach, with the exception of the intra-abdominal portion, there is no serosa associated with the esophagus.

N classification
- N0 – no regional lymph node metastases
- N1 – regional lymph node metastases

In the UICC classification, as distinct from the Japanese system, the regional nodes are described as mediastinal or perigastric for all tumors except those arising within the cervical esophagus. In this latter case, involved cervical nodes including supraclavicular nodes are regarded as N1 disease. It is in the area of classification of lymph node metastases that the largest differences exist between the UICC system and the Japanese system. These differences and their importance are discussed below.

M classification
- M0 – no evidence of distant metastases
- M1 – distant metastases, including distant lymph nodes

The UICC have published a new version of their TNM classification which contains some important changes for esophageal carcinoma.[5]

The main change has been a subclassification of M1 diseases as follows:

Upper-third tumors
- M1a – cervical lymph node metastases
- M1b – all other metastases

Middle-third tumors
- M1a – not applicable
- M1b – all metastatic disease

Lower-third tumors
- M1a – celiac lymph node metastases
- M1b – all other metastatic disease

As a consequence, stage IV disease (cf **Table 1.1**) has been subdivided into:

- IVA – M1a disease
- IVB – M1b disease

TNM stage grouping   The TNM stage groupings are shown in Table 1.1. While stage grouping brings together patients of similar prognosis, the actual figures reported vary quite considerably from series to series. Typical figures for stage I disease would be 60–70% 5-year survival rate, stage IIA disease 40–70%, stage IIB disease 25–40%, and stage III disease 15–25%. For patients with stage IV

Table 1.1 UICC stage grouping for esophageal carcinoma based on the 1987 TNM classification[4]

STAGE 0	STAGE I	STAGE IIA	STAGE IIB	STAGE III	STAGE IV
Tis N0 M0	T1 N0 M0	T2 N0 M0	T1 N1 M0	T3 N1 M0	M1
		T3 N0 M0	T2 N1 M0	T4 N0 M0	
				T4 N1 M0	

disease, overall few will survive 5 years. However, a patient can be classified as stage IV disease on the basis of positive celiac axis nodes alone. When treated with radical three-field lymphadenectomy, the 5-year survival rate for these patients can be as high as 19%.[6] This paradox illustrates some of the problems with the classification of lymph node metastases in the UICC TNM system.

UICC anatomic subsites In addition to providing the definitions for the TNM stage of tumors, the UICC system classifies the esophagus into four regions. These definitions of these regions have been drawn from the Japanese guidelines (*vide infra*).

 i.   The cervical esophagus (Japanese terminology – Ce) extending from the lower border of the cricoid cartilage and ending at the sternal notch, approximately 18 cm from the upper incisor teeth.
 ii. The upper thoracic esophagus (Japanese terminology – Iu) extending from the thoracic inlet to the level of the tracheal bifurcation, approximately 24 cm from the upper incisor teeth.
 iii. The mid-thoracic esophagus (Japanese terminology – Im) extends over the proximal half of the esophagus between the tracheal bifurcation and the esophagogastric junction; approximately between 24 and 32 cm from the upper incisor teeth.
 iv. The lower thoracic and abdominal esophagus (Japanese terminology – E) covering the distal half of the esophagus between the tracheal bifurcation and the esophagogastric junction; approximately 32–40 cm from the upper incisor teeth.

Japanese classification

In common with much of their surgical oncology, the Japanese have devoted great time and effort to produce a staging classification for esophageal car-cinoma. While this is not as detailed or descriptive as the Japanese rules for the study of gastric carcinoma, it is still substantially more intricate than the three-variable UICC TNM system.[7]

Tumor location As described above, the UICC used the Japanese guide lines to draw up the 1987 definitions of tumor location. There are a number of minor differences in nomenclature, but the anatomic landmarks used are identical. The classification provides for a separate subclassification of the lower thoracic esophagus from the abdominal esophagus (Ei and Ea respectively), but is otherwise identical.

Tumor depth The Japanese classification for depth of tumor invasion uses a seven-point system:

 i.   EP – tumor confined to the epithelium
 ii. MM – tumor confined to the muscularis mucosae
 iii. SM – tumor confined to the submucosa
 iv. MP – tumor confined to the muscularis propria
 v.   A1 – tumor through the muscularis propria and possibly invading the adventitia
 vi. A2 – definite adventitial invasion
 vii. A3 – invasion of neighboring tissues/organs

Using 5-year survival as a guide to the usefulness of this more detailed system, compared with the simpler T stage of the UICC system, then few advantages are seen. The survival of EP and MM tumors are almost identical (58 versus 56% at 5 years), as are the survival of MP and A1 (30 versus 25% at 5 years) tumors. On this basis it would seem that the use of the T stage of the UICC system provides as much prognostic information as does the more complex Japanese classification of depth of invasion.

Nodal metastases There are two methods used to describe lymph nodes and lymph node metastases. The first uses a topographic system to provide precise information regarding the anatomic location of lymph nodes. The second is a method for grouping nodes into categories of prognostic importance. Even in Japan there is no consensus as regards the topographic system for describing the location of lymph nodes relevant to the esophagus. The Japanese Society for Esophageal Diseases[7] has proposed a numeric system extending the system used for the classification of gastric neoplasms to the thorax and neck. This is described and illustrated in **Table 1.2** and **Figure 1.1**. In contrast, Akiyama[8] has proposed a system based upon lymph node groups in seven anatomic drainage sites (cervical, superior, middle, and lower mediastinal, superior gastric, celiac trunk, and common hepatic regions). This classification was based upon Akiyama's vast personal experience and the lymphatic drainage studies of Tanabe *et al.*[9] and Haagensen.[10] The detailed lymph node groups in Akiyama's system are described in **Table 1.3**. There is no consensus as to which system offers the best prognostic information and neither system has been widely adopted outside of Japan.

The Japanese guidelines divide lymph node metastases into five groups.

- N−, no nodal metastases
- N1+, paraesophageal nodal metastases
- N2+, other mediastinal and perigastric nodal metastases

- N3+, abdominal lymph node metastases other than perigastric nodes
- N4+, more distant nodes, including cervical nodes

The precise classification of any individual nodal metastasis would depend upon the location of the primary tumor, as shown in **Table 1.4**. Typical overall 5-year survival rates for these groups would be 40%, 20%, 15%, 6%, and 2% respectively.

How should lymph node metastases be described?

While the fourth edition of the UICC TNM classification has brought this system much closer to the Japanese classification, it is in the area of grouping of lymph node metastases that discrepancies, and indeed controversy, still feature. There are two major areas of debate, firstly should a topographic lymph node station map be used and if so, what should be the basis for this map? Secondly, how should the various tiers or groups of lymph nodes be described?

There is no consensus with which to answer the first point. As described above, neither of the two Japanese systems has gained widespread international acceptance. All would be in agreement that ideally such a system should be produced and agreed upon internationally to allow accurate

Table 1.2 Topographic classification of esophageal lymph node groups as described by the Japanese Society for Esophageal Diseases[3] and the Japanese Research Society for Gastric Cancer[65]

\ THORACIC AND CERVICAL NODAL GROUPS		ABDOMINAL NODAL GROUPS	
NO.	DEFINITION	NO.	DEFINITION
100	Lateral cervical lymph nodes	1	Right cardiac lymph nodes
101	Cervical paraesophageal nodes	2	Left cardiac lymph nodes
102	Deep cervical lymph nodes	3	Lesser curvature lymph nodes
103	Retropharyngeal lymph nodes	4	Greater curvature lymph nodes
104	Supraclavicular lymph nodes	5	Suprapyloric lymph nodes
105	Upper thoracic paraesophageal nodes	6	Subpyloric lymph nodes
106	Thoracic paratracheal lymph nodes	7	Left gastric artery lymph nodes
107	Carinal lymph nodes	8	Common hepatic artery nodes
108	Middle thoracic paraesophageal nodes	9	Celiac axis lymph nodes
109	Pulmonary hilar lymph nodes	10	Splenic hilar lymph nodes
110	Lower thoracic paraesophageal nodes	11	Splenic artery lymph nodes
111	Diaphragmatic lymph nodes	12	Hepatoduodenal ligament nodes
112	Posterior mediastinal lymph nodes	13	Retropancreatic nodes
		14	Mesenteric lymph nodes
		15	Middle colic artery nodes
		16	Para-aortic lymph nodes

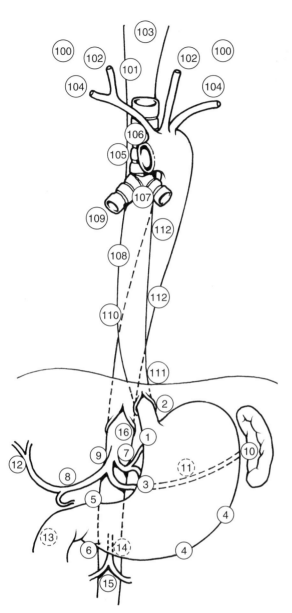

Figure 1.1 Topographic classification of esophageal lymph node groups, as described by the Japanese Society for Esophageal Diseases. Numbers indicate lymph node groups.

Table 1.3 Topographic description of esophageal lymph node groups as described by Akiyama[8]

ANATOMICAL DRAINAGE SITE	LYMPH NODE GROUP
Cervical lymph nodes	Deep lateral nodes (spinal accessory chain) Deep external nodes Deep internal nodes (recurrent nerve chain)
Superior mediastinal nodes	Recurrent nerve chain Paratracheal nodes Brachiocephalic artery nodes Paraesophageal nodes Infra-aortic arch nodes
Middle mediastinal nodes	Tracheal bifurcation nodes Pulmonary hilar nodes Paraesophageal nodes
Lower mediastinal nodes	Paraesophageal nodes Diaphragmatic nodes
Superior gastric lymph nodes	Pericardiac nodes Lesser curvature nodes Left gastric artery nodes
Celiac axis nodes	
Common hepatic artery nodes	

comparison of data from different centers. However, the problem with the Japanese system is that few have the resources to apply such a detailed system. To enable such a system to be used, the lymph nodes must be dissected from the specimen by the operating surgeon before the specimen is fixed if the topographic classification is

to be accurate. If a suitable, internationally agreed topographic system could be devised, then this may well be regarded in the future as the "gold standard", as all other nodal staging information could be derived from such a system. However, for the near future, other systems will remain the standard.

The UICC system has the simplest possible classification of lymph node metastases: they are either absent (N0) or they are present (N1). The question that has to be asked is does such a simple system provide the optimal amount of prognostic information that could be obtained from a descriptive system of lymph node metastases? It has to be remembered that the UICC system regards all nodal metastases other than perieso-phageal or perigastric nodes as M1 disease. This is in contrast to the five-tier Japanese system of classification, in which only the most advanced nodal disease is regarded as M1 disease. While there is little doubt that patients with very advanced disease fare very badly, there is a group of patients who are probably incorrectly

Table 1.4 Japanese classification of the grouping of lymph nodes according to the level of the primary tumor. The numbers refer to the classification described in Table 1.2 and Figure 1.1. The lymph node groups indicated in brackets are those not always dissected at operation

LOCATION OF TUMOR	LYMPH NODE GROUPINGS			
	N1	N2	N3	N4
Cervical esophagus	101	102, 104	100, 103, 105, 106, 107, 108	Beyond group 3
Upper thoracic esophagus	105	106, 107, 108, 112	101, 110, 111, 1, 2, (104), (109)	Beyond group 3
Middle thoracic esophagus	108	105, 106, 107, 110, 111, 112, 1, 2	3, 7, (104), (109)	Beyond group 3
Lower thoracic esophagus	110	108, 111, 112, 1, 2, 3, 7	105, 106, 107, (109)	Beyond group 3
Abdominal esophagus	1, 2	110, 111, 3, 7, 9, (10), (11)	108, 5, 8, (112), (4)	Beyond group 3

classified as M1 disease in the UICC system and these are patients with nodal metastases one tier more distant than paraesophageal or perigastric nodes, for example the celiac axis nodes. Following radical lymphadenectomy, Akiyama et al.[11] have reported a 5-year survival rate of 19% in patients with positive celiac nodes, while others have demonstrated survival figures far in excess of what would be expected in M1 disease. Therefore, the next revision of the UICC TNM system should probably include a second nodal tier (N2) before regarding lymph node metastases as M1 disease.

The other aspect of the classification of nodal metastases that should be considered in a staging system for esophageal carcinoma is the number of nodal metastases and the ratio of involved to non-involved nodes. Akiyama et al.[11] and Siewert's group[12] from Munich have shown that both the absolute number of involved lymph nodes and the ratio of involved to non-involved lymph nodes provide additional information to that provided by the standard TNM classification. In the context of a radical en-bloc resection with lymphadenectomy, the critical numbers seem to be seven or more involved nodes, or a ratio of involved to non-involved nodes of >0.2.

Summary – staging systems for esophageal carcinoma

In summary, the only system with a measure of international agreement is the UICC TNM classifica-

tion, and this should form the basis for all reporting of patients with esophageal carcinoma. However, with respect to the classification of lymph node metastases, the UICC system is oversimplified and a further revision to reclassify some nodal metastases from M1 disease to an N2 tier seems desirable. To provide additional information the total number of nodes resected and the number of involved nodes should also be recorded in the final histopathology report. It also seems to be highly desirable that a record is kept of the location of the involved nodes, but a standard nodal mapping system remains to be defined.

Preoperative staging

The process of preoperative staging of esophageal carcinoma starts with the initial clinical assessment and proceeds through investigations of increasing complexity. As with most gastrointestinal malignancies, the clinical detection of signs of the disease almost invariably indicates very advanced disease. The vast majority of patients require investigation to provide accurately the staging information that is required. The technology utilized in obtaining staging information is evolving rapidly. On this basis, only the most up-to-date information has been used to describe the application and results of the investigations described below. Throughout the following discussions it should be remembered that there is a very close relationship between depth of tumor invasion and the presence or absence of lymph node metastases (**Figure 1.2**)

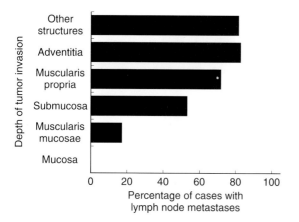

Figure 1.2 The incidence of lymph node metastases, according to the depth of invasion of esophageal carcinoma.[11]

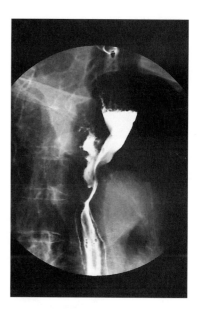

Figure 1.3 A barium swallow from a patient with a very advanced upper-third squamous carcinoma of the esophagus. The predicted T stage on the basis of this swallow alone was T4, confirmed on subsequent CT scanning.

which inevitably influences statements made regarding the overall accuracy of any particular preoperative staging modality. Indeed, by classifying all T1 and T2 tumors as N0 and all T3 and T4 tumors as N1, an overall staging accuracy of 67% can be obtained;[13] staging information must therefore be cautiously interpreted in the light of our knowledge of tumor behavior. One further point that deserves emphasis early in this discussion is that data derived from study of patients with squamous carcinoma of the esophagus may not be absolutely translated to a population of patients with distal third adenocarcinomas. This point is emphasized in a study from Germany in which preoperative staging using EUS was able to predict the ability to be able to perform a UICC R0 resection in 92% of esophageal adenocarcinomas, but was nearly 15% less accurate for patients with squamous carcinomas.[14]

Contrast radiology

For many practitioners the concept that simple contrast radiology can provide useful staging information is overlooked. While it is not a very sensitive investigation, the finding of a long (>8 cm) stricture[15] or a stricture with a change in the esophageal axis[16] is likely to indicate a T4 lesion (**Figure 1.3**). The ability of contrast radiology to easily delineate the height, length, and extent of an esophageal stricture make it, in the eyes of many physicians, a mandatory part of the work-up of a patient with esophageal cancer.

Upper gastrointestinal endoscopy

A detailed classification of the endoscopic findings of esophageal carcinoma has been proposed by the Japanese Society for Esophageal Diseases.[16a] This system is based on the concept of dividing esophageal cancers into either superficial lesions confined to the submucosa (pTis and pT1), or advanced tumors invading the muscularis propria and beyond (pT2–pT4). The superficial lesions are subdivided into three subgroups (types 0–I to 0–III) and the advanced lesions as types 1 to 4. The system is applied according to the macroscopic endoscopic appearances of the esophageal tumor. The tumor patterns are shown diagrammatically in **Figure 1.4**. Dittler, working in Munich, has prospectively studied the correlation between the JSED classification and UICC TNM staging.[17] The overall accuracy was 89%, with a sensitivity of 78% and a specificity of 93%. Although there was a weaker correlation between the JSED type 1 and 2 and the finding of a T2 cancer (**Table 1.5**), this simple staging classification provides a reasonably reliable source of staging information, particularly when the very strong association between tumor depth and the incidence of lymph node metastases is appreciated (**Figure 1.2**).

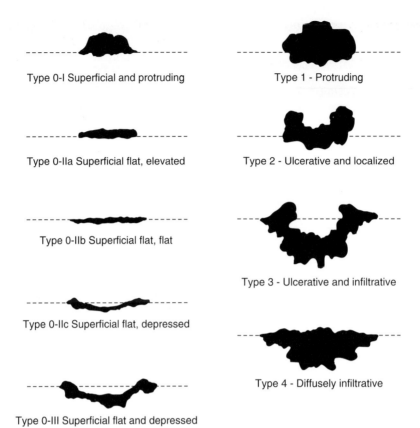

Figure 1.4 The macroscopic endoscopic classification of esophageal tumors, as proposed by the Japanese Society for Esophageal Diseases.[16a]

Table 1.5 The correlation between the Japanese Society for Esophageal Disease classification of endoscopic appearances (Figure 1.3) of esophageal carcinomas,[16a] and the UICC T stage of 209 esophageal cancers[17]

T CATEGORY	ENDOSCOPIC CLASSIFICATION	SENSITIVITY (%)	SPECIFICITY (%)	ACCURACY (%)
T1	Class 0 Class 1 Class 2 Class 4	83	97	95
T2	Class $\frac{1}{2}$ Class 0 Class 3	52	96	90
T3	Class 3 Class 2 Class 4	82	85	83
T4	Class 4 Class 3	83	90	88

Computed tomographic scanning

Since its introduction to clinical practice, there have been enormous improvements in the resolution of computed tomography (CT) scanners. The 1990s have seen the widespread introduction of fast helical scanners which have considerably improved image quality and have enabled far greater detail to be seen on reconstructions. As a consequence of these improvements, historic data regarding the accuracy of CT scanning must be interpreted with caution.

CT scanning has been the mainstay of staging esophageal carcinoma for more than 15 years in most units around the world. How accurate is the information obtained and have the newer generation of helical scanners added to our ability accurately to stage esophageal carcinoma? The second question can be answered easily – the data are simply not available and further studies are required.

CT scanning for T staging esophageal carcinomas With current technology, CT scanning cannot differentiate the individual layers of the esophageal wall. Therefore, the questions that could potentially be answered by CT scanning are: is the tumor contained within the esophageal wall (T1 and T2); does the tumor breach the esophageal wall (T3); and does the tumor invade other organs (T4)?

Overall, the accuracy of CT scanning in assessing T stage is between 50 and 65%,[18,19] but this may fall to as low as 36% for T1 and T2 tumors.[18]

One particularly important piece of information in staging esophageal cancer is determining as to whether there is invasion of other structures such as aorta, bronchus, or pericardium. This can be predicted using criteria of either mass effect or the loss of fat planes. Thompson and Halvorsen[20] reviewed current data in 1994 and found that CT scanning was considerably more accurate in determining the invasion of other structures than the overall accuracy of CT scanning in assessing T stage (94–97%; **Table 1.6**). However, a study from Munich showed an accuracy of just 50% for the assessment of mediastinal invasion;[21] therefore, while CT scanning can provide invaluable information it would, on the basis of current data, be wrong to deny a patient treatment for a so-called inoperable carcinoma purely because a CT scan indicated probable local mediastinal invasion. It should also be remembered that the interpretation of esophageal cancer staging CT scans is highly observer-dependent and that, even with experienced radiologists, there is considerable interobserver variation.[22]

One interesting development made possible with the advent of helical scanners is the measurement of tumor volume.[23] This may prove to be useful in assessing the response to chemotherapy, but further studies are required before a definitive statement can be made.

CT scanning for N staging esophageal carcinomas While, in contrast to endoluminal ultrasound, CT scanning potentially has the ability to visualize all relevant lymph node groups, its ability to determine the presence or absence of tumor involvement is based upon the single criterion of lymph node size. Most authors would regard a lymph node of >10 mm diameter as being potentially involved with tumor.

The overall accuracy of CT scanning in assessing lymph node involvement is low (50–60%), but this is due in large measure to a low sensitivity. The CT finding of potentially involved nodes of >10 mm diameter is 90–95% specific for lymph node metastases.[20]

CT scanning for M staging esophageal carcinomas The liver and the lung are the two most common sites for non-lymphatic metastatic spread of esophageal carcinoma. It is difficult to make definitive statements regarding

Table 1.6 A comparison of CT assessment of mediastinal invasion with surgical findings in patients with esophageal carcinoma[20]

AREA OF INVASION	SENSITIVITY (%)	SPECIFICITY (%)	ACCURACY (%)
Trachea/bronchus	93	98	97
Aorta	88	96	94
Pericardium	94	94	94

the overall accuracy of CT scanning in assessing distant metastases given that many patients will not undergo either resection or biopsy of the potential metastasis.

With respect to liver metastases, CT scanning is highly specific but will miss a proportion of smaller or capsular metastases, giving an overall sensitivity of 70–80%.

One area of distant spread particularly relevant to the distal third esophageal adenocarcinoma are peritoneal metastases. While gross disease may be picked up on CT imaging, small deposits are very often missed. When compared with laparoscopy (*vide infra*), CT scanning is inferior in detecting both peritoneal and hepatic metastases.[24] Even with a new latest-generation helical CT scanner, the accuracy with which liver metastases are detected is about 60% in our department; again it is the small, subcapsular lesions that are missed. We believe that the newer helical scanners may be slightly more sensitive in detecting peritoneal disease than the older scanners, but this will require confirmation.

Magnetic resonance imaging (MRI)

There are few data regarding MRI scanning in esophageal cancer that show it to be superior in any respect to conventional CT scanning. MRI appears to be very similar in its ability to detect mediastinal invasion,[25,26] and suffers from all the limitations of CT scanning. There is no difference in its ability to detect lymph node metastases,[21] with an overall accuracy of little more than 50%.

However, as with all technologies, constant advances are being made and an MRI endoscope has been introduced which may offer the potential advantage of high-resolution 3D tumor reconstruction.[27] In a small number of patients (seven), endoscopic MRI was 100% accurate for both T and N stage; these advances will be watched with interest.

There is, however, some evidence that the latest generation of MRI scanners are more accurate in detecting liver metastases than helical CT scanners. These data come predominantly from the field of colorectal cancer and have not been documented for upper gastrointestinal cancer. There is no doubt that more data will soon be appearing and this may well alter the staging approach in patients with esophageal or gastric malignancy.

One other area where MRI may offer advantages over CT scanning is in the reassessment of patients following neoadjuvant treatment. It appears from preliminary studies that some of the newer MRI sequences may be able to distinguish inflammatory change from viable tumor. At present, the use and indication for MRI in this setting remains speculative and experimental, but potentially developments in this area could be extremely important.

In summary, with currently available data there is no convincing evidence that the use of the more complex and time-consuming technique of MRI adds any further to the information obtainable from standard CT scanning in patients with esophageal cancer. However, the new developments should be watched with interest.

Endoluminal ultrasound scanning (EUS)

It is now nearly 20 years since the introduction of endoscopes equipped with ultrasound transducers.[28,29] Although echoendoscopy is now a very widely utilized technique, it has not enjoyed the almost universal use of techniques such as CT scanning for the assessment of upper gastrointestinal malignancies. The reasons for this are unclear, but without doubt cost and a lack of awareness of the role of this staging modality have both contributed to the situation.

Echoendoscopes can be broadly divided into two groups: firstly, the dedicated echoendoscopes which contain both optical and ultrasonic imaging equipment; and secondly "blind" ultrasound probes. This second group can be broken down again into dilating instruments and microinstruments which are designed to pass through the working channel of a conventional endoscope. The dedicated echoendoscopes are by far the most widely used, and indeed the precise role for the "blind" instrument remains to be fully clarified.

The standard echoendoscopes are based upon a mechanical rotating sector scanner and work at frequencies of 7.5 and 12 MHz. A number of smaller blind probes function at a frequency of 20 MHz.

At a frequency of 7.5 MHz, the echoendoscope has a depth of penetration of 9 cm with a resolution of 0.2 mm. The higher 12-MHz frequency gives an improved resolution of 0.1 mm, but the depth of penetration is reduced to 3 cm.

The wall of the gastrointestinal tract is demonstrated using the 7.5- or 12-MHz frequencies as a five-layered structure of alternate hyper- and hypoechogenicity.[30] The five layers are as follows:

1. Hyperechoic – superficial mucosa
2. Hypoechoic – deep mucosa
3. Hyperechoic – submucosa
4. Hypoechoic – muscularis propria
5. Hyperechoic – esophageal adventitia, gastric serosa

With the 20-MHz probes, the resolution is increased such that the wall of the gastrointestinal tract is seen as a nine-layered structure.[31] The mucosa is seen as a four-layered structure with the fourth of the nine layers (hypoechoic) representing the muscularis mucosae. The muscularis propria is represented as a three-layered structure: the innermost circular muscle fibers (hypoechoic); the interface of the circular and longitudinal layers (hyperechoic); and the hypoechoic longitudinal muscle fibers. The extra definition afforded in the mucosa should better allow the identification of muscosal (T1) carcinomas,[32] although a formal comparative study of 12-MHz and 20–25-MHz probes has not been performed.

EUS for T staging esophageal carcinomas There is little doubt that, overall, EUS is a very accurate method for assessing the depth of invasion of esophageal carcinoma. The accuracy reported in the literature ranges from 73% to 92%, with a mean of 85%.[18] The technique is slightly more accurate for T3 and T4 (90–92%) tumors than for T1 and T2 (80–85%) tumors.

One area of increasing interest is the accuracy of re-staging patients following neoadjuvant chemotherapy or chemoradiotherapy. In this context, EUS has been disappointing and indeed, appearances suggestive of T3 tumors in patients with complete or near-complete responses have been reported (**Figure 1.5**).[33] There is little doubt that further study and evaluation of staging modalities in this situation is required.

Many patients with Barrett's esophagus are entered into endoscopic surveillance programs, and a proportion are found to have either high-grade dysplasia or an early esophageal adenocarcinoma. What is the role of EUS in evaluating these patients? Unfortunately, although the data are limited, it appears that EUS cannot identify many of the early tumors and, because of the wall thickening found in Barrett's esophagus, significantly over-

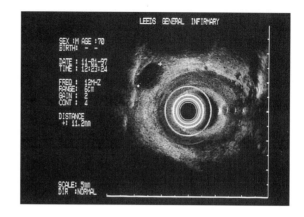

Figure 1.5 EUS appearance of a distal-third esophageal adenocarcinoma following neoadjuvant chemoradiotherapy. The appearances are the same as the pretreatment EUS examination and indicate a T3N1 tumor. The resected focus showed only a tiny remaining focus of intramucosal carcinoma, indicating the difficulty of restaging patients following neoadjuvant therapy.

stages both high-grade dysplasia and carcinoma.[34] As a consequence, the routine use of EUS in this small but increasingly important group of patients cannot be recommended.

EUS for N staging esophageal carcinomas The assessment of lymph node metastases with EUS in patients with esophageal carcinoma is obviously limited to the periesophageal and perigastric and celiac nodes because of the range of penetration of the instrument used. The endosonographic features predictive of lymph node metastases are, in order of increasing importance: echo-poor internal structure; sharply demarcated borders; rounded contour; and size >10 mm. These features are additive, and when all four are present EUS is virtually 100% accurate.[35] The overall accuracy for the EUS assessment of lymph node metastases is 70–90%[18] and is most accurate for paraesophageal and infra-aortic nodes.[36] Because of the nature of the examination of EUS, the accuracy in predicting N1 disease is greater (85–90%) than its ability to correctly predict N0 disease (65–80%).[18,35] The use of EUS to assess lymph node metastases must also take into account the fact that half the patients with a submucosal carcinoma and the vast majority of patients with a T2 or T3 tumor will have lymph node metastases (**Figure 1.2**).[11]

EUS and the high-grade esophageal stricture Using standard EUS instruments, the esophageal tumor can be traversed and useful imaging information obtained in 70–75% of cases. In 25–30% of cases, the stricturing of the esophagus is such that a standard instrument can be passed. When confronted with this situation there are a number of alternative strategies.

i. *Abandon the examination and infer staging information from the extent and degree of stricturing.* Some 90% of patients with a stricture prohibiting the passage of a conventional EUS instrument will have stage III or stage IV disease,[37] and it may be seen as unlikely that further useful information could be obtained from EUS examination.

ii. *Dilate the stricture and use a conventional EUS instrument.* This approach has little to commend it, as the risk of perforation is unacceptable and may be as high as 24%.[38,39]

iii. *Use a modified echoendoscope with a smaller diameter.* There are several instruments available which, by omitting the optics, have been manufactured with a smaller diameter (7–8 mm). These endoscopes can be passed through strictures over a guide wire and seem to be as accurate as conventional EUS instruments.[40] However, even with these narrower instruments, 10% of patients will require preliminary dilatation to approximately 33 Fr to permit the passage of the echoendoscope. Given the advanced nature of most of the esophageal tumors presenting with a high-grade stricture and the need to purchase a dedicated instrument, the precise value of this approach remains unclear.

iv. *Use a miniature EUS probe passed through the working channel of a conventional flexible endoscope.* While in principle this approach has much to commend it, with current technology the instrumentation is not sufficiently powerful to produce a beam that will penetrate advanced tumors.[41] It is not therefore in widespread use.

Given these alternative options, most practitioners simply abandon the procedure and utilise other staging methods to provide additional staging information in the presence of a high-grade esophageal stricture.

Percutaneous cervical ultrasonography

In Japan, one of the most common staging investigations for patients with esophageal carcinoma is a cervical ultrasound examination to look for enlarged lymph nodes. In a series of 209 patients, Tachimori *et al.*[42] found palpable cervical nodes in 26 patients. In 83 patients who went on to radical esophagectomy, the sensitivity and accuracy of ultrasonography was 79% and 94%, respectively.[42] Van Overhagen *et al.*[43] also found ultrasonography a useful technique, complementary with CT scanning in assessing cervical lymph nodes. It would seem to be reasonable to consider neck ultrasonography in patients with middle or upper-third carcinomas in whom a cervical nodal dissection might be contemplated. The applicability and usefulness of this technique for patients with distal-third adenocarcinomas has not been evaluated.

Comparison of staging methodologies

Much of the literature has asked the somewhat obvious question, what is the best preoperative staging modality for patients with esophageal carcinoma? In fact, the modalities described above are complementary: the question should in fact be, by what means can I obtain the most accurate overall staging information?

The clinical examination, barium meal, and endoscopy will provide the starting point for the accumulation of staging information and will be performed in virtually all patients with esophageal carcinoma. Assuming that the patient is not moribund, further more detailed information will be required. What modalities should then be employed? Many studies have compared EUS and CT scanning and these are summarized in **Table 1.7**. However, as stated above, the wrong question has been asked: the two modalities are complementary. While EUS is without doubt more accurate in assessing local T and local N stage, it is unable to provide the evidence of distant spread afforded with CT scanning. When information from CT scanning and EUS examination are combined, the overall accuracy of the staging information obtained rises from 64% to 86%.[19] Therefore, a reasonable strategy is to carry out thoracoabdominal CT scanning followed by EUS examination if no evidence

Table 1.7 Published comparisons of EUS and CT scanning in the preoperative staging of patients with esophageal carcinoma

REFERENCE	NO. OF PATIENTS	EUS T STAGE % (accuracy)	CT T STAGE % (accuracy)	EUS N STAGE % (accuracy)	CT N STAGE % (accuracy)
Tio et al.[44]	74	89	59	80	51
Botet et al.[19]	42	95	60	88	74
Ziegler et al.[45]	37	89	51	67	51
Grimm et al.[46]	49	89	62	–	–
Heintz et al.[47]	22	77	64	86	50
Schüder et al.[48]	22	86	57	81	48
Vilgrain et al.[49]	51	73	–	50	48
Greenberg et al.[50,*]	28	85	15	80	58
Holden et al.[51,*]	15	87	40	73	33

*Papers refer to both lower-third and gastroesophageal junction tumors.

of distant metastases or very advanced thoracic disease has been demonstrated. At present, MRI adds little to this overall assessment, but consideration should be given to percutaneous cervical ultrasound examination of neck nodes, particularly in cases of upper-third tumors.

Laparoscopic and thoracoscopic staging

Having obtained the non-invasive preoperative staging information, various treatment decisions will have been made: there may be evidence of advanced incurable disease with widespread metastases and the patient considered for palliation alone; there may be bulky local disease or evidence of nodal spread and neoadjuvant treatment may be considered or the patient may be considered a suitable candidate for primary potentially curative surgery. The currently available preoperative staging modalities are not perfect, and if one accepts the premise that the only place for surgical resection is in the patient in whom "cure" is a possibility, then further information may possibly be obtained from laparoscopy or thoracoscopy prior to resection.

Laparoscopy

The rationale behind the use of laparoscopy is to select patients in whom conventional non-invasive imaging has suggested resectable disease and identify those with "occult" liver or peritoneal metastases, in order to avoid unnecessary laparotomy. The data regarding the usefulness or otherwise of laparoscopy in patients with esophageal carcinoma

must be interpreted with caution. Virtually all of the published papers come from Europe or the USA where the predominant cancer is now lower-third adenocarcinoma. Many of the papers also mix true cancers of the esophagus together with carcinomas of the cardia and gastroesophageal junction; these cancers spread and behave in a different manner to true esophageal malignancies.[52] Despite these caveats, what is the evidence supporting the use of laparoscopy? One of the first reports was that of Watt et al. from Glasgow.[24] In a series of 90 patients, laparoscopy was significantly more accurate than CT scanning in detecting hepatic or peritoneal metastases and Watt concluded that it was a useful investigation. Further data from Glasgow have continued to support the view that laparoscopy is a useful staging modality, but the precise gains over conventional imaging techniques are not completely clear.[53] O'Brien et al. from Cork, Ireland found that the addition of laparoscopy prevented unnecessary laparotomy/thoracotomy in 20 of 110 cases of esophageal and gastric cancers, but interestingly reported that peritoneal metastases were not seen in any patient with squamous carcinoma of the esophagus.[54] Krasna and colleagues[55] have suggested in a small study of 19 patients that laparoscopy is more accurate in determining abdominal lymph node status than conventional imaging with six of 19 patients having unsuspected celiac nodal metastases. In a study from Holland, Bemelman et al.[56] demonstrated that laparoscopy changed the staging information in nine of 56 patients (17%), but again this was a mixed study of both esophageal and proximal gastric cancers. The addition of ultrasound to the laparoscopy increased the number of unsuspected liver metastases detected.[57]

From the published data, there appears little doubt that laparoscopy will alter the staging information in patients with distal-third esophageal cancers and proximal gastric cancers in approximately 20% of cases. However, what is far less clear is the role of laparoscopy in patients with more proximal esophageal tumors: more data are required before routine laparoscopy can be recommended.

The logical use of laparoscopy would be in the group of patients with lower-third tumors or tumors straddling the cardia that appear to be advanced on less invasive imaging. There seems to be little justification for performing laparoscopy in patients with a tumor staged as T1 on CT and EUS examination, but the patient with a bulky T3/T4 tumor may well benefit from pretreatment laparoscopy.

Thoracoscopy

Routine thoracoscopy prior to esophageal resection has been advocated as a useful additional staging modality, but relatively few studies have fully evaluated this technique. A study of 49 patients from the USA suggested that thoracoscopy correctly staged 88% of patients.[58] The value of the technique however was less clear. While three patients had a previously staged T4 tumor reclassified as T3, two patients had a T4 tumor completely missed.

On the basis of the very limited published data, together with my own, limited, experience of thoracoscopy it is difficult to justify the advocation of this technique.

Pathologic staging

The histopathologic examination of the resected esophageal specimen is without doubt one of the most important aspects of the staging of patients with esophageal carcinoma. There are a number of specific features that all those involved with esophageal surgery need to ensure are recorded on the pathology report. Not only is useful prognostic information obtained but very useful "quality control" information can be obtained for the surgeon, i.e., number of resected nodes and clear lateral margins, etc.

Histologic classification of tumor type

Squamous cell carcinoma The grade of neoplasm (well, moderate or poorly differentiated) seems to have little effect if any upon prognosis.[59,60] The pattern of invasion and the presence of an inflammatory response to the tumor seem to have some prognostic impact,[59] but compared with the TNM classification the effect is weak. One very important prognostic factor for esophageal carcinoma is the presence of multifocal intramural esophageal metastases, which may be of more influence than the presence of lymph node metastases.[61]

Adenocarcinoma For adenocarcinoma there are few data, but those available would suggest that the grade and type of tumor adds nothing to the prognostic information provided by TNM staging.[62]

Classification of lymph node metastases

The question as to how the pathologist should classify lymph node metastases returns the argument stated in detail above as to which staging system should be used. Certainly, the total number of nodes examined and the number of nodes containing tumor should be recorded. The anatomic location of positive nodes should also be recorded: in an ideal situation a detailed mapping system such as that of Akiyama would be used, but it is more likely that a simpler system will be employed recording the broad anatomic location of the involved nodes. Given the current debate regrading the evolution of the TNM classification, it would seem that for future comparisons the minimum standard which should be employed would divide the nodes into the following groups which will allow for more detailed classification later:

- celiac nodes
- hepatic artery nodes
- perigastric nodes
- periesophageal – infracarinal
- periesophageal – supracarinal
- cervical nodes
- other more distant nodes

Lateral resection margins

The concept that the pathologist should examine the proximal and distal resection margin of an esophagectomy specimen is universal; the lateral or circumferential margin has however received far less attention, but is equally likely to be a very important prognostic factor. In a small study of 50 patients Sagar *et al.*[63] looked at the influence of an involved lateral margin and found, not unsurprisingly, that at 36 months 11 of the 20 patients with a positive lateral margin had developed local recurrence compared with just four of the remaining 30 patients. This is the only study examining this one factor and further data are required, but in the meantime it would seem prudent to record the circumferential margin status on the pathology report.

Staging strategy for esophageal carcinoma

Integrating all the data described above, what would be the "gold standard" staging pathway for patients with esophageal carcinoma? This pathway is based on currently published data and takes into account the potential developments in the field of MR imaging. Where the recommendation is based on experimental evidence then this is indicated. Obviously, the general fitness and treatment options suitable for any individual patient must be taken into account when staging patients with esophageal cancer.

The overall approach is shown in **Figure 1.6**. There is no doubt that this protocol will be modified and refined over the next few years as more data regarding the utility of MRI and laparoscopy become available. Although this point of view will be controversial, it is very difficult to justify the routine use of laparoscopy in patients with esophageal carcinoma. The use of laparoscopy is likely to be confined to the patient with a bulky lower-third carcinoma probably encroaching upon the cardia; for other locations, there is little data to justify its general use.

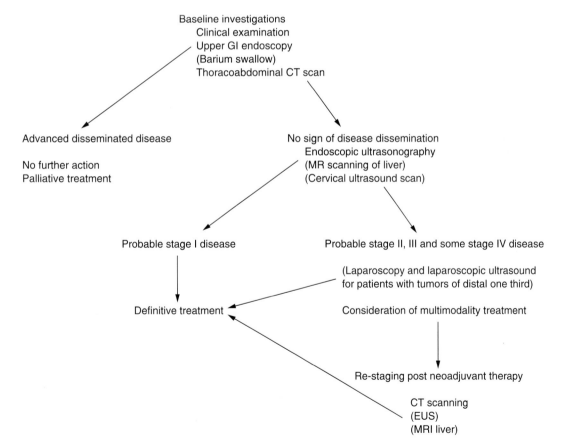

Figure 1.6   Suggested staging protocol for patients with esophageal carcinoma. Staging modalities whose value is unproven or difficult to justify in all cases are indicated by parentheses.

GASTRIC CANCER

In separating the description of the staging of upper gastrointestinal cancer into two sections for esophageal and gastric cancer, a somewhat arbitrary distinction has been made that in many areas the two diseases can be assessed in a similar fashion. Despite this, there are enough substantial differences in both staging systems and staging methodology to warrant separate descriptions. It must however be remembered that for tumors straddling the gastroesophageal junction it is almost impossible truly to separate the two pathologies. This section describes the approaches to staging patients with gastric carcinoma and highlights areas of debate and controversy.

Staging systems

As for esophageal carcinoma, there is great debate worldwide as to the optimal staging system for describing gastric cancer. Again, there are competing systems and similarly there is particular controversy as to how best to classify lymph node metastases. The merits and weaknesses of the individual systems will be discussed and a compromise proposed. Given the very great interest in the results of surgery for gastric cancer in Japan, it is now more pressing than ever that a worldwide standard is agreed to facilitate international collaboration and comparison. The classification systems only apply to carcinoma and not to other gastric tumors such as lymphoma, where different systems are used. The assessment of patients with gastric lymphoma is discussed elsewhere in this book.

TNM classification

The fourth edition of the TNM classification was published in 1987,[4] and describes the methods for classifying gastric carcinomas.

The location of the tumor should be described where possible to the third of the stomach in which the bulk of the tumor sits. Some tumors will occupy more than one-third of the stomach, and patients with linitis plastica cannot easily have the tumor location so classified. The thirds of the stomach are divided by subdividing the greater and lesser curvatures at two equidistant points; these points are then joined to give:

- upper third: includes the cardia and fundus
- middle third: includes most of the corpus
- lower third: includes the pylorus and antrum

T stage The primary tumor is classified into six categories:

- T0 – no evidence of primary tumor
- Tis – carcinoma *in situ*: an intraepithelial tumor with no evidence of lamina propria invasion
- T1 – tumor invades lamina propria or submucosa
- T2 – tumor invades muscularis propria (T2a) or subserosa (T2b)
- T3 – tumor penetrates the serosa without invasion of adjacent structures
- T4 – tumor invades adjacent structures

N stage The nodal status is described in three categories:

- N0 – no regional nodal metastases
- N1 – metastases in perigastric nodes within 3 cm of the tumor
- N2 – metastases in perigastric nodes more than 3 cm from the tumor or in left gastric, hepatic splenic or celiac nodes

More distant nodes such as those in the liver hilum or para-aortic area are classified as distant metastases.

However, the UICC have published a new version of their TNM classification which contains some important changes for gastric carcinoma.[5]

The major change in the classification of gastric carcinoma is in the description of the N stage of tumors, moving from a three-tier to a four-tier system as follows:

- N0 – no nodal disease
- N1 – 1–6 involved regional nodes
- N2 – 7–15 involved regional nodes
- N3 – >15 involved regional nodes

The stage groupings for gastric cancer have also altered (**Table 1.8**) compared with the 1987 TNM Classification (**Table 1.9**).

M stage As with all tumors, M1 indicates the presence of distant metastases, including more distant nodal disease.

Typical 5-year survival rates would be: stage I, 90%; stage II, 60–70%; stage III, 30%; and stage IV, 5%.

Japanese classification

As for esophageal carcinoma, the Japanese have proposed a very detailed and precise system for

Table 1.8 UICC stage grouping for gastric carcinoma based on the 1997 TNM classification[5]

STAGE 0	STAGE I	STAGE II	STAGE III	STAGE IV
Tis N0 M0	T1 N0 M0 (IA)	T1 N2 M0	T2 N2 M0 (IIIA)	T4 N1-3 M0
	T1 N1 M0 (IB)	T2 N1 M0	T3 N1 M0 (IIIA)	T1-3 N3 M0
	T2 N0 M0 (IB)	T3 N0 M0	T4 N0 M0 (IIIA)	Any T, Any N, M1
			T3 N2 M0 (IIIB)	

Table 1.9 UICC stage grouping for gastric carcinoma based on the 1987 TNM classification[4]

STAGE 0	STAGE I	STAGE II	STAGE III	STAGE IV
Tis N0 M0	T1 N0 M0 (IA)	T1 N2 M0	T2 N2 M0 (IIIA)	T4 N2 M0
	T1 N1 M0 (IB)	T2 N1 M0	T3 N1 M0 (IIIA)	Any T, Any N, M1
	T2 N0 M0 (IB)	T3 N0 M0	T4 N0 M0 (IIIA)	
			T3 N2 M0 (IIIB)	
			T4 N1 M0 (IIIB)	

the classification of patients with gastric carcinoma. The first Japanese edition of the *General Rules for Gastric Cancer Study* was published in 1962. Now, with many corrections and improvements it is in its 12th edition. Although parts of the 10th edition were translated into English,[64] the 12th edition was the first to be fully translated. This 12th edition was published in 1995, and is a key reference source for any surgeon/oncologist with an interest in gastric cancer.[65] While the key features of the Japanese system will be described here, the reader should study the full volume.

Tumor location In common with the TNM system, the location of the tumor is described as being within one of the three portions of the stomach: C – upper third; M – middle third; and A – lower third. If more than one portion is involved, it should be described according to the sections in which the tumor is contained, e.g., CM indicates a tumor extending from the upper third into the middle third of the stomach.

Macroscopic tumor type The Japanese system has a detailed descriptive component to detail the macroscopic appearance of the primary tumor. The system is as follows, and although initially appearing complex and unwieldy, underpins much of the staging information used in Japan (**Figures 1.7** and **1.8**).

Type 0 Superficial, flat tumors with or without minimal elevation or depression. Early gastric cancer (T1 lesion irrespective of nodal status) is a concept introduced by the Japanese and generally these lesions are described as subtypes of type 0.

Type 0 is subdivided again into five subcategories (**Figure 1.7**):

- Type 0 I: protruded type
- Type 0 IIa: superficial elevated type
- Type 0 IIb: flat type
- Type 0 IIc: superficial depressed type
- Type 0 III: excavated type

Type 1 Polyploid tumors sharply demarcated from the surrounding mucosa, usually attached on a wide base.

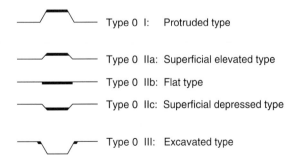

Type 0 I: Protruded type

Type 0 IIa: Superficial elevated type

Type 0 IIb: Flat type

Type 0 IIc: Superficial depressed type

Type 0 III: Excavated type

Figure 1.7 The macroscopic classification of type 0 gastric cancer, according to the Japanese Research Society for Gastric Cancer.

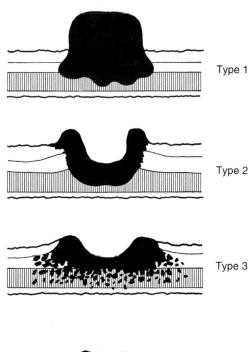

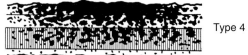

Figure 1.8   The macroscopic classification of types 1–4 gastric cancer, according to the Japanese Research Society for Gastric Cancer.

Type 2   Ulcerated carcinomas with sharply demarcated and raised margins.

Type 3   Ulcerated carcinomas without definite limits, infiltrating into the surrounding wall.

Type 4   Diffusely infiltrating carcinomas in which ulceration is usually not a marked feature.

Type 5   Non-classifiable carcinomas that cannot be classified into any of the above types.

T stage   The T stage of the Japanese system is very close to that of the UICC TNM system. There are a number of subtle differences, but these have little impact on the overall T1 through to T4 classification. However, it is important to mention at this stage the Japanese concept of early gastric cancer (EGC). An early gastric cancer is a tumor confined to the mucosa or submucosa, irrespective of lymph node status, that is to say any T1 tumor. According to the Japanese, any other tumor must by definition

be an advanced gastric cancer; this is often a source of confusion as many Western surgeons would not regard a T2 N0 cancer as advanced.

N stage   The classification of lymph nodes and nodal metastases is the area in which the greatest differences exist between the UICC TNM system and the TNM system. The Japanese system classifies the lymph nodes according to a station map described in **Table 1.2** and **Figure 1.9**.

Having classified the lymph nodes to stations, lymph node metastases are described according to both the location of the involved nodes and the primary tumor (**Table 1.10**). The tiers of nodal involvement are from N0 through to N4.

P stage   Peritoneal metastases are classified as:
- P0 – no peritoneal metastases
- P1 – metastases to adjacent peritoneum only
- P2 – a few distant peritoneal metastases
- P3 – numerous distant metastases

The stage groupings for patients with gastric cancer classified according to the Japanese system (**Table 1.11**) are different from the UICC stage groupings, and it is therefore difficult to directly compare data published using the different systems.

Lymph node metastases

As is apparent from the descriptions of the two competing staging systems, it is in the classification of lymph node metastases that the greater differences are to be found. The TNM system has the advantage of being simple but is very arbitrary: what is 3 cm in the fresh specimen may well be far less in the fixed specimen examined by the pathologist. It also takes little account of the overall number of lymph node metastases and the precise location of the involved nodes; the latter point being very important in assessing prognosis.[66] Despite these criticisms, there is a reasonably good correlation between the UICC nodal status and 5-year survival.

The Japanese system is detailed and very time-consuming for surgeons and pathologists, particularly given the average nodal yield with a D2 gastrectomy is 50–60. It provides the most detailed possible picture of nodal disease and enables all other staging systems to be derived from the information recorded. The definition of nodal stations are inextricably linked to the extent of the lymphadenectomy performed at operation. In the ideal

Table 1.10 The classification of nodal metastases according to the 12th edition of the Japanese Classification of Gastric Carcinoma. ▢ stations represent N1 nodes, ▢ stations N2 nodes, ▢ stations N3 nodes and ▢ stations N4 nodes

LYMPH NODE NUMBER		TUMORS INVOLVING THE WHOLE STOMACH	TUMORS OF THE ANTRUM	TUMORS OF THE MID STOMACH	TUMORS OF THE PROXIMAL STOMACH	ADDITIONAL NODES IF TUMOR INVADES ESOPHAGUS
1	right cardia					
2	left cardia					
3	lesser curve					
4sa	short gastric					
4sb	left gastroepiploic					
4d	right gastroepiploic					
5	suprapyloric					
6	infrapyloric					
7	left gastric artery					
8a	anterior hepatic artery					
8p	posterior hepatic artery					
9	celiac artery					
10	splenic hilum					
11	splenic artery					
12	hepatoduodenal ligament					
13	retropancreatic					
14A	superior mesenteric artery					
14V	superior mesenteric vein					
15	middle colic					
16a2,b1	para-aortic					
16a1,b2	para-arotic					
17	anterior pancreatic					
18	inferior pancreatic					
19	infra-diaphragmatic					
20	esophageal hiatus					
105	upper esophagus					
106	tracheal					
107	tracheal bifurcation					
108	middle esophagus					
109	pulmonary hilum					
110	lower esophagus					
111	supradiaphragmatic					
112	posterior mediastinum					

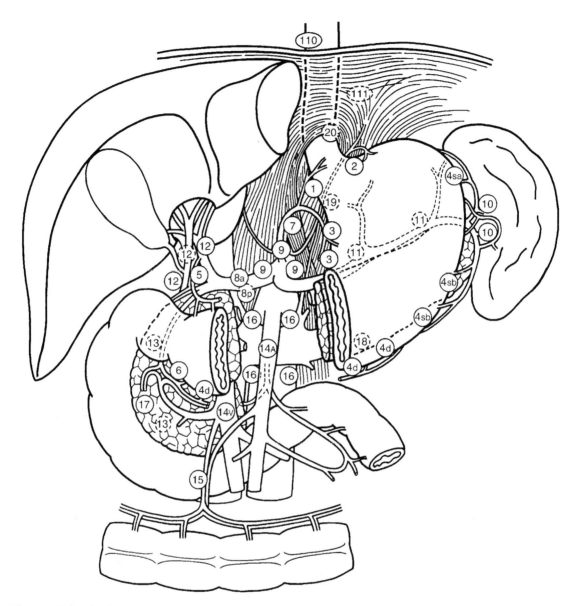

Figure 1.9 The lymph node station numbers of the stomach, according to the Japanese Research Society for Gastric Cancer.

situation, the Japanese system has much to commend it, but the time and fiscal considerations have discourged many surgeons and pathologists from employing this approach.

A third alternative strategy has recently received much attention in an attempt to improve upon the rather arbitrary nature of the UICC system and the complexity of the Japanese system. Instead of relying upon the location of the involved nodes, the nodal status of any individual patient is described using either the absolute number of involved nodes or the proportion of involved to the number of nodes retrieved. There are a number of immediate problems with this strategy: firstly, and perhaps most important, is that this method of describing lymph node metastases is only applicable to operative specimens and could not be applied preoperatively; secondly, that sufficient numbers of nodes must be both retrieved and analyzed to make a valid calculation; and finally, as with the

Table 1.11 Stage grouping for patients with gastric cancer according to the 12th edition of the Japanese Classification of Gastric Carcinoma. This is for comparison with the UICC stage grouping and makes no reference to the P stage of the Japanese system. All tumors greater than P1 T3 N0 represent IVb disease

	N0	N1	N2	N3
T1	Ia	Ib	II	IIIa
T2	Ib	II	IIIa	IIIb
T3	II	IIIa	IIIb	IVa
T4	IIIa	IIIb	IVa	IVb

UICC system, no account is made of the location of the involved nodes. Despite these criticisms, the assessment of the number of involved nodes appears to provide useful additional information in the assessment of prognosis in patients who have undergone gastric resection.

There is no consensus as to which of these systems should be used in describing lymphatic metastases in patients with gastric cancer; short of the very detailed Japanese system, it would seem to be a reasonable compromise to recommend the use of the UICC system together with a record of the number of nodes involved and the total number retrieved in patients undergoing operative treatment.

Which system should be used?

There is no correct answer to this question. The Japanese are adamant that their very detailed system provides much useful information that just would not be recorded if the much simpler UICC system were to be adopted. The rest of the world has, by and large, used the UICC system. The only consensus that can currently be recommended is that for the purposes of international comparison, the UICC system should be used for all international publications. However, further refinements and revisions of the UICC system will be needed over the next few years to take into account the criticisms of the Japanese, many of which are valid. The minimum data set for staging gastric cancer must therefore be the UICC system, but as there is a gradual move worldwide to define operations for gastric cancer according to the Japanese rules, it is likely that the topographic lymph node classifica-

tion that they have defined will assume greater importance.

Preoperative staging

As with esophageal carcinoma, any staging information obtained must be interpreted in the light of our knowledge of the behavior of gastric cancer. The T stage of the tumor is the single most important determinant of outcome and by inference, an accurate definition of T stage will give possibly the greatest prognostic information. The importance of the T stage in assessing other factors such as nodal metastases and peritoneal spread cannot be overestimated. There is an almost linear relationship between depth of tumor invasion and the incidence of lymph node metastases (**Figure 1.10**) and indeed with the simple expedient of classifying any T1 or T2 carcinoma as node-negative and any T3 or T4 cancer as node-positive, then an accuracy of 70–75% could be achieved (data derived from Soga et al.[67] and Kodama et al.[68]). It is therefore against this background that any staging modality should be judged. In the face of a reasonably accurate T stage estimation, then an accuracy of 70% or less in the estimation of nodal involvement is poorer than would be achieved by "chance." It also must be remembered that the chance of peritoneal metastases is very low indeed in T1 and T2a tumors, and again this will inevitably color the interpretation of the usefulness or otherwise of any staging modality given the enormous importance both clinically and prognostically of this finding. In the following paragraphs the standard modalities used for staging gastric carcinoma are

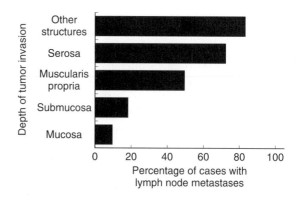

Figure 1.10 The incidence of lymph node metastases according to the depth of invasion of gastric carcinoma.[67,68]

described; while all have specific indications, their blanket use without thought for tumor biology leads to overinvestigation with little benefit to either the patient or clinician.

Professor Maruyama from the National Cancer Center Hospital in Tokyo has developed a simple computer program which utilizes the large database of patient information from the NCCH.[69] The program, when given information regarding a number of simple clinical parameters, provides the likelihood of nodal metastases in any of the 16 nodal groups, together with information on the likely pattern of recurrence. While the database is Japanese, it has been validated in European patients,[70] and its use may well help in the preoperative work-up of patients with gastric carcinoma (**Figure 1.11**).

Endoscopy

No clinician would dispute the role of flexible upper gastrointestinal endoscopy in the diagnosis of gastric cancer; its role in staging is, outside Japan, not widely recognized. One of the most striking features to a Western observer is the reliance placed upon the endoscopic appearance of gastric cancers in their staging, and in particular of early gastric cancers.

The endoscopic classification of gastric cancers is based upon the macroscopic classification described above. The primary role for using endoscopy is in the assessment of early lesions. Sano and colleagues[71] studied 206 early gastric cancers and 32 "early-like" advanced cancers, subsequently treated by radical surgery. The endoscopic assessment was based upon the macroscopic appearance of the tumors using indigo-carmine dye spraying. Particular attention was paid to the pattern of mucosal folds around the lesion (**Figure 1.12**). The overall accuracy of the endoscopic staging was 69%. The accuracy in predicting a mucosal cancer was 87% and a submucosal cancer 60%. The impressive feature of this study is that the accuracy of predicting a mucosal cancer is as good as, if not better than, that of endoscopic ultrasonography. There is considerable support within the Japanese literature for the use of endoscopic staging of gastric cancer.

While radical surgery underpins much of the Japanese approach to the treatment of gastric cancer over the past 5–10 years, interest has grown in the use of endoscopic resection for small mucosal early gastric cancers. To accomplish this safely, the preoperative staging system must be able to identify a subgroup of patients with a very low chance of nodal metastases. This information is derived primarily from the endoscopic assessment of the tumor. What factors are important in deciding that the risk of nodal metastases is very low? Yamoa and colleagues[72] studied 1196 patients with mucosal gastric cancers and identified three independent risk factors: (i) lymphatic invasion; (ii) histologic tumor ulceration; and (iii) size $\geqslant 30$ mm. When none of these risk factors was present, the risk of nodal metastases was 0.36% (one of 277 patients).

Sano and colleagues[73] have also produced a list of features of an early gastric cancer which suggest that the risk of nodal metastases is very low:

- mucosal cancer
- size <15 mm
- no ulceration/ulcer scars
- well-differentiated tumors

In combining these data, it would be reasonable to offer endoscopic resection to patients with a small (<1.5 cm), well-differentiated mucosal tumor with no evidence of ulceration. The single most important factor is the lack of submucosal involvement; the risk of nodal metastases is 20% if the submucosa is involved, and therefore if the resected specimen shows any suspicion of submucosal involvement the patient should proceed to radical surgical treatment.

CT scanning

CT scanning for T staging gastric cancers   Unlike EUS examination and to a lesser extent MRI, CT scanning is unable to distinguish the layers of the gastric wall, severely limiting its ability to assess T stage. While CT scanning can demonstrate tumor spread outwith the wall of the stomach, its ability to demonstrate invasion often relies on the loss of fat planes which may be lost for other reasons in the thin patients with gastric cancer. Various methods, such as the examination of the patient prone and distension of the stomach with water, have been advocated to increase the accuracy of the CT staging of gastric cancer, but the evidence to support this hypothesis is not substantial. The overall accuracy of CT scanning in assessing T stage is between 40 and 50%,[74] but the clinical importance of this figure is a little unclear given CT scanning's inability to distinguish the

```
PROGNOSIS AND LN-METASTASES OF THE PATIENTS WITH SAME BACKGROUND
treated by resection in National Cancer Center Tokyo, 1969-1983


          PATIENT                 X11111111      JF
    ---------------------------------------------------------------
          SEX and AGE             M    67 (+5/-5)
          TYPE and DEPTH          2C   PM
          LOCATION                M    A
          MAX DIAMETER            6.5 cm  (+2.5/-2.5)
          HISTOLOG TYPE           MOD

[ DEPTH OF INVASION ] SM                    PM              S1
---------------------------------------------------------------------
TYPE OF CANCER          2C                 B3              B3
5 YEAR SURV RATE       88.2%              76.6%           55.9%
GREENWOOD 5% ERR       22.1%              23.7%           16.2%
NUMBER OF CASES         12                 13              44

[ LYMPH NODE METASTASIS ]   meta/dissect (meta% in group)
---------------------------------------------------------------------
    LN- 1      0/12 (  0.0%)      0/13 (  0.0%)     11/43 ( 25.0%)
    LN- 2      0/ 1 (  0.0%)      0/ 0 (  0.0%)      0/11 (  0.0%)
    LN- 3      2/12 ( 17.0%)      6/13 ( 46.0%)     27/44 ( 61.0%)
    LN- 4      3/12 ( 25.0%)      4/13 ( 31.0%)     23/44 ( 52.0%)
    LN- 5      0/12 (  0.0%)      1/13 (  8.0%)      1/44 (  2.0%)
    LN- 6      2/12 ( 17.0%)      2/13 ( 15.0%)     10/44 ( 23.0%)
    LN- 7      1/12 (  8.0%)      3/13 ( 23.0%)     13/44 ( 30.0%)
    LN- 8      0/12 (  0.0%)      2/13 ( 15.0%)      9/44 ( 20.0%)
    LN- 9      0/12 (  0.0%)      0/12 (  0.0%)      8/43 ( 18.0%)
    LN-10      0/ 1 (  0.0%)      0/ 0 (  0.0%)      0/11 (  0.0%)
    LN-11      0/ 4 (  0.0%)      0/ 6 (  0.0%)      1/20 (  2.0%)
    LN-12      0/ 5 (  0.0%)      1/ 8 (  8.0%)      1/16 (  2.0%)
    LN-13      0/ 2 (  0.0%)      0/ 1 (  0.0%)      0/ 5 (  0.0%)
    LN-14      0/ 1 (  0.0%)      0/ 1 (  0.0%)      0/ 4 (  0.0%)
    LN-15      0/ 1 (  0.0%)      0/ 1 (  0.0%)      0/ 1 (  0.0%)
    LN-16      0/ 3 (  0.0%)      1/ 1 (  8.0%)      2/13 (  5.0%)
---------------------------------------------------------------------
[ CAUSE OF DEATH ]
LIVING NOW       11 ( 92.0%)        9 ( 69.0%)       22 ( 50.0%)
UNKNOWN           0 (  0.0%)        0 (  0.0%)        2 (  5.0%)
PERIT DISSEMI     0 (  0.0%)        2 ( 15.0%)        4 (  9.0%)
HEPATIC META      0 (  0.0%)        0 (  0.0%)        2 (  5.0%)
LOCAL RECURR      0 (  0.0%)        0 (  0.0%)        5 ( 11.0%)
DISTANT META      0 (  0.0%)        2 ( 15.0%)        3 (  7.0%)
RECURRENCE        0 (  0.0%)        0 (  0.0%)        0 (  0.0%)
DIRECT DEATH      0 (  0.0%)        0 (  0.0%)        0 (  0.0%)
OTHER CANCER      0 (  0.0%)        0 (  0.0%)        1 (  2.0%)
OTHER DISEASE     1 (  8.0%)        0 (  0.0%)        5 ( 11.0%)
---------------------------------------------------------------------
[ CURABILITY AT SURGERY ]
ABS CURATIVE     11 ( 92.0%)       10 ( 77.0%)       27 ( 61.0%)
REL CURATIVE      1 (  8.0%)        2 ( 15.0%)       12 ( 27.0%)
REL NON-CURA      0 (  0.0%)        0 (  0.0%)        3 (  7.0%)
ABS NON-CURA      0 (  0.0%)        1 (  8.0%)        2 (  5.0%)
---------------------------------------------------------------------
```

Figure 1.11   A typical "print-out" from Professor Maruyama's computer program used to predict spread and behavior of patients with gastric carcinoma.

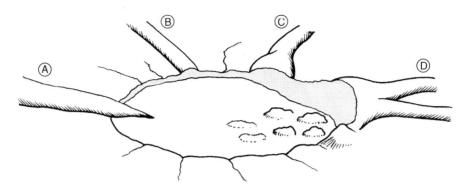

Figure 1.12   The morphologic assessment of fold convergence used in the endoscopic staging of early gastric cancers. Types A and B are associated with mucosal cancers, type C with submucosal cancers, and the fold merging seen in type D with tumors invading the muscularis propria.[71]

layers of the gastric wall. What is perhaps more important is the ability to detect T4 disease with invasion of other viscera. Halvorsen *et al.*[75] reported that CT scanning failed to detect pancreatic invasion in eight of 11 cases, giving a sensitivity of just 27%; very similar figures were reported by Andaker *et al.*[76] It has been our recent experience that helical scanning has produced some improvement in CT scanning's ability to detect T4 disease. In a series of 105 patients, the sensitivity and specificity for mesocolonic and colonic invasion were 76% and 95%, but for pancreatic invasion sensitivity fell to 50% with 99% specificty.

CT scanning for N staging gastric cancers   There is little doubt from the literature that CT scanning, even with the latest generation of spiral scanners, is a very inaccurate method for the assessment of lymph node metastases in patients with gastric cancer. The sensitivity has been reported as being between 48% and 91%, with most reports being at the lower end of this range.[74,76] It has been our experience that, for perigastric nodes, the sensitivity of CT scanning is 24%, very similar to the experience of others,[76] but that for N2 nodes the sensitivity almost doubled to 43%.

In contrast to this poor sensitivity, when a "cut-off" of ≥10 mm in size is used to indicate an involved node, the specificity of CT scanning approaches 100%, both in our department and others.[76] Others have suggested that the finding of nodes of ≥20 mm in diameter are more likely to be reactive rather than neoplastic.[74]

Because with CT scanning we are limited to the single criterion of node size to ascribe any individual node as involved, it is difficult to see how improvements in scanner resolution will increase the overall accuracy which is at present little better than 50%. Moreover, it has been our experience that, even with the latest generation of helical scanners, this is so.

CT scanning for M staging gastric cancers   With gastric cancer the two areas of distant metastasis of most concern to the surgeon considering operative intervention are peritoneal and liver deposits. The early experience with CT scanning suggested that its ability to detect peritoneal disease was very low, often relying on inferences from the finding of ascites. Our recent experience suggests that the newer generation of scanners has produced improvements in this area with a sensitivity and specificity of 71% and 93% respectively; however, there was a significant incidence of false positives (30% of the total positives).

Regarding CT scanning's ability to detect liver metastases, the picture is clearer and suggests that a very significant proportion of the lesions are missed. Liver metastases are relatively uncommon at presentation (8–10%) in patients with gastric cancer and so absolute numbers are small. However, it has been our experience (and of others) that 40–50% of liver lesions are missed on CT scanning alone.[24] Most of these lesions are small and peripheral and therefore may be detectable by either laparoscopy or laparoscopic ultrasound (*vide infra*).

In conclusion, the overall impression of CT scanning is of a rather inaccurate, but specific, staging tool. It provides some useful information to guide the surgeon towards other staging modalities such as laparoscopy, but on its own – with the exception of the patient with widespread dissemination of disease – it should not be the sole modality upon which management decisions are made.

MRI scanning

The role of MRI in the preoperative staging of patients with gastric carcinoma is far from clear. Motion artefact and other technical problems have limited the application of MRI in the study of patients with gastric cancer and the number of published series is very small. Early reports suggested that it added little to the assessment provided by CT scanning.[77] In contrast to CT scanning, MRI does have the ability to distinguish the individual layers of the gastric wall and it has been suggested that MRI scanning can accurately (88% overall accuracy) predict the depth of tumor and serosal invasion.[78] These data were from a small, non-comparative study and require verification. A further potential advantage of MRI scanning may be an improved ability to image perigastric lymph nodes, but again further detailed studies are required.[79]

In an interesting development, Inui and colleagues[27] explored the possibility of the use of endoscopic MRI. While technical problems limited its use to just 14 of 24 cases, it had an accuracy of 89% in predicting the T stage of gastric cancers.

Despite these interesting developments, there seems to be little justification for the routine use of MRI in staging patients with gastric cancer outside the research and development setting. As mentioned above, when discussing the use of MRI in staging esophageal cancer, there is some evidence that the latest generation of MRI scanners may facilitate the more accurate detection of liver metastases, but to date there are no data regarding this for patients with gastric cancer.

EUS

The principles of endoscopic ultrasonography have been described in the section on staging of patients with esophageal carcinoma. The techniques used and the interpretation of the data are similar but it must be remembered that, as opposed to the esophagus, the wall of the stomach has a serosal layer. There are a number of limitations to the use of EUS in staging patients with gastric cancer. Firstly,

although not of the same magnitude as for patients with esophageal cancer, a proportion of patients have non-traversable lesions (about 15%). Secondly, there are a number of areas of the stomach where it is technically difficult to obtain high-quality images; these are the high lesser curve and the prepyloric antrum. Thirdly, it can be difficult to distinguish between a bulky T2 lesion and a T3 lesion with serosal invasion. Finally, as for esophageal cancer, there are no absolute criteria for the definition of involved lymph nodes.

With these limitations in mind, the evidence surrounding the use of EUS to stage gastric cancer is presented below.

EUS for T staging gastric cancers Aside from the recent developments with endoscopic MRI, which at present remain highly experimental, EUS is the only modality able to give "accurate" information regarding the T stage of gastric cancer. The question that needs answering is just how accurate is EUS. It must also be remembered that the T stage information obtained from screening is probably the most crucial in terms of making clinical decisions for the patient.

A large number of studies have reported the accuracy of EUS staging of gastric carcinoma and these are summarized in **Table 1.12** (data taken from the review by Pollack et al.[80]). Using data taken from the larger studies, Pollack examined the accuracy of EUS across the UICC T stage categories and found that EUS was most accurate for T1 and T3 tumors and, as with the esophagus, least accurate for T2 tumors (**Table 1.13**). The tendency with EUS is to overstage T2 tumors and understage T3 tumors.[81] In terms of making management decisions, it would appear that EUS can reliably distinguish T3 and T4 lesions. In addition, at the other end of the spectrum is may be possible with high-resolution, high-frequency EUS to distinguish mucosal cancers which may be candidates for

---

Table 1.12 The accuracy of EUS in staging gastric carcinomas based on published series. (Adapted from Pollack et al.[80] and Rösch et al.[81]

	NO. OF PATIENTS	T STAGE (%)	N STAGE (%)
T Stage	2610	77	
N Stage	1118		69

Table 1.13 The accuracy of EUS in staging gastric cancer. (From Pollack et al.[80])

STAGE	NO. OF CASES	ACCURACY (%)
T1	483	86
T2	301	64
T3	500	91
T4	143	80
N0	282	85
N1	311	71
N2	232	65

local endoscopic resection from submucosal candidates which are not;[82] however, these data are newly acquired and will need larger studies for their confirmation.

EUS for N staging of gastric cancers There is no doubt that EUS is less accurate for the estimation of N stage than for T stage in gastric cancer. The overall accuracy is about 70% (**Table 1.12**). It is most accurate for the estimation of N0 status and least accurate in its ability to demonstrate involved N2 nodes. However, compared with CT scanning's overall accuracy of little better than 50% for the estimation of nodal status, EUS remains the best staging modality available for this parameter. It is difficult to envisage how modifications to the technique of EUS will improve its ability to evaluate the nodal status of patients with gastric cancer.

Comparison of staging methodologies

As in the case of esophageal carcinoma, it is an artificial discussion to consider which staging modality is "best" for the patient with gastric carcinoma. The two modalities are complementary and have a different pattern of strengths and weaknesses. This was elegantly demonstrated by Botet et al. in 1991,[74] who showed that the overall accuracy of CT scanning was 45% of cases, rising to 73% of cases when combined with the findings of EUS examination. However, because of its greater accuracy in assessing T and local N stage and the low incidence of distant metastases in patients presenting with gastric carcinoma, the use of EUS alone was similar in accuracy to CT and EUS.

In its current state of development, MRI scanning has little to add to the routine staging of patients with gastric cancer, but new developments should be watched with interest.

Laparoscopic staging

Laparoscopy and intraoperative ultrasound

The role of laparoscopy in the routine staging of patients with gastric carcinoma remains controversial, and while much data have been published, no clear consensus has emerged (**Table 1.14**). Unlike esophageal cancer, there is still a role for palliative resection in patients with advanced symptomatic disease and while other treatment modalities are gaining acceptance, their use is not universal. Much of the data regarding staging laparoscopy for patients with gastric carcinoma have come from centers with a high incidence of very advanced disease; in Japan where more than 60% of the cancers are EGCs, staging laparoscopy is very rare. The other difficulty regarding the evaluation of staging laparoscopy is that much of the published data have mixed cases of gastric and esophageal carcinoma, making an independent analysis extremely difficult. The major series of published data are shown in **Table 1.14**; a striking feature is the extreme variability of the results reported.

What then is the evidence regarding staging laparoscopy? There is no doubt that disease that would preclude curative surgical resection and, unappreciated by preoperative CT scanning, is detected in 20–30% of Western patients.[91,97] However, it is clear that from preceding discussions the optimal "non-invasive" staging is obtained with a combination of helical CT and endoscopic ultrasound examination, and there is no large series looking at the added utility of laparoscopy in this setting. Most of the disease thus detected is unexpected peritoneal metastases occurring in patients with T3/T4 tumors; unexpected liver metastases are uncommon (4%[91]) when modern helical CT scanning has been employed prior to laparoscopy. Although only commented on in a few papers,[87] there is no doubt that to maximize the yield from staging laparoscopy, the lesser sac needs to be entered. This in itself poses few difficulties, but potentially can make subsequent radical surgery technically more difficult if there is a delay between laparoscopy and definitive surgery.

What is unclear from published data is the precise relationship between the usefulness of staging laparoscopy and the stage of the tumor as derived from EUS and CT examination. It is my own personal belief that the role of staging laparoscopy is in

Table 1.14 Results of staging laparoscopy for gastric and esophageal neoplasms. Peritoneal metastases and liver metastases refer to the proportion of patients in whom they were found when conventional (usually CT) imaging had failed to detect them. Resectability refers to the proportion of patients in whom laparoscopy had suggested that the lesion was resectable and was found to be so at subsequent laparotomy. Treatment altered refers to the number of patients in whom a significant change in management was made, e.g., no operation. Overall accuracy refers to the results of laparoscopy together with conventional imaging (CT). n.s. = not specified

REFERENCE	YEAR	NO. OF PATIENTS	LOCATION OF TUMORS	PERITONEAL METASTASES (%)	LIVER METASTASES (%)	RESECTABILITY (%)	TREATMENT ALTERED (%)	OVERALL ACCURACY (%)
Asencio et al.[83]	1997	71	71 gastric (n.b. only 37 patients had a CT scan)	30	25	97	41	80
Bemelman et al.[84]	1995	56	38 esophageal 18 gastric	3	2	100	6	98
Bonavina et al.[85]	1997	50	14 esophageal 36 gastric	11	3	100	10	92
Burke et al.[86]	1997	111	111 gastric	37	n.s	100	22	94
Charukhchyan and Lucas[87]	1998	502	502 gastric	n.s	n.s	43 (93% with lesser sac examination)	n.s.	95 (with lesser sac examination)
D'Ugo et al.[88]	1997	100	100 gastric	n.s	n.s	n.s	21	72
Dagnini et al.[89]	1986	369	280 esophageal 89 gastric no patient had CT scan	5	10	95	20	96
Kriplani and Kapur[90]	1991	40	40 gastric	10	10	87	40	92
Lowy et al.[91]	1996	71	71 gastric	25	4	93	23	93
Molloy et al.[92]	1995	244	244 cardia and esophagus	31	10	72	42	n.s
O'Brien et al.[93]	1995	145	110 carcinoma of gastroesophageal junction, 30 esophageal	16	1.4	n.s	9	92
Possik et al.[94]	1986	360	360 gastric no patient had CT scan	35	17	80	34	83
Stell et al.[95]	1996	103	103 gastric	8	6	81	17	96
Van Dijkum et al.[96]	1997	64	64 esophageal	n.s	n.s	n.s	6	n.s

the evaluation of patients with T3 or T4 tumors as judged by CT and EUS. Given the very low incidence of distant metastases, and the almost unheard of finding of peritoneal metastases in patients with T1 or T2a disease, it is difficult to believe that the routine use of laparoscopy is justifiable in these patients.

The addition of laparoscopic ultrasound to laparoscopy will certainly increase the ability to detect liver metastases. In a series of 111 patients with advanced gastric cancer, the use of laparoscopic ultrasound detected liver metastases in 8% of cases that were not seen on preoperative imaging.[57] It therefore seems appropriate to recommend the use of laparoscopic ultrasonography to laparoscopy in the preoperative evaluation of patients with advanced gastric cancer in whom the finding of liver metastases would obviate the need for a laparotomy.

In summary, laparoscopy/laparoscopic ultrasound will provide additional and important staging information in a significant minority of patients with advanced gastric cancer. The precise role of laparoscopy/laparoscopic ultrasonography will vary from center to center according to many factors, such as the stage mix of the patients being treated, and the other staging modalities available locally.

In my own practice we would perform an initial helical CT scan. If there was no evidence of disseminated disease on this examination, we would proceed to endoscopic ultrasound examination. If the combined staging suggested stage I, II or IIIa disease, we would then proceed to surgery. If however the likely stage were IIIb or IV, then most patients will be laparoscoped with selective use of laparoscopic ultrasonography. Using this policy, the incidence of open/close exploratory laparotomies is between 1 and 2%. We do not routinely enter the lesser sac and certainly with increasing use of endoscopic ultrasound we have not found unexpected posterior fixity to present a clinical problem.

Peritoneal cytology

The routine use of intraoperative cytology is widespread in Japan. At the start of the operation for an advanced gastric cancer, 100–150 ml of warm saline are instilled into the peritoneal cavity. Following gentle agitation, 40–50 ml of the saline solution is recovered and sent for cytologic examination. The recovered saline is centrifuged and

examined for the presence of neoplastic cells. In patients with serosal invasion, peritoneal cytology is positive in 12–38% of cases.[98,99]

The finding of neoplastic cells is not unsurprisingly associated with a poorer prognosis, as has recently been demonstrated in Dutch patients by Bonenkamp *et al.* (**Figure 1.13**).[98] The influence of positive peritoneal cytology has not as yet been incorporated formally into either the Japanese or UICC staging systems.

It could easily be postulated that patients with positive peritoneal cytology, but no other residual disease, would be good candidates for postoperative intraperitoneal chemotherapy. This approach is being actively studied by several groups, but as yet no results have been published.

Pathologic staging

Histologic classification/staging

The American pathologist Stout commented in 1953 that "histological classification was valueless and that a knowledge of the gross appearance and spread of tumours was of more value in assessment of prognosis."[100] This view has persisted for many years and there is widespread belief among clinicians and pathologists that histologic grading of gastric cancers adds nothing further to the assessment of prognosis over and above what may be derived from the TNM stage of the tumor. We have demonstrated that the only

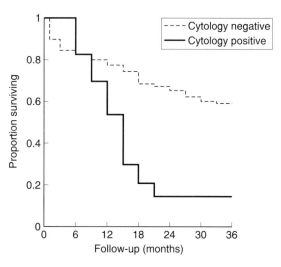

Figure 1.13 The prognostic value of positive cytology findings from abdominal washings in patients with gastric cancer.[98]

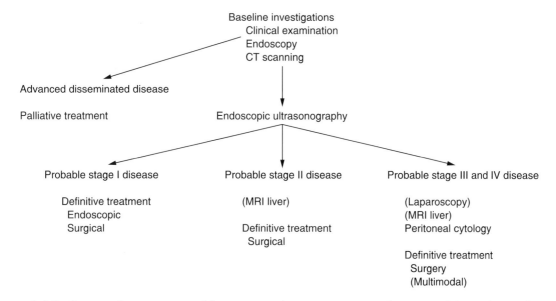

Figure 1.14 Suggested staging protocol for patients with gastric carcinoma. Staging modalities whose value is unproven or difficult to justify in all cases are indicated by parentheses.

histologic staging system to add to the prognostic information provided by the TNM classification is the Goseki classification.[101,102] Goseki and colleagues[102] based their system on two features of gastric cancer: the structural features of tubular differentiation, and the functional status of mucus production.

The Lauren classification[103] has been one of the most widely applied histologic grading systems, particularly in epidemiologic studies. While this system may have its applications in such broad epidemiologic studies, there is no evidence that the Lauren classification can add to the prognostic information that is provided by TNM staging. In the original description of the Lauren system there was an 8% difference in survival between the intestinal and diffuse groups at three years (43% versus 35% respectively).[103] However, when the Lauren classification was applied by other authors to larger series of patients, no difference in 5-year survival was found.[104]

Staging strategy for gastric carcinoma

The overall strategy for staging the patient with gastric carcinoma will inevitably vary from unit to unit, and will be highly dependent upon the available resources and, in particular, the case mix seen. There is no doubt that one of the reasons for differing strategies between Japan and the West is the different proportions of early gastric cancer. **Figure 1.14** shows a recommended staging protocol for the patient with cancer which takes into account currently published data, but does not reflect skills and resources that may not be available in many Western units, such as the very skilled endoscopic assessment found in Japan. Despite the recent enthusiasm for laparoscopic staging of patients with gastric cancer, it is very difficult to justify its routine use. As liver metastases are relatively uncommon in patients with gastric carcinoma, the use of laparoscopy should be confined to patients with a significant risk of peritoneal spread, that is stage III or stage IV disease.

REFERENCES

1. Committee on TNM classification. *TNM classification of malignant tumours.* Geneva, International Union Against Cancer, 1968: 25–6.
2. Committee on TNM classification. *TNM classification of malignant tumours.* International Union Against Cancer, 2nd edition, Geneva, 1974: 39–42.

3. Committee on TNM classification. *TNM classification of malignant tumours*. International Union Against Cancer, 3rd edition, Geneva, 1978: 57–61.

4. Committee on TNM classification. *TNM classification of malignant tumours*. International Union Against Cancer, 4th edition, Berlin: Springer, 1987: 40–2.

5. Sobin LH and Wittekind C (eds) *TNM Classification of Malignant Tumours*, 5th Edition. New York: John Wiley & Sons, Inc., 1997.

6. Akiyama H, Tsurumaru M, Udagawa H & Kajiyama Y. Radical lymph node dissection for cancer of the thoracic oesophagus. *Ann Surg* 1994; **220**: 364–72.

7. Japanese Society for Esophageal Diseases. Guidelines for clinical and pathologic studies on carcinoma of the esophagus. *Jpn J Surg* 1976; **6**: 70–86.

8. Akiyama H. *Surgery for Cancer of the Esophagus*. Baltimore: Williams & Wilkins, 1990.

9. Tanabe G, Baba M, Kuroshima K *et al.* Clinical evaluation of esophageal lymph flow based on the RI uptake of removal regional lymph nodes following lymphoscintigraphy. *J Jpn Surg Soc* 1986; **87**: 315–23.

10. Haagensen CD. *The Lymphatics in Cancer*. Philadelphia: WB Saunders, 1972: 60–84.

11. Akiyama H, Tsurumaru M, Udagawa H & Kajiyama Y. Systemic lymph node disection for esophageal carcinoma – effective or not? *Dis Esoph* 1994; **7**: 2–13.

12. Roder JD, Busch R, Stein HJ, Fink U & Siewert JR. Ratio of invaded to removed lymph nodes as a predictor of survival in squamous cell carcinoma of the oesophagus. *Br J Surg* 1994; **81**: 410–13.

13. Rösch T, Classen M & Dittler HJ. *Gastroenterologic Endosonography*. Stuttgart: Georg Thieme Verlag, 1992.

14. Rösch T, Lorenz R, Zenker K *et al.* Local staging and assessment of resectability in carcinoma of the esophagus, stomach and duodenum by endoscopic ultrasonography. *Gastrointest Endosc* 1992; **38**: 460–7.

15. Sugimachi K, Watanabe M, Sadanaga N *et al.* Pre-operative estimation of complete resection for patients with oesophageal carcinoma. *Surg Oncol* 1994; **3**: 327–34.

16. Akiyama H, Kogure T & Itai Y. The esophageal axis and its relationship to the resectability of carcinoma of the esophagus. *Ann Surg* 1972; **190**: 100.

16a. Japanese Society for Esophageal Diseases. *Guidelines for the Clinical and Pathological Studies on Carcinoma of the Esophagus*. 8th Edition, Tokyo, Kanebara, 1992.

17. Dittler HJ, Pesarini AC & Siewert JR. Endoscopic classification of esophageal cancer: correlation with T stage. *Gastrointest Endosc* 1992; **38**: 662–7.

18. Hölscher AH, Dittler HJ & Siewert JR. Staging of squamous esophageal cancer: accuracy and value. *World J Surg* 1994; **18**: 312–20.

19. Botet JF, Lightdale CJ, Zauber AG, Gerdes H, Urmacher C & Brennan MF. Preoperative staging of esophageal cancer: comparison of endoscopic US and dynamic CT. *Radiology* 1991; **181**: 419–25.

20. Thompson WM & Halvorsen RA. Staging esophageal carcinoma II: CT and MRI. *Semin Oncol* 1994; **21**: 447–52.

21. Lehr L, Rupp N & Siewert JR. Assessment of the resectability of esophageal carcinoma by computed tomography and magnetic resonance imaging. *Surgery* 1988; **103**: 344–8.

22. Goei R, Lamers RJ, Engelshove HA & Oei KT. Computed tomographic staging of esophageal carcinoma: a study on interobserver variation and correlation with pathological findings. *Eur J Radiol* 1992; **15**: 40–4.

23. Liang EY, Chan A, Chung CS & Metreweli C. Short communication: oesophageal tumour volume measurement using spiral CT. *Br J Radiol* 1996; **69**: 344–7.

24. Watt I, Stewart I, Anderson E, Bell G & Anderson JR. Laparoscopy, ultrasound and computer tomography in cancer of the oesophagus and gastric cardia: a prospective comparison for detecting intraabdominal metastases. *Br J Surg* 1989; **76**: 1036–40.

25. Takashima S, Takeuchi N, Shiozaki H *et al.* Carcinoma of the esophagus: CT vs. MR imaging in determining resectability. *Am J Roentgenol* 1991; **156**: 297–302.

26. Quint LE, Glazer GM & Orringer MB. Esophageal imaging by MR and CT: study of normal anatomy and neoplasms. *Radiology* 1985; **156**: 727–31.

27. Inui K, Nakazawa S, Yoshino J *et al.* Endoscopic MRI: preliminary results of a new technique for visualization and staging of gastrointestinal tumours. *Endoscopy* 1995; **27**: 480–5.

28. DiMagno EP, Buxton JL, Regan PT *et al.* Ultrasonic endoscope. *Lancet* 1980; **i**: 629–31.

29. Strohm WD, Philip J, Hagenmuller F *et al.* Ultrasonic tomography by means of an ultrasonic fiberendoscopy. *Endoscopy* 1980; **12**: 241–4.

30. Kimmey MB, Martin RW, Haggitt RC *et al.* Histologic correlates of gastrointestinal ultrasound images. *Gastroenterology* 1989; **96**: 433–41.

31. Wiersema MJ & Wiersema LM. High resolution 25-MegaHertz ultrasonography of the gastrointestinal wall: histologic correlates. *Gastrointest Endosc* 1993; **39**: 499–504.

32. Simuzu Y, Tsukagoshi H, Nakazato T *et al.* Clinical evaluation of endoscopic ultrasonography (EUS) in the diagnosis of superficial esophageal carcinoma. *Jpn J Clin Pathol* 1995; **43**: 221–6.

33. Dittler HJ, Rösch Th, Fink U, Siewert JR & Classen M. Endosonographic restaging of carcinoma of the esophagus and cardia following radio and chemotherapy. *Gastrointest Endosc* 1992; **38**: 241–4.

34. Falk GW, Catalano MF, Sivak MR, Rice TW & Van Dam J. Endosonography in the evaluation of patients with Barrett's esophagus and high grade dysplasia. *Gastrointest Endosc* 1994; **40**: 207–12.

35. Catalano MF, Sivak MV, Rice T, Gragg, LA & Van Dam J. Endosonographic features predictive of lymph node metastasis. *Gastrointest Endosc* 1994; **40**: 442–6.

36. Chandawarakar RY, Kakegawa T, Fujita H, Yamana H, Toh Y, Fujitoh H. Endosonography for preoperative staging of specific nodal groups associated with esophageal cancer. *World J Surg* 1996; **20**: 700–2.

37. Catalano MF, Van Dam J & Sivak MV. Malignant esophageal strictures: staging accuracy of endoscopic ultrasonography. *Gastrointest Endosc* 1995; **41**: 535–9.

38. Van Dam J, Rice TW, Catalano MF, Kriby T & Sivak MV. High grade malignant stricture is predictive of esophageal tumour stage. Risks of endosonographic evaluation. *Cancer* 1993; **71**: 2910–17.

39. Rösch T, Dittler JH, Fockens P, Yasuda K & Lightdale C. Major complications of endoscopic ultrasonography: results of a survey of 42,105 cases. *Gastrointest Endosc* 1993; **39**: A341.

40. Binmoeller KF, Seifert H, Seitz U, Izbicki JR, Kida M & Soehendra N. Ultrasonic esophagoprobe for TNM staging of highly stenosing esophageal carcinoma. *Gastrointest Endosc* 1995; **41**: 547–52.

41. Saisho H, Sai K, Tsuyuguchi T, Yamaguchi T, Matsutani S & Ohto M. A new small probe for ultrasound imaging via conventional endoscope. *Gastrointest Endosc* 1995; **41**: 141–3.

42. Tachimori Y, Kato H, Watanabe H & Yamaguchi H. Neck ultrasonography for thoracic esophageal carcinoma. *Ann Thorac Surg* 1994; **57**: 1180–3.

43. Van Overhagen H, Lameris JS, Berger MY *et al.* Improved assessment of supraclavicular and abdominal metastases in oesophageal and gastro-oesophageal junction carcinoma with the combination of ultrasound and computed tomography. *Br J Radiol* 1993; **66**: 203–8.

44. Tio TL, Coene PPLO, den Hartog Jager FCA & Tytgat GNT. Preoperative TNM classification of esophageal carcinoma by endosonography. *Hepatogastroenterology* 1990; **37**: 376–8.

45. Ziegler K, Sanft C, Zeitz M *et al.* Evaluation of endosonography in TN staging of oesophageal carcinoma. *Gut* 1991; **32**: 16.

46. Grimm H, Maydeo A, Hamper K, Maas R, Noar M & Soehendra N. Results of endoscopic ultrasound and computed tomography in preoperative staging of esophageal carcinoma: a prospective controlled study. *Gastrointest Endosc* 1991; **37**: 279.

47. Heintz A, Hölme U, Schweden F & Junginger T. Endosonographie versus Computertomographie bei der praoperativen Stadienbeurteilung von Ösophaguscarcinomen. *Z. Gastroenterol* 1991; **29**: 49.

48. Schüder G, Koch B, Seitz G, Hildbrandt U, Ecker KW & Feifel G. Endosonograpisches Staging beim Ösophaguscarcinom – ein prospektiver Vergleich mit herkommlichen bildgebenen Verfahren. *Z. Gastroenterol* 1990; **28**: 534.

49. Vilgrain V, Mompoint D, Palazzo L *et al.* Staging of esophageal carcinoma: comparison of endoscopic US and dynamic CT. *Am J Roentgenol* 1990; **155**: 277.

50. Greenberg J, Durkin M, An Drunen M & Aranha GV. Computed tomography or endoscopic ultrasonography in preoperative staging of gastric and esophageal tumours. *Surgery* 1994; **116**: 701–2.

51. Holden A, Mendelson R & Edmunds S. Preoperative staging of gastro-oesophageal junction carcinoma: comparison of endoscopic ultrasound and computed tomography. *Aust Radiol* 1996; **40**: 206–12.

52. Tachimori Y, Kato H, Watanabe H, Sasako M, Kinoshita T & Maruyama K. Difference between carcinoma of the lower esophagus and the cardia. *World J Surg* 1996; **20**: 507–10.

53. Molloy RG, McCourtney JS & Anderson JR. Laparoscopy in the management of patients with cancer of the gastric cardia and oesophagus. *Br J Surg* 1995; **82**: 352–4.

54. O'Brien MG, Fitzgerald EF, Lee G, Crowley M, Shanahan F & O'Sullivan GC. A prospective comparison of laparoscopy and imaging in the staging of esophagogastric cancer before surgery. *Am J Gastroenterol* 1995; **90**: 2191–4.

55. Krasna MJ, Flowers JL, Attar S & McLaughlin J. Combined thoracoscopic/laparoscopic staging of esophageal cancer. *J. Thorac Cardiovasc Surg* 1996; **111**: 800–6.

56. Bemelman WA, van Delden OM, van Lanschot JJ *et al.* Laparoscopy and laparoscopic ultrasonography in staging of carcinoma of the esophagus and gastric cardia. *J Am Coll Surg* 1995; **181**: 421–5.

57. Feussner H, Kraemer SJ & Siewert JR. The technique of laparoscopic ultrasound study in diagnostic laparoscopy (in German) *Langenbecks Archiv fur Chirurgie* 1994; **379**: 248–54.

58. Krasna MJ, Reed CE, Jaklitsch MT, Cushing D & Sugarbaker DJ. Thoracoscopic staging of esophageal cancer: a prospective multiinstitutional trial. *Ann Thorac Surg* 1995; **60**: 1337–40.

59. Sarbia M, Bittinger F, Porschen R, Dutkowski P, Willers R & Gabbert HE. Prognostic value of histopathologic parameters of esophageal squamous carcinoma. *Cancer* 1995; **76**: 922–7.

60. Lieberman MD, Shriver CD, Bleckner S & Burt M. Carcinoma of the esophagus. Prognostic significance of histologic type. *J Thorac Cardiovasc Surg* 1995; **109**: 130–8.

61. Kuwano H, Watanabe M, Sadanaga N *et al.* Univariate and multivariate analyses of the pronostic significance of discontinuous intramural metastasis in patients with esophageal carcinoma. *J Surg Oncol* 1994; **57**: 17–21.

62. Hölscher AH, Bollschweiler E, Bumm R, Bartels H, Höfler H & Siewert JR. Prognostic factors of resected adenocarcinoma of the oesophagus. *Surgery* 1995; **118**: 845–55.

63. Sagar PM, Johnston D, McMahon MJ, Dixon MF & Quirke P. Significance of circumferential resection margin involvement after oesophagectomy. *Br J Surg* 1993; **80**: 1386–8.

64. Japanese Research Society for Gastric Cancer. General rules for the study of gastric cancer. *Jpn J. Surg* 1981; **11**: 127–45.

65. Japanese Research Society for Gastric Cancer. *Japanese Classification of Gastric Carcinoma.* 1st English Edition. Tokyo: Kanehara, 1995.

66. Sasako M, McCulloch P, Kinoshita T & Maruyama K. New method to evaluate the therapeutic value of lymph node dissection for gastric cancer. *Br J Surg* 1995; **82**: 346–51.

67. Soga J, Kobayashi K, Saito J, Fuijimaki M & Muto T. The role of lymphadenectomy in curative surgery for gastric cancer. *World J Surg* 1979; **3**: 101–8.

68. Kodama Y, Sugimachi K, Soejima K, Matsusuka T & Inokuchi K. Evaluation of extensive lymph node dissection for carcinoma of the stomach. *World J Surg* 1981; **5**: 241–8.

69. Maruyama K, Kinoshita T, Sasako M & Okabayashi K. New technologies in gastric cancer surgery: computer system to make operation plan and intraoperative staining of regional lymph nodes for complete dissection. *Dev Oncol* 1990; **59**: 107–18.

70. Bollschweiler E, Boettcher K, Hoelscher AH *et al.* Preoperative assessment of lymph node metastases in patients with gastric cancer: evaluation of the Maruyama computer program. *Br J Surg* 1992; **79**: 156–60.

71. Sano T, Okuyama Y, Kobori O, Shimuzu T & Morioka Y. Early gastric cancer: endoscopic assessment of depth of invasion. *Digest Dis Sci* 1990; **35**: 1340–4.

72. Yamoa T, Shirao K, Ono H *et al.* Risk factors for lymph node metastasis from intramucosal gastric carcinoma. *Cancer* 1995; **77**: 602–6.

73. Sano T, Kobori O & Muto T. Lymph node metastasis from early gastric cancer: endoscopic resection of tumour. *Br J Surg* 1992; **79**: 241–4.

74. Botet JF, Lightdale CJ, Zauber AG *et al.* Preoperative staging of gastric cancer: comparison of endoscopic ultrasound and dynamic CT. *Radiology* 1991; **181**: 426–32.

75. Halvorsen RA, Yee J & McCormick VD. Diagnosis and staging of gastric cancer. *Semin Oncol* 1996; **23**: 325–35.

76. Andaker L, Morales O, Hojer H, Backstrand B, Borch K & Larsson J. Evaluation of pre-operative computed tomography in gastric malignancy. *Surgery* 1991; **109**: 132–5.

77. Oberstein A, Bockhorn H & Meves M. The value of computerised and magnetic resonance imaging for staging esophageal and cardiac cancer in comparison with conventional diagnosis. *Bildgebung* 1989; **56**: 91–6.

78. Matsushita M. Oi H, Murakami T *et al.* Extraserosal invasion in advanced gastric cancer: evaluation with MR imaging. *Radiology* 1994; **192**: 87–91.

79. Isozaki H, Okajima K, Nomura E *et al.* Preoperative diagnosis and surgical treatment for lymph node metastasis in gastric cancer (Japanese). *Jpn J Cancer Chemother* 1995; **23**: 1275–83.

80. Pollack BJ, Chak A & Sivak MV. Endoscopic ultrasonography. *Semin Oncol* 1996; **23**: 336–46.

81. Rösch T. Endosonographic staging of gastric cancer: a review of the literature results. *Gastrointest Endosc Clin N Amer* 1995; **5**: 549–57.

82. Yanai H, Fulimura H, Suzumi M *et al.* Delineation of the gastric muscularis mucosae and assessment of depth of invasion of early gastric cancer using a 20 MHz endoscopic ultrasound probe. *Gastrointest Endosc* 1993; **39**: 505–12.

83. Asencio F, Aguilo J, Salvador JL *et al.* Video-laparoscopic staging of gastric cancer. A prospective multicenter comparison with noninvasive techniques. *Surg Endosc* 1997; **11**: 1153–8.

84. Bemelman WA, van Delden OM, van Lanschot JJ *et al.* Laparoscopy and laparoscopic ultrasonography in staging of carcinoma of the esophagus and gastric cardia. *J Am Coll Surg* 1995; **181**: 421–5.

85. Bonavina L, Incarbone R, Lattuda E, Segalin A, Cesana B & Peracchia A. Preoperative laparoscopy in management of patients with carcinoma of the esophagus and of the esophagogastric junction. *J Surg Oncol* 1997; **65**: 171–4.

86. Burke EC, Karpeh MS, Conlon KC & Brennan MF. Laparoscopy in the management of gastric adenocarcinoma. *Ann Surg* 1997; **225**: 262–7.

87. Charukhchyan SA & Lucas GW. Laparoscopy and lesser sac endoscopy in gastric carcinoma operability assessment. *Am Surg* 1998; **64**: 160–4.

88. D'Ugo DM, Persani R, Caracciolo F, Roconi P, Coco C & Picciocchi A. Selection of locally advanced gastric carcinoma by preoperative staging laparoscopy. *Surg Endosc* 1997; **11**: 1159–62.

89. Dagnini G, Caldironi MW, Marin G, Buzzaccarini O, Tremolada C & Ruol A. Laparoscopy in abdominal staging of esophageal carcinoma. Report of 369 cases. *Gastrointest Endosc* 1986; **32**: 400–2.

90. Kriplani AK & Kapur BM. Laparoscopy for preoperative staging and assessment of operability in gastric carcinoma. *Gastrointest Endosc* 1991; **37**: 441–3.

91. Lowy AM, Mansfield PF, Leach SD & Ajani J. Laparoscopic staging for gastric cancer. *Surgery* 1996; **119**: 611–14.

92. Molloy RG, McCourtney JS & Anderson JR. Laparoscopy in the management of patients with cancer of the gastric cardia and oesophagus. *Br J Surg* 1995; **82**: 352–4.

93. O'Brien MG, Fitzgerald EF, Lee G, Crowley M, Shanahan F & O'Sullivan GC. A prospective comparison of laparoscopy and imaging in the staging of esophagogastric cancer before surgery [see comments]. *Am J Gastroenterol* 1995; **90**: 2191–4.

94. Possik RA, Franco EL, Pires DR, Wohnrath DR & Ferreira EB. Sensitivity, specificity, and predictive value of laparoscopy for the staging of gastric cancer and for the detection of liver metastases. *Cancer* 1986; **58**: 1–6.

95. Stell DA, Carter CR, Stewart L & Anderson JR. Prospective comparison of laparoscopy, ultrasonography and computed tomography in the staging of gastric cancer [see comments]. *Br J Surg* 1996; **83**: 1260–2.

96. van Dijkum EJ, de Wit LT, van Delden OM *et al.* The efficacy of laparoscopic staging in patients with upper gastrointestinal tumors. *Cancer* 1997; **79**: 1315–9.

97. Conlon KC & Karpeh MS, Jr. Laparoscopy and laparoscopic ultrasound in the staging of gastric cancer. *Semin Oncol* 1996; **23**: 347–51.

98. Bonenkamp JJ, Songun I, Hermans JN & van de Velde CJ. Prognostic value of positive cytology findings from abdominal washings in patients with gastric cancer. *Br J Surg* 1996; **83**: 672–4.

99. Teramoto T, Onda M, Tokunaga A *et al.* Evaluation of peritoneal lavage smears and gastric wall brushing smears in gastric cancer surgery (Japanese). *Jpn J Cancer Chemother* 1994; **21**: 2260–2.

100. Stout AP. Armed Forces Institute of Pathology. F65. *Tumours of the stomach, fasicle 21.* Washington, DC, 1953.

101. Martin IG, Dixon MF, Sue-Ling H, Axon ATR & Johnston D. Histological grading can predict survival in gastric cancer: an assessment of the prognostic value of the Goseki grading system. *Gut* 1994; **35**: 758–63.

102. Goseki N, Takizawa T & Koike M. Differences in the mode of extension of gastric cancer classified by histological type: new histological classification of gastric carcinoma. *Gut* 1992; **33**: 606–12.

103. Lauren P. The two histological main types of gastric carcinoma. *Acta Pathol Microbiol Scand* 1965; **64**: 31–49.

104. Hawley PR, Westerman P & Morson BC. Pathology and prognosis of carcinoma of the stomach. *Br J Surg* 1970; **57**: 877–83.

2

BARRETT'S ESOPHAGUS, INTESTINAL METAPLASIA AND ADENOCARCINOMA

JOHN V. REYNOLDS

INTRODUCTION

Barrett's esophagus is a condition in which the normal squamous mucosa of the esophagus is replaced by columnar epithelium resembling intestinal-type mucosa.[1] The condition was first described in 1906 by Tileston, a pathologist, who noted the close resemblance of the mucosa around "peptic ulcers of the esophagus" to gastric mucosa.[2] In 1950, Norman Rupert Barrett, an English cardiothoracic surgeon, erroneously characterized esophageal ulcers as resulting from a congenitally short esophagus that pulled a tubular stomach into the mediastinum, mistaking the ulcerated, columnar-lined esophagus for an intrathoracic stomach.[3] Allison and Johnstone in 1953 identified that the intrathoracic viscus was clearly esophagus and not stomach[4] and suggested that ulcers in the columnar-lined esophagus should be called "Barrett's ulcers," thus generously perpetuating this eponym. Both Barrett and Allison assumed that the esophageal columnar lining was congenital in origin. This was first challenged in 1960, when Goldman and Beckman proposed that Barrett's epithelium is most likely acquired in response to esophageal injury.[5] Considerable experimental and clinical evidence now support this proposal, including the high prevalence of Barrett's esophagus among patients with severe reflux esophagitis, the mid-life median age of diag-nosis and its rarity in childhood, and its association with other conditions promoting reflux, including scleroderma, treated achalasia, and following major esophagogastric resections.

The importance of Barrrett's epithelium lies in its malignant potential.[6,7] The association of intestinal epithelium containing goblet cells with Barrett's esophagus was first reported in 1951 by Bosher and Taylor,[8] and a year later Morson and Belcher[9] described this association with adenocarcinoma. Goblet cells staining positive for acid mucopolysaccharide and Alcian blue are characteristic of what is now called specialized intestinal metaplasia (SIM), which in addition may contain villous projections, paneth, and enterochromaffin cells.[10] Although Paull *et al.*[11] in their seminal report on the histologic spectrum of Barrett's esophagus in 1976 identified two other types of metaplasia in addition to SIM, neither gastric–fundic epithelium nor junctional epithelium appears to have premalignant potential and SIM represents the true Barrett's premalignant pathologic phenotype. The progression of SIM to low-grade dysplasia and high-grade dysplasia and ultimately invasive adenocarcinoma has been well described in subsequent years, although an understanding of the molecular and biochemical events in this model of tumorigenesis is in its infancy.

Barrett's esophagus is identified endoscopically by a rich-pink, velvety appearance in the lower esophagus replacing the pale, pink-gray squamous mucosa. This pattern is typically circumferential, but it may be present in tongues of mucosa in the squamous lining. The condition has been arbitrarily defined as ≥3 cm of this macroscopic phenotype above the esophagogastric junction, which is most often identified endoscopically by the proximal margin of the gastric folds or the point where the tubular stomach expands into the sac-like stomach. There are considerable technical problems however in determining endoscopically where the end of a dynamic structure such as the esophagus ends and the stomach begins, and this is subject to considerable imprecision.

The definition of Barrett's esophagus based on this macroscopic phenotype is necessarily arbitrary. The principal purpose of this definition was to avoid false-positive biopsies of stomach especially in patients with hiatus hernia and severe reflux esophagitis. This traditional understanding of what Barrett's esophagus denotes is currently of little value, since it has become clear that SIM can occur in macroscopic Barrett's epithelium extending <3 cm into the lower esophagus, or in macroscopically normal and thus endoscopically inconspicuous biopsies taken from below the gastroesophageal junction.[12] It is also evident that short segments of SIM can be associated with adenocarcinoma of the esophagus, esophagogastric junction, and gastric cardia.[13,14]

This author favors the modern view that SIM over any length is abnormal and probably associated with malignant potential, and that a new nomenclature and classification is required.[1] The focus of this article is to tie in the emerging knowledge in this area with the existing literature on traditional Barrett's esophagus, and to highlight the key management strategies as they relate to the diagnosis, treatment and prevention of adenocarcinoma of the lower esophagus, esophagogastric junction, and gastric cardia.

THE RISING INCIDENCE OF ADENOCARCINOMA OF THE ESOPHAGUS AND GASTRIC CARDIA

Attention has focused on Barrett's esophagus and SIM in recent years largely due to the alarming increase in incidence of adenocarcinoma of the esophagus and proximal stomach. In 1991, Blot

et al.[15] reported on the trends for esophageal and gastric cancer from 1976 to 1987 identified through the population-based cancer registries that constitute the National Cancer Institute's Surveillance, Epidemiology and End Results Program. The incidence rate for adenocarcinoma of the esophagus increased by 100% among men during this time, while the rates for squamous cell cancer were stable. In marked contrast to previous reports, the rates of adenocarcinoma of the esophagus exceeded rates of squamous cell cancers among white men below the age of 55 in the period 1984–1987. A similar trend was observed in the proximal stomach, and by 1987 adenocarcinoma of the cardia represented 47% of gastric cancers. By 1987, the annual age-adjusted incidence rate for adenocarcinoma of the esophagus and gastric cardia combined was 5.1 per 100 000 white men, ranking it as one of the 15 most common cancers in the United States. For both cancers, the rate of increase during the 1970s and 1980s, approximately 5–10% per year, surpassed that of any other cancer. A rising incidence of these cancers was also observed in Europe.[16–18]

This trend is also highlighted in other recent important studies. Pera et al.[19] from the Mayo Clinic reported on the increased incidence of adenocarcinoma of the esophagus and esophagogastric junction in the residents of Olmstead County, Minnesota between 1975 and 1989. Seventeen residents developed squamous cell cancer, eight developed adenocarcinoma of the esophagus, and 14 developed adenocarcinoma of the esophagogastric junction. Comparing this period with the period 1935–1971, the annual incidence of esophageal adenocarcinoma for Olmstead County increased from 0.13 to 0.74 per 100 000 person-years, and that of junctional adenocarcinoma from 0.25 to 1.34 per 100 000 person-years. Daly et al.[20] compared data on 4368 cases accessioned by the National Cancer DataBase in 1988 with 5256 cases accessioned in 1993. Incidence of adenocarcinoma of the esophagus increased from 33% in 1988 to 43% in 1993, while that of lower-esophageal tumors increased from 41% to 48%. The experience of large specialist units, such as the recent report from the Johns Hopkins Hospital, confirms this dramatic rise in esophageal adenocarcinoma in white men.[21]

"TRADITIONAL" BARRETT'S ESOPHAGUS: THE RISK OF ADENOCARCINOMA

Barrett's esophagus with SIM is the only recognized risk factor for esophageal adenocarcinoma. The likelihood of adenocarcinoma developing in an individual is unclear. Past studies have varied widely and are confused by slight changes in definition and contamination with prevalence data, but in general relate to a minimum of 3 cm of columnar-lined epithelium in the lower esophagus. The studies do not include patients with shorter segments of columnar epithelium and are not specific for SIM. In six retrospective series, the cancer incidence ranged from 1/55 to 1/141 patient-years with an average or 1/161 patient-years of follow-up.[22–27] In six prospective studies where SIM was present in between 68 and 100% of cases, the incidence of adenocarcinoma ranged from 1/52 to 1/208 years of patient follow-up, an average of 1/104.[28–33] For adult patients with Barrett's esophagus, the annual rate of cancer development is between 0.5% and 1%.

Short-segment Barrett's esophagus

The increasing recognition that many patients who had esophagectomies for adenocarcinoma at the esophagogastric junction had SIM identified in the resected specimen led Spechler and colleagues at the Beth Israel Hospital in Boston prospectively to evaluate SIM at the squamocolumnar junction.[12] They studied 142 patients undergoing elective endoscopic examination in a general endoscopy unit. Two biopsy specimens were taken from the squamocolumnar junction (the Z line) in the distal esophagus, irrespective of its appearance and location. Two patients (1%) were found to have endoscopically apparent Barrett's esophagus, i.e., SIM >3 cm above the gastroesophageal junction. Among 14 patients with no endoscopic evidence of Barrett's esophagus, 26 (18%) were found by hematoxylin and eosin (H&E) staining to have SIM at the gastroesophageal junction, and 114 (80%) had no evidence of intestinal metaplasia. In 9/26 (36%) with SIM at the junction, the squamocolumnar and gastroesophageal junctions appeared as a straight line at the same level. In 17/26 (65%), columnar epithelium extended up to 3 cm in the distal esophagus and appeared as a wavy or zigzag line, occasionally with tiny tongues extending into the lower esophagus. Thus, the prevalence rate of short-segment Barrett's esophagus in an unselected population of patients was more than 10-fold higher than that observed for endoscopically apparent Barrett's esophagus in that unit. In a subsequent report, the frequency of SIM was found to increase with the extent of columnar lining in the esophagus.[34] However, even in patients with no columnar lining in the esophagus (i.e., the Z line coincided with the anatomic esophagogastric junction), SIM was found at the squamocolumnar junction in 15% of these patients. Of note, and in keeping with the trend for adenocarcinoma at this site, all patients with SIM were white.

In a similar study, Johnston et al.[35] reported that 16 of 170 patients (9.4%) without Barrett's esophagus (defined as ≥ 2 cm of columnar-lined epithelium) had short segments of SIM. Twelve of these patients (7%) had SIM limited to the esophagogastric junction. The epidemiologic features were similar to those of Barrett's patients, with a white male predominance. In this study the presence of short segments of SIM correlated with symptoms of regurgitation. Clark et al.[36] confirmed similar findings in 9% of unselected patients.

These studies relied on H&E staining alone to detect intestinal metaplasia. Alcian blue at pH 2.5 detects goblet cells and is more sensitive than H&E and highly specific for the histological diagnosis of SIM.[37] The additional advantage of staining with Alcian blue is to identify patients missed with H&E staining alone. In 158 consecutive patients, Nandurkar et al.[38] reported that SIM was detected in 46 (36%) patients using a combination of H&E and Alcian blue staining, whereas it would only have been detected in 23 (15%) if H&E alone was used. In a similar study, Trudgill et al.[39] identified intestinal metaplasia in 21 of 120 (18%) of patients undergoing endoscopy. The prevalence of intestinal metaplasia increased from 20% to 30% as the distance from the proximal margin of the gastric folds increased from <1 cm to between 2 and 3 cm. Metaplasia was associated with increasing age but, in contrast to the above studies but consistent with the Spechler series, SIM was not associated with symptomatic, endoscopic, or histologic markers of gastroesophageal reflux disease (see **Table 2.1**).

Although the evidence to date linking SIM with reflux disease is inconsistent, recent intriguing research suggests that reflux-induced changes of inflammation and metaplasia of the epithelium of

Table 2.1 Reported and personal experience* of the prevalence of SIM and dysplasia

AUTHOR AND REFERENCE	NUMBER	STAINING	**PREVALENCE OF SIM	PREVALENCE OF DYSPLASIA
Spechlar[1]	156	H+E	18%	0.64%
Nandurkar[38]	158	H+E, Alcian Blue	36%	na
Trudgill[39]	120	H+E, Alcian Blue	18%	na
Johnston[35]	170	H+E, ± Alcian Blue	9.4%	0%
Morales[51]	104	H+E, Alcian Blue	21%	0%
DeMeester[36]	241	H+E, Alcian Blue	14%	12%
Sharma[49]	59	H+E, Alcian Blue	na	8.5%
Reynolds*	199	H+E, Alcian Blue	18%	0%

**Prevalence of SIM excluding classical Barrett's
na denotes not assessed

the cardia of the stomach is tightly associated with SIM and may be the first indicator of the effects of duodenogastric reflux disease.[40,41] In 334 consecutive patients with foregut symptoms, De Meester and co-workers reported that cardiac epithelium was found in 246 (74%) and evidence of inflammation (carditis, characterized by the presence of eosinophil or plasma cell infiltration of the lamina propria and hyperplasia of the mucous cells in the foveolar region) occurred in 96% of these cases.[40] Intestinal metaplasia only occurred in association with carditis and was seen in 29 (12%) of these patients. Carditis and SIM was strongly associated with the hallmarks of gastroesophageal reflux disease, including increased esophageal acid exposure, a defective lower esophageal sphincter, and erosive esophagitis. The authors maintain that cardiac metaplasia of squamous epithelium resulting from injury or reflux is the only way that cardiac mucosa occurs in the junctional region, and that its presence is always abnormal and is a sensitive indicator of reflux. The change to SIM appears to be continuous where the cardiac cells initially undergo enlargement and distension with neutral (Alcian blue-negative) mucin. This is followed by a change in the mucin type to acid mucin, producing cardiac mucous cells that show variably positive staining with Alcian blue. This is followed by the appearance of well-formed goblet cells which have a rounded mucin globule that is strongly Alcian blue-positive and separated from the cell surface by eosinophilic cytoplasm. Intestinalization of cardiac mucosa appears to give the mucosa an increased ability to withstand damage by refluxed gastric contents, as

the fully intestinalized mucosa commonly shows minimal inflammation and reactive change. Although an attractive concept, this intriguing hypothesis remains controversial and requires further confirmatory validation (see **Table 2.2**).

Short-segment Barrett's esophagus and adenocarcinoma

Adenocarcinoma of the esophagogastric junction and gastric cardia is about twice as common as esophageal adenocarcinoma. It has much in common with esophageal adenocarcinoma, including an association with reflux symptoms, a predominance in white males, an increasing incidence, and similar tumor histology.

Schnell et al.[14] described four patients with short tongues of columnar epithelium extending 0.5–2 cm upward from the esophagogastric junction. At endoscopy, none had a viable tumor, but an adenocarcinoma in specialized epithelium was found in each patient. Hamilton et al.[42] noted Barrett's epithelium in 39 of 61 cases (64%) undergoing resection for adenocarcinoma of the esophagus or junction. In this series, approximately 45% of the esophageal adenocarcinomas were found in association with Barrett's mucosa <3 cm long. Clark et al.[43] found Barrett's epithelium in 42% (13/31) of junction and 79% (38/48) of esophageal adenocarcinomas. The SIM was dysplastic in 36 of 38 esophageal tumors, and in 10 of 13 tumors of the cardia. In a study from the Mayo Clinic of 24 patients with esophagogastric junction tumors (defined by the authors as a tumor with its midpoint located within 2 cm of the esophagogastric junction), Cameron et al.[44] noted SIM in 10/24

Table 2.2 Reported and personal experience* of SIM and association with reflux symptoms, endoscopic oesophagitis, histological oesophagitis, carditis and *H. Pylori* infection

AUTHOR AND REFERENCE	AREA	REFLUX SYMPTOMS	ENDOSCOPIC OESOPHAGITIS	HISTOLOGICAL OESOPHAGITIS	CARDITIS	*H. PYLORI*
Spechlar[12]	Boston	ns	ns	S	na	na
Nandurkar[38]	Sydney	ns	ns	S	S	ns
Trudgill[39]	Sheffield	ns	ns	ns	na	na
Johnston[35]	Maryland	S	ns	ns	na	na
Morales[51]	Arizona	ns	ns	na	na	S
DeMeester[36]	Los Angeles	All had reflux	na	na	na	ns
Reynolds*	Dublin	S	S	na	S	ns

ns denotes not significant
S denotes significant
na denotes not assessed

cases (42%) of junction tumors compared with 100% in cases of esophageal adenocarcinoma. Only five cases had classical Barrett's esophagus with SIM >3 cm, and the remainder had shorter segments. SIM was present in 67% of cases with tumors <6 cm but in only 17% of larger tumors, suggesting that enlarging tumors may overgrow and obliterate the columnar epithelium from which they arise and that the overall association of SIM with adenocarcinoma for tumors in this area is underestimated. Moreover, where tumors have arisen from short lengths of SIM, this metaplastic mucosa would be much more rapidly eroded than traditional Barrett's epithelium with SIM >3 cm. This study showed that adenocarcinoma of the esophagogastric junction is associated with short segments of specialized epithelium at least as frequently as long segments.

The dysplasia and cancer risk of patients identified with short segments of intestinal metaplasia is not known. The assumption is that the risk of mutagenesis and progression to adenocarcinoma would correlate with the length of SIM, and thus traditional Barrett's esophagus with long-segment disease would carry a greater risk, and this is borne out by several studies.[45,46] Since short-segment SIM appears to be at least 10 times more common than SIM >3 cm, however, adenocarcinoma of the esophagogastric junction may be seen more frequently simply because there are more in the general population. Available data suggest that the prevalence of dysplasia in short-segment Barrett's esophagus is approximately 8–9%, and the incidence about 6%, and that adenocarcinoma can develop, but is

rare.[47,48] Defining short-segment Barrett's esophagus as <3 cm of Barrett's-appearing epithelium above the gastroesophageal junction at endoscopy, Sharma et al.[49] reported that five of 59 patients had low-grade dysplasia (LGD) at initial endoscopy, for a prevalence of 8.5%; none had high-grade dysplasia (HGD). Thirty-two patients had follow-up endoscopy over a mean period of 37 months. Five patients developed dysplasia on follow-up, three low-grade and two high-grade, an incidence of dysplasia of 5.7% per year, and one patient with HGD progressed to adenocarcinoma. Weston et al.[50] reported that the prevalence of dysplasia at diagnosis in short-segment Barrett's esophagus as 8.1% compared with 24.4% in patients with traditional Barrett's. The prevalence of adenocarcinoma was 15% for patients with Barrett's esophagus and 0% for short-segment Barrett's esophagus. Dysplasia developed during follow-up (12–40 months) in two of 26 patients with short-segment Barrett's esophagus and in six of 29 with traditional Barrett's esophagus. Two cases of HGD and one mucosal adenocarcinoma developed in patients with traditional Barrett's, but this was not observed in short-segment Barrett's esophagus. Drewitz et al.[33] prospectively studied 170 patients with SIM, 47 of whom had short segments of SIM. One case with short-segment SIM developed adenocarcinoma in a 5-year follow-up period, compared with three cases in the group with SIM >3 cm.

Many tumors at the esophagogastric junction have developed in the cardia. The prevalence of SIM is 35–42% in patients with adenocarcinoma of the cardia. In Spechler's study,[12] nine of 26 patients with SIM had it confined to the esophagogastric junction, and this probably corresponds to SIM of the cardia. The malignant potential of SIM restricted to the cardia is unknown. In a study of 104 patients undergoing elective endoscopy, 24 were found to have SIM of the cardia,[51] though dysplasia was not evident. There was a strong association between SIM of the cardia and *Helicobacter pylori* infection. This may be a little surprising since epidemiologic studies have failed to show an association between cardia tumors and *H. pylori*.[52,53] Cameron *et al.*[44] also noted that SIM above the junction was not seen in their series of patients with squamous cell cancer of the esophagus, but was commonly found below the junction in this population of patients. At the time of writing, there is no report of dysplastic epithelium in true cardia biopsies. One would anticipate that SIM of the cardia would carry malignant potential, and long-term studies will be required to determine the incidence of dysplasia and adenocarcinoma developing in such areas.

CURRENT UNDERSTANDING OF PATHOPHYSIOLOGICAL, MOLECULAR AND BIOCHEMICAL MECHANISMS IN BARRETT'S ESOPHAGUS

Physiologic mechanisms

Barrett's esophagus develops as a consequence of severe prolonged gastroesophageal reflux. In a canine model, a mucosal defect in the lower esophagus is repaired by columnar epithelium in the presence of long term acid stimulation, or by physiologic levels of acid when accompanied by bile.[54–57] In animal models, combining the prolonged exposure of the esophageal mucosa to acid and alkali with the subcutaneous administration of a carcinogenic agent has reproduced the development of complications such as adenocarcinoma.[58,59]

The source of the cell of origin of columnar epithelium in Barrett's esophagus remains unclear. Bremner *et al.*[57] originally thought that metaplasia resulted from proximal migration from the cardia. The recent work from the same group suggesting that the metaplastic process begins in the cardia in response to reflux would support this thesis.[40]

There is perhaps more compelling evidence that the progenitor cell of Barrett's epithelium is derived from squamous epithelium. Gillen *et al.*[55] demon-

strated in an experimental model that columnar epithelium develops in a mucosal defect above a squamous barrier. The experiments of Li *et al.*,[56] which showed that both regenerating columnar and squamous epithelium are in continuity with the ducts of esophageal glands, support the concept of a multipotential esophageal gland stem cell. In humans, Shields *et al.* demonstrated, by using scanning and transmission electron microscopy, the presence of distinctive cells at the junction of squamous and Barrett's epithelium that express cytokeratins of both squamous and columnar mucosa.[60,61] This multilayered epithelium has light microscopic features of both squamous and columnar epithelium. These studies are in keeping with a multipotential cell giving rise to SIM, analogous to the squamous to columnar metaplasia that occurs in the cervix.

The factors governing the development of SIM are probably multifactorial, but the clearest physiologic association is with severe reflux disease. The changes in Barrett's esophagus are characterized by decreased lower esophageal sphincter pressure, increased frequency and duration of esophageal acid exposure, reduced symptom severity index, and delayed esophageal acid clearance compared with patients with severe esophagitis in the absence of Barrett's epithelium.[62–64] In case control studies, patients with Barrett's epithelium develop symptoms at an earlier age, have a longer duration of symptoms, and are more prone to complications such as stricture and ulcer formation.[65] It is now well recognized that patients with complicated Barrett's esophagus reflux considerably greater amounts of acid and bile than uncomplicated cases.[66–69] The mixed reflux of gastric and duodenal juices is more harmful to the esophageal mucosa than gastric juice alone. Patients with Barrett's metaplasia have a significantly higher prevalence of abnormal esophageal bilirubin exposure than patients with erosive esophagitis. Studies using ambulatory bilirubin monitoring reveal that duodenogastric reflux increases complications, and bile in combination with acid can cause severe mucosal injury. Duodenogastric contents contain bile acids, trypsin, and lysolecithin. Animal studies suggest that duodenogastric reflux (DGR) at bile concentrations of >1 mmol/l, usually causes the most serious esophageal damage in synergy with acid.

Molecular mechanisms

In a manner comparable with the well-characterized polyp–cancer sequence in the pathogenesis of colorectal cancer, there is now increasing evidence that the development of carcinoma in Barrett's esophagus follows a similar defined sequence, with histomorphologic progression from SIM to low-grade and high-grade dysplasia, and ultimately adenocarcinoma. However, while the biochemical and molecular events involved in tumor progression in the colon have been the subject of intense investigation,[70,71] relatively little is known about the molecular events involved in the pathogenesis of the Barrett's cancer sequence.

Studies of esophageal tumors have been hampered by the heterogeneity of cells within the samples, thus limiting the sensitivity of even microdissected samples. The available data suggest however a similar accumulation of genetic aberrations involving particularly proto-oncogenes that act as positive regulators of cell division or as inhibitors of differentiation, and tumor suppressor genes that inactivate the products of genes that negatively regulate growth or that induce differentiation or apoptosis. In both colon cancer and Barrett's esophagus, losses of 17p and 5q alleles results in deletions of the genes encoding p53 and the adenomatous polyposis gene (*APC*) gene. However, in colon cancer, it appears that 5q allelic losses precede 17p allelic losses, whereas in Barrett's epithelium the reverse occurs.[72–74] In human esophageal cancers, loss of heterozygosity involves multiple tumor suppressor genes, with 93% of lesions showing deletion of at least one of the four gene loci for retinoblastoma (*Rb*), p53, *APC* or deleted in colorectal cancer (*DCC*); also in 71% of cases this is evident in multiple (two or more) loci.[74]

Overexpression of receptors with tyrosine kinase activity is also common, including the proto-oncogene *Src*, the epidermal growth factor receptor and the oncoprotein c-erbB2, as well as the ligands epidermal growth factor (EGF) and transforming growth factor-alpha (TGF-α).[75–80] Although coexpression of mitogenic ligand and receptor suggests an aberrant autocrine loop, it is not possible to determine whether it is reflective rather than implicit in the carcinogenic pathway. Ultimately, the intracellular cascade leading to cell division and differentiation is subject to a multiplicity of other regulatory factors. Assay techniques have relied upon immunostaining and the practical application of research into tyrosine-specific protein kinase activity has been disappointing to date. EGF, for instance, may show differences in distribution between Barrett's epithelium and that of normals, but no relationship between mucosal subtype of metaplasia, i.e., intestinal versus gastric, nor degrees of dysplasia, have been observed.[76] Studies evaluating EGF-receptor and TGF-α have suffered from small numbers in each of the histologic subtypes.[76,77] Although enhanced expression of both occurs in SIM compared with controls, there has been no demonstrable semi-quantitative difference in intensity of staining between varying degrees of dysplasia nor between dysplasia and carcinoma[77,80] Similarly, the oncogene c-*erbB-2* has been found to be elevated in Barrett's mucosa but only slightly elevated in Barrett's adenocarcinoma.[78,79]

These molecular changes may correlate with both increased epithelial cell proliferation, measured by the expression of proliferating cell nuclear antigen (PCNA), Ki67, c-*myc* or nucleolar organizer regions (NOR), and with abnormal nuclear content, or aneuploidy. Aneuploidy probably represents the presence of multiple genetic lesions and an increased genomic instability. Such a phenotype may be associated with loss of *p53*, as well as other suppressor genes. Aneuploidy observed by flow cytometry is observed in about 70% of patients with esophageal adenocarcinoma. Prospective studies suggest that abnormal ploidy is a prerequisite to the development of high-grade dysplasia or cancer, regardless of the initial histologic phenotype, as patients with normal nuclear ploidy do not progress in short periods of follow-up.[81,82] Only two-thirds of patients with flow-cytometric abnormalities progress histologically, but with no indicators of who might in turn progress from high-grade dysplasia to cancer or follow a more rapid time course to progression. Other studies have shown either no correlation between ploidy and grade of dysplasia, or indeed, a discordance.[83,84] At present, it is unclear whether flow-cytometric abnormalities of the cell cycle are complementary risk factors or merely serve as confirmatory markers.

Most attention in Barrett's research has focused on the short arm of chromosome 17, the site of the *p53* gene.[85] In high-grade dysplasia, loss of the *p53* gene is observed in 93% of patients, but in only 43% for the *APC* gene. Loss of the *APC* gene is always associated with loss of the *p53* gene. It appears that 17p allelic losses are associated with a greater incidence of development of aneuploidy which is common in dysplasia and cancer, an increase in the rate of genomic instability and in the probability of allele loss at other chromosomal locations, and are thus early events in the progression of Barrett's to adenocarcinoma.[72,86,87]

Quantitative studies have used the p53 protein as a surrogate marker for mutations. Although mean protein levels increase with histomorphologic progression,[88] not all mutated *p53* genes will produce excess protein or protein with an increased half-life. Moreover, a single monoclonal antibody may not identify all species of abnormal protein from the wild-type product; nor is protein overexpression always associated with allele loss and an increased risk.[89] Thus, numerous examples of discordance of *p53* genotype and phenotype are reported. A negative immunostain may still be accompanied by loss of function of *p53*, especially when a stop codon mutation results in abrogation of protein production while the wild-type allele is lost. Using immunocytochemistry, Ramel *et al.*[88] found *p53* expression in only 53% of adenocarcinomas, 45% of cases with high-grade dysplasia, 15% with low-grade dysplasia, and 5% with non-dysplastic epithelium. Although there is a clear trend to higher expression with malignant progression, the lack of expression of *p53* in a larger proportion of the tumors indicates its low sensitivity for high-risk patients. In order to discern if overexpression of the protein is a marker of increased risk of carcinogenesis, prospective surveillance studies are required.

Polymerase chain reaction (PCR) methodology has demonstrated the same *p53* mutations in both diploid and aneuploid cell populations of patients with high-grade dysplasia and adenocarcinoma. This corroborates the hypothesis that *p53* is implicit in clonal evolution of Barrett's progression and that mutations of this and possibly other loci on the 17p chromosome are early events. However, only two-thirds of patients at the histomorphologic end-point of carcinoma show mutations with the primers used. In contrast, studies of 17p loss of heterozygosity in similar multiple cell populations showed detectable losses in diploid cells in 91% of patients with Barrett's high-grade dysplasia or cancer,

suggesting both that loss of heterozygosity is a more sensitive marker at this time and that these events occur prior to aneuploidy.[87]

It thus seems that, at this time, extreme caution must be recommended to applying our current molecular understanding to management decisions, in particular with respect to patients with dysplasia. In the future it is hoped that major breakthroughs in this area may help select patients with high-grade dysplasia who may safely be kept under surveillance rather than subjected to high-risk resectional surgery. The answer to a core question, why some patients respond to reflux disease by metaplasia, may also have an explanation in the genome.[90,91]

Biochemical mechanisms

Several histomorphologic studies demonstrate considerable microscopic heterogeneity in Barrett's epithelium, with frequent coexistence in areas adjacent to esophageal, junctional and cardia adenocarcinoma of different types of metaplasia and dysplasia.[7,92] This suggested that these tumors arose from Barrett's epithelium. A recent report provided biochemical evidence to strengthen this link by demonstrating a common pattern in adenocarcinoma of the esophagus and cardia and Barrett's epithelium.[93] These authors demonstrated that Barrett's epithelium expresses biochemical markers of intestinal-type differentiation, namely sucrase–isomaltase and crypt cell antigen. The biochemical profile was common to cardia metaplasia (no goblet cells but intestinal proteins), SIM, dysplasia, and adenocarcinoma. Intestinal proteins were not expressed in normal esophagus, esophageal submucosal glands, and esophageal squamous cell cancer or stomach mucosa. This suggests that intestinal differentiation is not the result of proliferating precursor cells. Thus, novel expression of intestinal-type proteins in Barrett's epithelium and adenocarcinoma suggests the existence of a specific program for this pathology and supports a stem-cell origin theory. The pattern of intestinal protein expression in adenocarcinoma of the esophagus without Barrett's epithelium is identical, and suggests a common oncogenic pathway with SIM as precursor. Moreover, intestinal protein expression on adenocarcinoma is independent of location in the esophagus or cardia, lending further weight to the emerging consensus that a distinction between adenocarcinoma of the esophagus and cardia is artificial.

MANAGEMENT ISSUES

Surveillance

Patients with Barrett's esophagus are advised to have regular endoscopic surveillance in an attempt to diagnose esophageal cancer at a premalignant or early stage, and thus offer the prospect of cure. This assumption has not been proven in a randomized trial, and it is likely to remain so. If the annual risk of cancer development were 1.3%, then a randomized trial to demonstrate the efficacy of endoscopic surveillance would require 5000 patients to be followed for 10 years. For patients with short segments of specialized intestinal metaplasia at the esophagogastric junction whose annual cancer risk appears to be substantially smaller than 1.3%, even larger numbers of patients and a longer duration of follow-up would be required for a study to demonstrate a significant benefit for surveillance. Thus, a controlled randomized trial to compare surveillance versus no surveillance in Barrett's esophagus would be a massive undertaking, and seems unlikely to be done. Provenzale et al.[94] explored the value of several different endoscopic surveillance strategies using a Markov model to construct a computer cohort simulation of 10 000 patients with Barrett's esophagus. The model was highly sensitive to the value chosen for the incidence of cancer in Barrett's esophagus, For an annual cancer incidence of 1–2%, endoscopic surveillance performed every 2–3 years was found to provide the greatest quality-adjusted life expectancy, whereas no surveillance was the preferred strategy if the cancer incidence fell below 0.5%. Although this may support endoscopic surveillance, the soft data employed in its construction have been criticized. Published incidence rates vary dramatically, and since recent prospective data suggest that incidence may be lower than initial estimates,[33] it may be that a surveillance program is difficult to sustain.

Although the cost-effectiveness of this process has not been validated in prospective studies, the lack of such studies does not preclude its clinical rationale and usefulness. For instance, Streitz et al.[95] reviewed a series of 77 patients who had adenocarcinoma in a Barrett's esophagus. Of these patients, 58 presented with symptoms of esophageal cancer in which Barrett's mucosa was identified incidentally, and 19 had adenocarcinoma discovered during endoscopic surveillance. There was a higher percentage of patients in the surveillance group with stages 0 or I cancer compared with the symptomatic group (58% versus 17%; $P = 0.006$). The 5-year actuarial survival rate in the surveillance group was also significantly better than in the symptomatic group (62% versus 20%; $P = 0.007$). It is rare for esophageal cancer to be diagnosed at an early and curable stage in the Western world, and there is no question that surveillance of patients with Barrett's esophagus offers the best chance of increasing early diagnosis.

The biggest challenge faced is that patients fulfilling the traditional criteria for Barrett's esophagus represent just the tip of the iceberg of those at risk of esophageal adenocarcinoma, and thus surveillance programs are unlikely to have a significant overall impact. For instance, Cameron et al.[96] compared population-based and autopsy prevalence of Barrett's esophagus in Olmstead County. The estimate of prevalence based on autopsy data (376/1000 patients) was markedly increased compared with clinical cases (23/100 000) suggesting that for every one case of Barrett's esophagus treated by a physician, there were 20 cases in the general population that went unrecognized. The prospects for screening become even more daunting if one accepts that short segments of specialized intestinal metaplasia also require surveillance. It seems that physicians identify fewer than 5% of the population with SIM, the group most at risk for developing esophageal adenocarcinoma. To decrease mortality from esophageal cancer we need a screening test to identify high-risk individuals in the population. Endoscopic examination with biopsies is an excellent screening, but it is unlikely that health care planners will sanction widespread use of this expensive test to screen for a condition that predisposes to an uncommon tumor. Balloon cytology, although 80% sensitive for high-grade dysplasia or carcinoma, is unfortunately a poor screening test for SIM, and Falk et al. identified goblet cells in only 15 of 63 patients.[97]

A further point against surveillance is that esophageal adenocarcinoma remains a relatively uncommon tumor, despite the marked increase in its incidence in the past 20 years. Even a 30-fold increase in this low rate represents a small risk for the individual patients, and esophageal cancer appears to be an uncommon cause of death for patients with Barrett's esophagus.[25,98,99] In a recent report from The Netherlands,[98] 155 patients seen between 1973 and 1986 (but not entered in a surveillance program) were traced in 1994. By this time, 79 had died, death being related to esophageal cancer in only two cases (2.5%). Three further cases had esophageal cancer, but died from unrelated causes. Other groups have found that the actuarial survival of patients with endoscopically obvious Barrett's esophagus did not differ significantly from age- and sex-matched control subjects in the general population.[25,27]

The cost-effectiveness of endoscopic surveillance for Barrett's esophagus might be improved if high-risk groups could be identified. Men, patients with Barrett's ulcers, and those with longer segments of intestinal metaplasia have a higher risk.[32] The most important marker of risk, however, is dysplasia.

Dysplasia represents unequivocal neoplastic change in the epithelium but confined within the basement membrane of the gland from which it arose. The criteria used by Riddell *et al.*[100] for dysplasia in inflammatory bowel disease are generally used. Dysplastic cell nuclei demonstrate variations in size and shape, and show hyperchromasia, enlargement, and elongation with a coarse chromatin pattern and wrinkling of the nuclear membrane. The nuclei also show loss of polarity, crowding, and stratification instead of their orderly arrangement at the bases of the columnar cells. Low-grade dysplasia is defined as nuclear dysplasia to a similar degree as an average tubular or villous adenoma of the colon. Nuclear stratification does not involve the full thickness of the epithelium. Similar changes may be seen in regenerative epithelium, but nuclear enlargement is less marked, chromatin remains finely dispersed, nuclei and nucleoli are regular, apoptosis is abundant, and the cytoplasm remains abundant and characteristically stains purple due to increased ribosomes and decreased secretions. In high-grade dysplasia, the architectural and cytologic changes are more severe. The dysplasia with nuclear stratification may extend through the full thickness of the epithelium, and very marked nuclear pleomorphism, rounding, and enlargement may be observed. By definition, in intramucosal adenocarcinoma, neoplastic cells

have penetrated through the crypt basement membrane and infiltrated the lamina propria, typically as single cells or in clusters. Although difficult to determine, because lymphatic channels are present within the esophageal mucosa, there is a small but definite risk of regional lymph node metastases in patients with intramucosal adenocarcinoma.

It is almost certain that adenocarcinoma does not develop in the absence of dysplasia in its evolution.[13,28,101,102] However, the diagnosis of dysplasia does not predict which lesions will progress to adenocarcinoma, and over what time course. Nor does the extent of dysplasia bear relationship to the presence or absence of a cancer. Specifically, there is a major dilemma of how to manage patients with high-grade dysplasia in the absence of an intramucosal carcinoma. Only about 40–50% of patients with high-grade dysplasia progress to cancer after 5 years of follow-up, yet the current recommendation is that they are offered high-risk resectional surgery.[102–105] It is widely accepted that pathologic diagnosis of the various forms of dysplasia on biopsy is difficult, that rigorous sampling protocols should be adhered to, and that a pathologist experienced in the diagnosis of gastrointestinal malignancies should be relied on to make the diagnosis.[106] Laser-induced fluorescence (LIF) spectroscopy may have a role in this respect.[107] Cancer in Barrett's esophagus is preceded by dysplasia that is not detectable through white-light endoscopy.

Dysplasia can thus be only recognized with biopsies and, because of its focal nature, extensive biopsy specimens are required for a reliable diagnosis. LIF refers to the use of light to detect or discriminate microscopically different types of tissue *in situ*. A low-power laser light is directed toward a tissue surface, inducing the tissue to fluoresce at wavelengths characteristic of its underlying chemical composition and/or microscopic structure. Because benign and malignant tissues are comprised of different biochemical substrates, or similar substrates in altered concentrations, the induced fluorescence spectra may be used to distinguish normal (benign) from disease (dysplastic or malignant) tissue. Panjehpour *et al.*[107] showed that this technique has high sensitivity and specificity for dysplasia.

The frequency of development of low-grade dysplasia in surveillance programs is unclear. In one study of 81 patients with Barrett's esophagus followed with endoscopic biopsy for a total of 289 patient-years, dysplasia developed in 28% of patients.[33] Of 10 patients with low-grade dysplasia in the initial biopsy, one progressed to adenocarcinoma in 4.3 years, two regressed after 3–5 years, and seven remained the same for 1.5–7 years. Two in three patients with HGD developed invasive cancer, and none of 58 patients with no dysplasia developed cancer. The authors concluded that only patients with dysplasia develop invasive adenocarcinoma, and that persistent HGD was a reliable marker for the subsequent development of adenocarcinoma.

The most recent guidelines for surveillance in Barrett's were provided through a Working Party Report presented at the World Congress of Gastroenterology in 1990.[108] The following recommendations were made:

1. *Endoscopy control*: endoscopic samples should comprise four large, deep biopsy specimens at intervals of 2 cm along the entire metaplastic mucosa of the esophagus, as well as one or two specimens from below the lower esophageal sphincter.
2. *Barrett's and no dysplasia*: surveillance should be at an interval of 12–24 months. This issue is most controversial, as the necessity of regular surveillance of Barrett's esophagus without dysplasia is questionable.
3. *Low-grade dysplasia*: these patients should have 3 months of medical therapy, followed by re-endoscopy. There is considerable difficulty in distinguishing low-grade dysplasia from mucosa regenerating in response to an inflammatory stimulus. If dysplasia is no longer evident, the above follow-up is appropriate. If dysplasia persists, the patient should continue medical therapy and endoscopy every 12 months.
4. *High-grade dysplasia*: if the dysplasia is extended to multiple foci, and the patient is fit, resectional surgery is recommended. In patients unfit for surgery, surveillance with an interval of at least 6 months is recommended.
5. *Carcinoma* in-situ *or adenocarcinoma*: if the patient is fit, resectional surgery should be offered.

At that time it seemed clear that patients with Barrett's esophagus should have regular surveillance, perhaps annually, the goal being to detect high-grade dysplasia or early carcinoma. The benefit of frequent surveillance is now clearly in doubt, and the costs are considerable. Surveillance at 2–5 years for patients with Barrett's may be more appropriate, akin to the now accepted elongated surveillance periods for patients with adenomatous colorectal polyps, provided there is no focal abnormality on endoscopy and no dysplasia on biopsy. For screening purposes, many would now suggest that endoscopic screening for Barrett's may be limited to patients with a long duration of symptoms or severe symptoms.[109,110] I would support the view that a consensus conference is needed in this area.[111]

Management of high-grade dysplasia

There is high incidence of invasive carcinoma in esophagectomy specimens when preoperative biopsies show only high-grade dysplasia. Edwards *et al.*[112] recently reviewed a collected series of 96 esophagectomy specimens among which 41% had evidence of invasive cancer in addition to high-grade dysplasia. In another report,[113] 38% of 16 patients resected for HGD had intramucosal carcinoma, but none had deeper invasion. In the Mayo Clinic series of esophagectomies for high-grade dysplasia,[114] 50% of 18 patients had invasive carcinoma. The overall 5-year survival rate was 67%. Cameron *et al.*[101] performed a detailed pathologic study of resected specimens for Barrett's esophagus and noted that two of 19 patients (10.5%) resected for HGD had a submucosal cancer in the resected specimen. Levine *et al.*[102] in the Seattle group missed no carcinoma in seven patients with HGD using a protocol requiring multiple large biopsies.

The length of time taken for high-grade dysplasia to progress to invasive adenocarcinoma is unresolved. Tygat and Hameeteman[115] reported the development and progression of dysplasia in five patients. In their series, endoscopic biopsy specimens showed dysplastic epithelium before the development of invasive adenocarcinoma, and low-grade dysplasia preceded high grade. Although low-grade dysplasia regression was observed in two patients, once dysplasia became high grade, it progressed to invasive adenocarcinoma in all cases within 1 year. In another series, such progression is reported in two of four cases.[116]

Miros et al.[31] concluded that only patients with dysplasia develop invasive adenocarcinoma, and that persistent HGD was a reliable marker for the subsequent development of adenocarcinoma. Although a significant percentage of patients with HGD will already have an adenocarcinoma, others develop it later.

Levine and colleagues,[102,103] proponents of endoscopic surveillance, have argued that a rigorous, systematic biopsy protocol might have differentiated high-grade dysplasia from early adenocarcinoma and prevented false-negative preoperative diagnoses of esophageal adenocarcinoma. In a group of patients who underwent esophagectomy for high-grade dysplasia, none had invasive cancer. Using a similar systematic biopsy protocol, Cameron et al.[117] reported a low incidence of undetectable carcinoma (1/13) after esophagectomy. Other series from proponents of this technique show progression to adenocarcinoma in 15 of 58 (26%) and in eight of 42 (19%) patients with high-grade dysplasia.[103,104] There is thus a body of opinion that, with a strict biopsy protocol and frequent surveillance, many patients may be spared an esophagectomy with its attendant risks.

However, there are several problems with this approach. The first relates to the complexity of this systematic biopsy approach. The "Seattle Protocol" developed by Levine, Reid and colleagues involves obtaining four-quadrant biopsy specimens at 2-cm intervals throughout the columnar-lined esophagus using "jumbo" biopsy forceps.[102,105] This required 148 esophagoscopies during 959 total patient-months of follow-up, or an average of one esophagoscopy per patient every 6.5 months. In 29 patients, 3848 biopsy specimens were sent for pathologic analysis. In one patient, 185 biopsies of a 3-cm segment of Barrett's epithelium were taken during five endoscopies over a 10-month period.

A further problem with this approach includes the difficulty in detecting early foci of adenocarcinoma, even with a systematic protocol. Tumors may develop away from the region of endoscopically abnormal mucosa, the focus of adenocarcinoma may be small and subject to sampling error, and the invasive component may undermine regenerated non-neoplastic epithelium.[117] Thus, in short-term follow-up, apparent progression or regression of high-grade dysplasia or early adenocarcinoma

may be due to sampling error. In this respect, although 22 of 29 patients remained without disease at a median follow-up period of 15 months, invasive carcinoma developed in seven patients in the Levine series at 2, 4, 5, 6, 20, 22 and 37 months' follow-up.[102,103] This suggests both that high-grade dysplasia can progress rapidly to adenocarcinoma, and also the possibility that early tumors were missed, even with this protocol.

Adenocarcinoma in association with high-grade dysplasia is usually detected at an early stage, with tumor penetration rarely deeper than the submucosa.[102,105,114] Although considered early disease, there is a significant incidence of lymph node positivity in esophageal adenocarcinoma that has penetrated into the submucosa. A recent report highlights the fact that the tumor may be at a more advanced stage. Heitmiller et al.[118] reported a series of 30 patients from the Johns Hopkins Medical Institutions who underwent esophagectomy for high-grade dysplasia. Thirteen patients (43%) were found to have invasive adenocarcinoma in the resected specimen. Of note, three of these patients (23%) with adenocarcinoma had locally advanced tumors (AJCC stage III). The lack of statistically significant differences in the number of preoperative esophagoscopies, number of biopsy specimens from Barrett's mucosa, and duration of endoscopic follow-up between this group and the 17 patients with no evidence of adenocarcinoma, suggest that the diagnostic and surveillance techniques did not account for the finding.

Endoscopic ultrasound has been postulated to have a potential role in the evaluation of patients with Barrett's esophagus and high-grade dysplasia. However, Falk et al.[119] reported that endoluminal ultrasound scanning did not differentiate between benign and malignant wall thickening of the esophagus in nine patients with high-grade dysplasia. Moreover, the accuracy for identifying T1 and T2 tumors is highly variable and dependent on operator experience.[120] It should however be recommended as a useful adjunct to decision making in patients with high-grade dysplasia, particularly if transmural thickening and abnormal nodal enlargement is identified.

At present, in my view the endoscopic diagnosis of high-grade dysplasia should prompt immediate consideration of esophagectomy, but the decision to proceed should be based on the risk of performing an esophagectomy in the individual patient and the consistency of the pathologic findings of endoscopically directed biopsies. Most patients with Barrett's mucosal changes are more vigorous and nutritionally fit than patients with symptomatic or obstructing carcinoma, and the mortality risk should be negligible.[112,118,121] This can only be achieved by specialist surgeons in specialist units.[121] If the choice is made not to operate, an enormous burden is placed on the surgeon, perhaps also a significant risk applied to the patient. As discussed previously, an improved molecular understanding of tumor progression in the esophagus may in future permit high-grade dysplasia to be categorized into low-risk and high-risk groups for progression to adenocarcinoma, with the former safely continued in endoscopic surveillance programs or treated using novel strategies short of resectional surgery (*vide infra*).

The management of adenocarcinoma in Barrett's esophagus is along established lines and is discussed elsewhere in this book. Excellent survival can be obtained for early-stage disease. Siewert *et al.*[122] reported an overall 5-year survival rate of 86% for patients with stage I and II disease. The overall 5-year survival rate following surgery reported from a European multicenter survey[123] for intraepithelial, intramucosal, and submucosal tumors was 92.8, 72.8, and 44.3%, respectively. Streup *et al.*[124] reported a survival rate of 72% following resection of tumors that did not have nodal metastases. The detection of early-stage cancer is possible only with surveillance, but unfortunately in most series of Barrett's adenocarcinoma only a small percentage of cases have been identified from surveillance programs.[125]

Medical therapy

Proton pump inhibitors (PPIs) are highly effective at controlling symptoms and healing esophagitis. Since patients with Barrett's esophagus have higher acid reflux than patients with severe esophagitis without Barrett's epithelium, and visceral sensitivity to acid may be somewhat impaired in patients with Barrett's epithelium, successful elimination of reflux symptoms does not does guarantee adequate control of acid reflux.[69,126,127] It is likely therefore that greater than standard doses of PPIs are needed in patients with Barrett's esophagus, and ideally ambulatory 24-h pH monitoring is necessary to document normalization of esophageal acid expo-

sure, as very high doses of PPIs may be required.[127–129] There is no clear consensus on optimum medical therapy for symptomatic or asymptomatic Barrett's, but since both represent severe reflux disease, the logic is that continued treatment with high-dose PPIs is required. PPIs should be also used where dysplasia is identified, particularly in the presence of a macroscopic abnormality, with repeat biopsies after 6 weeks to 3 months. The goal of medical therapy should never be to promote regression of Barrett's epithelium, which does not appear to occur even with normalization of esophageal pH.[128] Although partial regressions have been reported in up to 3% of cases,[131,132] and the appearance of squamous islands are often seen in patients on long-term PPIs,[128–130] there are so many difficulties and biases in accurately determining this finding that most of the data are unconvincing.

There are several current concerns about prolonged medical therapy in patients with Barrett's esophagus. The first revolves around the fact that the major increase in esophageal and proximal gastric adenocarcinoma is occurring at the same time, and at approximately the same rate as the use of antisecretory drugs. Experimental models have shown that rats exposed to pure duodenal refluxate (following total gastrectomy and esophagoduodenostomy) in the absence of gastric juice develop adenocarcinomas in significantly greater numbers than animals who have their stomach, in particular the parietal cell component, retained and an esophagoduodenostomy bypass.[133] This cannot be directly extrapolated to humans, but it does suggest a potential role for antisecretory drugs in the development of adenocarcinoma.

In humans, there is evidence that long-term PPIs are associated with an increase in plasma gastrin, as well as increased enterochromaffin-like cell density and atrophic gastritis. Klingenberg-Knol *et al.*[134] found an annual increase of atrophy of 6.25% during long-term treatment with omeprazole, which contrasts with the annual increase of 1.2% in an untreated population from the same country with comparable age and prevalence of *H. pylori* infection reported by Kiupers *et al.*[135,136] These investigators confirmed such results in two different cohorts of patients with reflux esophagitis with either omeprazole or fundoplication.[137] Among 72 patients treated with fundoplication, atrophic gastritis did not develop in any of the 31 who were infected with *H. pylori* at baseline, or in the 41 who were not infected. In 105 patients treated with omeprazole for 5 years, none of whom had atrophic gastritis at baseline, atrophic gastritis developed in 18 of 59 infected with *H. pylori* and two of 46 who were not infected. It would thus seem logical to cure *H. pylori* before embarking on long-term therapy with PPIs. The problem is that the efficacy of PPIs decreases after the infection is cured and the gastric mucosa healed, and the damage induced by the mucosa may worsen. Moreover, reinfection with *H. pylori* is not uncommon and it is becoming clear that continued surveillance, both serologic and of the corpus, is necessary in patients on long-term medical therapy.[135] At this stage we are learning of the risk of atrophic gastritis, and since conceptually the sequence from atrophic gastric cancer may take 15 years, extreme caution should be exercised.

Patients with Barrett's esophagus have a significantly higher prevalence of increased exposure to duodenal juice than patients with erosive esophagitis or with no mucosal injury. Esophageal exposure to duodenal contents occurs at all pH values, and Kauer *et al.*,[66] in analyzing the cumulative period during which the esophagus is exposed to duodenal juice report that the pH of the esophagus was between 4 and 7 for 87% of that time. The authors considered that acid suppression with a change in the pH of gastric juice may keep bile salts in solution and, in the presence of reflux, enhance injury to the esophagus through bile crossing the cell membrane and damaging the mucosa. At a low pH, bile salts tend to precipitate out of solution and are thus of minimal effect. This thesis, if proven, would lend even stronger weight to the suggestion that anti-reflux surgery, which re-establishes the barrier between the stomach and the esophagus, is the preferred therapy in Barrett's patients.

Anti-reflux surgery

Anti-reflux surgery provides long-term relief of symptoms and healing of mucosal inflammation. Given the marked defects in esophageal physiology that exist, anti-reflux surgery is an excellent option for long-term control, and effective symptom control is reported in 70–85% of cases.[138–143] The advent of laparoscopic fundoplication has widened the acceptance and use of anti-reflux surgery.[144] The long-term results should equal that achieved by the traditional open operation. Fundoplication should theoretically be considerably superior to medical therapy as definitive therapy. The hospital stay is 2–3 days, and lost working time is minimal. Fundoplication restores the physiology of the lower esophageal sphincter, prevents reflux and improves esophageal clearance. The superiority of anti-reflux surgery over histamine antagonists has been proven in a randomized trial, and long-term side effects are few.[145] Given that Barrett's esophagus represents extreme gastroesophageal reflux disease, and the concerns about long-term use of PPIs, anti-reflux surgery offers a physiologic solution and is a logical option in suitable patients and should be considered early.

Like medical therapy, anti-reflux surgery should never be offered to promote regression of Barrett's epithelium. An initial report by Brand *et al.*[146] that anti-reflux surgery could lead to regression of Barrett's epithelium led to considerable enthusiasm. They described rapid reversion of columnar epithelium in four of 10 patients. Williamson *et al.*[147] described partial regression in four of 37 patients following anti-reflux surgery, while Skinner *et al.*[148] reported regression in only two of 23 patients. Experimental studies documented regeneration of columnar epithelium with squamous islands after anti-reflux surgery. Combining several anti-reflux series, six of 190 patients had complete reversal of Barrett's esophagus at follow-up of 2–7 years. In the UK, Sagar *et al.*[149] reported that 24 of 56 patients had partial or complete regression of Barrett's esophagus (median preoperative length 8 versus 4 cm postoperatively; $P < 0.01$). Complete regression with histologic confirmation of squamous epithelium throughout the tubular esophagus occurred in five patients. Ortiz *et al.*[150] reported partial regression of Barrett's epithelium in eight of 32 patients following anti-reflux surgery, though the significance of partial regression was unclear. Unfortunately, in most series of anti-reflux surgery in Barrett's esophagus the risk of progression to dysplasia and cancer persists. In Sagar's series, nine of 56 patients showed progression of Barrett's mucosa and carcinoma developed in one patient. Although rare, carcinoma may develop after successful control of reflux.[151,152]

Despite the clear need for continued endoscopic surveillance of patients following successful anti-reflex surgery, there is some suggestion that such surgery may modulate the natural history of Barrett's esophagus and provide some protection against the development of dysplasia and carcinoma. McCallum et al.[153] analyzed the longitudinal follow-up of patients with Barrett's esophagus in the registry of the American College of Gastroenterologists. Ten patients in the medically treated group (19.7%) developed dysplasia and one developed carcinoma while on therapy, while only two developed dysplasia following anti-reflux surgery (3.4%). In a prospective randomized study, dysplasia developed in six (five low-grade, one high-grade) of 27 (22%) patients on medical therapy and in only one patient following anti-reflux surgery.[150] This patient was shown to have had an ineffective anti-reflux operation. Of note, in the series by Sagar et al.,[149] all patients who had regression of Barrett's mucosa following surgery had control of symptoms, but the patient who developed adenocarcinoma within the mucosa had persistent symptoms for 9 years after his anti-reflux operation. The final piece of evidence to suggest that surgery may alter the natural history comes from consideration of the time scale in which cancer develops. Tygat and Hameeteman[115] demonstrated that the time for cancer to supervene once dysplasia developed was approximately 3 years, though when adenocarcinoma develops after anti-reflux surgery, it is almost always before 3 years. In a series of 118 patients who had anti-reflux surgery for Barrett's esophagus between 1960 and 1990, three cancers developed over an 18-year follow-up, and all occurred within the first 3 years.[154] This early clustering, rather than random distribution throughout the follow-up period, suggests that the point of no return in the dysplasia–adenocarcinoma sequence had already been passed before the time of surgery.

An area that has received little attention is whether the identification and treatment of severe esophagitis in the absence of Barrett's esophagus (BE) may have an impact on the incidence of BE and adenocarcinoma. Dr Tom McMeester, a surgical leader in this area, has for many years pleaded an aggressive diagnostic approach and early and effective treatment for patients with esophagitis greater than grade II.[155] Since most of these patients will have lifelong dependence on medication, surgery would appear to be the preferred option.

Novel strategies

In view of the controversy about the appropriate management of high-grade dysplasia, and the significant risks of esophagectomy, alternatives have been sought to treat high-grade dysplasia and perhaps early adenocarcinoma in the often elderly unfit patients with Barrett's esophagus. Up to 50% of patients with high-grade dysplasia will not progress to adenocarcinoma during follow-up of up to 44 months. The working hypothesis is that Barrett's esophagus can be reversed if esophageal acid exposure can be normalized, either by anti-reflux surgery or PPIs, and the Barrett's mucosa ablated by endoscopic destructive techniques. With a major component of the reflux eliminated, squamous epithelium can repopulate the distal esophagus. This was validated in experimental models, suggesting again that re-epithelialization occurs from a multipotential stem cell that differentiate normally in the absence of reflux.[56,156] Regression and in some cases total reversal of Barrett's esophagus has been accomplished with Nd:YAG, argon, and KTP laser.[157–159] Photodynamic therapy has reversed Barrett's epithelium using different photosensitizers including 5-aminolevulinic acid.[160–162] Overholt and Panjehpour[162] have reported on the treatment of Barrett's dysplasia or early carcinoma with photodynamic therapy. Fourteen patients had superficial cancer, 17 high-grade dysplasia, and five low-grade dysplasia. The hematoporphyrin derivative sodium porfimer was injected and 48 h later photodynamic therapy was applied. Omeprazole was given for 3 months. After therapy, 10 patients had normal squamous and 19 had Barrett's mucosa without dysplasia. Barr et al.[161] used photodynamic therapy and the oral photosensitizing agent, 5-aminolevulinic acid, an agent with a short half-life that concentrates in the dysplastic epithelium and omeprazole 40 mg daily. Eradication was achieved in five patients with high-grade dysplasia, with follow-up between 26 and 44 months. In two patients, squamous mucosa developed within glands of Barrett's mucosa, again supporting the pluripotential cell thesis. Sampliner et al.[163] reported on the reversal of segments of Barrett's esophagus in 10 patients treated with high-dose omeprazole and endoscopic multipolar electrocoagulation.

There are considerable problems with the approach. The Nd:YAG laser and photodynamic therapy produce a significant depth of injury in the wall of the esophagus, and these therapies may be associated with significant complications including structuring. All modalities of therapy are costly and require multiple sessions. The criteria for eradication should be that, endoscopically, Barrett's epithelium is not visualized, a rigorous biopsy follow-up shows no evidence of intestinal metaplasia, and the incidence of cancer is decreased in long-term follow-up. For all therapies, residual intestinal metaplasia has been present and may occur and may be present underlying islands of squamous epithelium. There are also reports of adenocarcinoma arising in squamous mucosa[162] that had been treated with photodynamic therapy to induce complete re-epithelialization. It is also not possible to prove that we have removed every final gland of intestinal metaplasia. Further difficulties are whether lifelong high-dose acid suppression is required. Moreover, the disappointing results of endoluminal ultrasound scanning to date suggest that this therapy is doomed to failure unless one is sure that there is no submucosal spread of tumor.

It is clear that for the future these novel strategies require validation. For the moment, they are investigational and are perhaps best studied in the high-risk group of patients, namely males, aged 50 years or more with dysplasia who, in an informed protocol, choose not to undergo surgery or are unfit for surgery.

REFERENCES

1. Spechler SJ & Goyal RK. The columnar-lined esophagus, intestinal metaplasia and Norman Barrett. *Gastroenterology* 1996; **110**: 614–21.
2. Tileston W. Peptic ulcer of the esophagus. *Am J Med Sci* 1906; **132**: 240–65.
3. Barrett N. Chronic peptic ulcer of the oesophagus and oesophagitis. *Br J Surg* 1950; **38**: 175–82.
4. Allison PR & Johnstone AS. The oesophagus lined with gastric mucous membrane. *Thorax* 1953; **8**: 87–101
5. Goldman MC & Beckman RC. Barrett syndrome: case report with discussion about concepts of pathogenesis. *Gastroenterology* 1960; **39**: 104–14.
6. Naef AP, Savory M & Ouzel L. Columnar-lined lower esophagus: an acquired lesion with malignant predisposition. *J Thorac Cardiovasc Surg* 1975; **70**: 826–35.
7. Haggitt RC, Tryzelaar J, Ellis FH *et al.* Adenocarcinoma complicating columnar epithelial-lined (Barrett's) esophagus. *Am J Clin Pathol* 1978; **70**: 1–5.
8. Bosher LH & Taylor FH. Heterotopic gastric mucosa in the esophagus with ulcer and stricture formation. *J Thorac Surg* 1951; **21**: 306–12.
9. Morson BC & Belcher JR. Adenocarcinoma of the esophagus and ectopic gastric mucosa. *Br J Cancer* 1952; **6**: 127–30.
10. Weinstein WM & Ippoliti AF. The diagnosis of Barrett's esophagus: goblets, goblets, goblets. *Gastrointest Endosc* 1996; **444**: 91–4.
11. Paull A, Trier JS, Dalton MD *et al.* The histologic spectrum of Barrett's esophagus. *N Engl J Med* 1976; **295**: 476–80.
12. Spechler SJ, Zeroogian JM, Antonioli DA *et al.* Prevalence of metaplasia at the gastroesophageal junction. *Lancet* 1994; **344**: 1533–6.
13. Hamilton SR & Smith RRL. The relationship between columnar epithelial dysplasia and invasive adenocarcinoma arising in Barrett's esophagus. *Am J Clin Pathol* 1987; **87**: 301–12.
14. Schnell TG, Sontag SJ & Chejfec G. Adenocarcinomas arising in tongues or short segments of Barrett's esophagus. *Dig Dis Sci* 1992; **37**: 137–43.
15. Blot WJ, Devesa SS, Kneller SS & Fraumeni JF, Jr. Rising incidence of adenocarcinoma of the oesophagus and gastric cardia. *JAMA* 1991; **265**: 1287–9.
16. Powell J & McConkey CC. Increasing incidence of adenocarcinoma of the gastric cardia and adjacent sites. *Br J Cancer* 1990; **62**: 440–3.
17. Reed PI. Changing pattern of oesophgeal cancer. *Lancet* 1991; **338**: 178.
18. Parker SL, Tong T, Bolden S *et al. Cancer Statistics* 1997; **CA 47**: 75.
19. Pera M, Cameron AJ, Trastek VF, Carpenter HA & Zinssmeister AR. Increasing incidence of adenocarcinoma of the oesophagus and oesophagogastric junction. *Gastroenterology* 1993; **104**: 510–13.
20. Daly JM, Karnell LH & Menck HR. National Cancer Data Base report on esophageal carcinoma. *Cancer* 1996; **78**: 1820–8.
21. Heitmiller RF & Sharma RR. Comparison of prevalence and resection rates in patients with esophageal squamous cell carcinoma and adenocarcinoma. *J Thorac Cardiovasc Surg* 1996; **112**: 130–6.
22. Ovaska J, Mieetinen M & Kivilaasko E. Adenocarcinoma arising in Barrett's esophagus. *Dig Dis Sci* 1989; **34**: 1336–9.

23. Williamson WA, Ellis FH, Gibb SP *et al.* Barrett's esophagus: prevalence and incidence of adenocarcinoma. *Arch Intern Med* 1991; **151**: 2212–16.

24. Achkar E & Carey W. The cost of surveillance for adenocarcinoma complicating Barrett's esophagus. *Am J Gastroenterol* 1988; **3**: 291–4.

25. Van der Veen AH, Dees J, Blankensteijn JD *et al.* Adenocarcinoma in Barrett's esophagus: an overrated risk? *Gut* 1989; **30**: 14–18.

26. Spechler SJ, Robbins AH, Rubins HB *et al.* Adenocarcinoma and Barrett's esophagus: an overrated risk? *Gastroenterology* 1984; **87**: 927–33.

27. Cameron AJ, Ott BJ & Payne WS. The incidence of adenocarcinoma in columnar-lined (Barrett's) esophagus. *N Engl J Med* 1985; **313**: 857–9.

28. Hammeeteman W, Tytgat NJ, Houthoff HJ *et al.* Barrett's esophagus: Development of dysplasia and adenocarcinoma. *Gastroenterology* 1989; **96**: 1249–56.

29. Bonelli L, GOSPE (Gruppo Operativo per lo Studio delle Precancerosi Esofagee). Barrett's esophagus: results of a multicentre survey. *Endoscopy* 1993; **25**(suppl.): 652–4.

30. Robertson CS, Mayberry JF, Nicholson DA *et al.*. Value of endoscopic surveillance in detection of neoplastic change in Barrett's esophagus. *Br J Surg* 1988; **75**: 760–3.

31. Miros M, Kerlin P & Walker N. Only patients with dysplasia progress to adenocarcinoma in Barrett's esophagus. *Gut* 1991; **32**: 1441–6.

32. Iftikhar SY, James PD, Steele RJC *et al.* Length of Barrett's esophagus: an important factor in the development of dysplasia and adenocarcinoma. *Gut* 1992; **33**: 1155–8.

33. Drewitz DJ, Sampliner RE & Garewal HS. The incidence of adenocarcinoma in Barrett's esophagus: a prospective study of 179 patients followed 4.8 years. *Am J Gastroenterol* 1997; **92**: 212–15.

34. Spechler SJ, Zeroogian JM, Wanh HH, Antonioli DA & Goyal RK. The frequency of specialized intestinal metaplasia at the squamocolumnar junction varies with the length of columnar esophagus lining the esophagus. *Gastroenterology* 1995; **108**: A224.

35. Johnston MH, Hammond AS, Laskin W & Jones M. The prevalence and clinical characteristics of short segments of specialized intestinal metaplasia in the distal esophagus on routine endoscopy. *Am J Gastroenterol* 1996; **91**: 1507–11.

36. Clark GW, Ireland AP, Peters JH *et al.* Short-segment Barrett's esophagus; a prevalant complication of gastroesophageal reflux disease with malignant potential. *J Gastrointest Surg* 1997; **1**: 113–22

37. Gottfield MR, McClave SA & Boyce HW. Incomplete intestinal metaplasia in the diagnosis of columnar lined esophagus (Barrett's esophagus). *Am J Clin Pathol* 1989; **92**: 741–6.

38. Nandurkar S, Talley NJ, Martin CJ, Ng THK & Adams S. Short segment Barrett's oesophagus: prevalence, diagnosis and associations. *Gut* 1997; **40**: 710–15.

39. Trudgill NJ, Suvarna SK, Kapur KC & Riley SA. Intestinal metaplasia at the squamocolumnar junction in patients attending for diagnostic gastroscopy. *Gut* 1997; **41**: 585–9

40. Oberg S, Peters JH, De Meester TR *et al.* Inflammation and specialized intestinal metaplasia of cardiac mucosa is a manifestation of gastroesophageal reflux disease. *Ann Surg* 1997; **226**: 522–32.

41. Riddell RH. The biopsy diagnosis of gastroesophageal reflux disease, "carditis," and Barrett's oesophagus, and sequelae of therapy. *Am J Surg Pathol* 1996; **20** (Suppl. 1): S31–50.

42. Hamilton SR, Smith RL & Cameron JL. Prevalence and characteristics of Barretts esophagus in patients with adenocarcinoma of the esophagus or esophagogastric junction. *Hum Pathol* 1988; **19**: 942

43. Clark GWB, Smyrk TC, Burdiles P *et al.* Is Barrett's metaplasia the source of adenocarcinoma of the cardia? *Arch Surg* 1994; **129**: 609–14

44. Cameron AJ & Lomboy CT, Pera MM & Carpenter HA. Adenocarcinoma of the oesophagogastric junction and Barrett's oesophagus. *Gastroenterology* 1995; **109**: 1541–6.

45. Cameron AJ & Lomboy CT. Barrett's esophagus: age, prevalence and extent of columnar epithelium. *Gastroenterology* 1992; **103**: 1241–5.

46. Ransom JM, Patel GK, Clift SA, Womble NE & Read RC. Extended and limited types of Barrett's esophagus in the adult. *Ann Thorac Surg* 1982; **33**: 19–27.

47. Loughney TM, Lazas DJ, Frishberg DP *et al.* Short segment Barrett's esophagus: Serial endoscopic and histologic assessment. *Gastroenterology* 1996: A181.

48. Conio M, Aste H & Bonelli L. "Short" Barrett's esophagus: a condition not to be underestimated. *Gastrointest Endosc* 1994; **40**: 111–13.

49. Sharma P, Morales TG, Bhattacharyya A, Garewal HS & Sampliner R. Dysplasia in short-segment Barrett's esophagus: a prospective 3-year follow-up. *Am J Gastroenterol* 1997; **92**: 2012–16.

50. Weston AP, Krmpotich P, Makdisi WF *et al.* Short segment Barrett's esophagus: clinical and histological features, associated endoscopic findings, and association with gastric intestinal metaplasia. *Am J Gastroenterol* 1996; **91**: 981–2.

51. Morales TG, Sampliner MD & Bhattacharyya A. Intestinal metaplasia of the gastric cardia. *Am J Gastroenterol* 1997; **92**: 414–18.

52. Parsonnett J, Friednet G, Vandersteen DP *et al.* *Helicobacter pylori* infection and the risk of gastric carcinoma. *N Engl J Med* 1991; **83**: 1734–9.

53. Talley NJ, Zinsmeister AR, Weaver A *et al.* Gastric adenocarcinoma and *Helicobacter pylori* infection. *J Natl Cancer Inst* 1991; **83**: 1734–9.

54. Hennessy TPJ, Edlich RF, Buchin RJ, Tsung MS, Provost M & Wangensteen OH. Influence of gastroesophageal incompetence on regeneration of esophageal mucus. *Arch Surg* 1969; **97**: 105–7.

55. Gillen P, Keeling P, Byrne PJ, West AB & Hennessy TPJ. Experimental columnar metaplasia in the canine oesophagus. *Br J Surg* 1988; **75**: 113–15.

56. Li H, Walsh TN, O'Dowd G, Gillen P, Byrne PJ & Hennessy TPJ. Mechanisms of columnar metaplasia and squamous regeneration in experimental Barrett's oesophagus. *Surgery* 1994; **115**: 176–81.

57. Bremner CG, Lynch VP & Ellis FH, Jr. Barrett's esophagus: congenital or acquired? An experimental study of esophageal mucosal regeneration in the dog. *Surgery* 1970; **68**: 209–16.

58. Attwood SEA, Smyrk TC, De Meester TR, Mirvish SS, Stein HJ & Hinder RA. Duodenoesophageal reflux and the development of esophageal adenocarcinoma in rats. *Surgery* 1992; **111**: 503–10.

59. Pera M, Trastek VF, Carpernter HA *et al.* Influence of pancreatic and biliary reflux on the development of esophageal adenocarcinoma. *Ann Thorac Surg* 1993; **55**: 1386–93.

60. Shields HM, Sawhney RA, Zwas F *et al.* Scanning electron microscopy of the human esophagus: application to Barrett's esophagus, a precancerous lesion. *Microsc Res Tech* 1995; **31**: 248–56.

61. Boch JA, Shields HM, Antonioli DA, Zwas F, Sawhney RA & Trier JS. Distribution of cytokeratin markers in Barrett's specialised columnar epithelium. *Gastroenterology* 1997; **112**: 760–5.

62. Vaezi MF, Singh S & Richter JE. Role of acid and duodenogastric reflux in esophageal mucosal injury: a review of animal and human studies. *Gastroenterology*, 1995; **108**: 1897–907.

63. Caldwell MTP, Lawlor P, Byrne PJ, Walsh TN & Hennessy TPJ. Ambulatory oesophageal bile reflux monitoring in Barrett's oesophagus. *Br J Surg* 1995; **82**: 657–60.

64. Johnson DA, Winters C & Spurling TJ. Esophageal acid sensitivity in Barrett's esophagus. *J Clin Gastroenterol* 1987; **9**: 23–7.

65. Eisen GM, Sandler MD, Murray S & Gottfried M. The relationship between gastroesophageal reflux disease and its complications with Barrett's oesophagus. *Am J Gastroenterol* 1997; **92**: 27–31.

66. Kauer WKH, Peters JH, DeMeester TR *et al.* Mixed reflux of gastric and duodenal juices is more harmful to the esophagus than gastric juice alone. *Ann Surg* 1995; **222**: 525–33.

67. Vaezi MF & Richter JE. Synergism of acid and duodenogastro-oeosphageal reflux in complicated Barrett's oesophagus. *Surgery* 1995; **117**: 699–704.

68. Gillen P, Keeling P, Byrne PJ *et al.* Implication of duodenogastric reflux in the pathogenesis of Barrett's oesophagus. *Br J Surg* 1988; **75**: 540–3.

69. Champion G, Richter JE, Vaezi MF, Singh S & Alexander R. Duodenogastric reflux: relationship to pH and importance in Barrett's esophagus. *Gastroenterology* 1994; **107**: 747–54.

70. Fearon ER & Vogelstein B. A genetic model for colorectal tumorigenesis. Cell 1990; **61**: 759–67.

71. Vogelstein B, Fearon ER, Hamilton SR *et al.* Genetic alterations during colorectal tumor development. *N Engl J Med* 1988; **319**: 525–32.

72. Blount PL, Meltzer SJ, Yin J, Huang Y, Krasna MJ & Reid BJ. Clonal ordering of 17p and 5q allelic losses in Barrett's dysplasia and adenocarcinoma. *Proc Natl Acad Sci USA* 1993; **90**: 3221–5.

73. Krishnadeth KK, Tilanus HW, van Blankenstein M *et al.* Accumulation of genetic abnormalities during neoplastic progression in the esophagus. *Gut* 1992; **33**: 439–43.

74. Huang Y, Boynston RF, Blount PL *et al.* Loss of heterozygosity involves multiple tumor suppressor genes in human esophageal cancers. *Cancer Res* 1992; **52**: 6525–30.

75. Kumble S, Omary MB, Cartwright CA & Triadafilopoulous G. Src activation in malignant and premalignant epithelia of Barrett's esophagus. *Gastroenterology* 1997; **112**: 348–56.

76. Jankowski J, Coghill G, Tregaskis B *et al.* Epidermal growth factor in the esophagus. *Gut* 1992; **33**: 1448–52.

77. Jankowski J, Murphy S, Coghill G *et al.* Epidermal growth factor receptors in the esophagus. *Gut* 1992; **33**: 439–43.

78. Hardwick RH, Shepherd NA, Moorghen M, Newcomb PV & Alderson D. c-*erbB-2* over expression in the dysplasia/carcinoma sequence of Barrett's esophagus. *J Clin Pathol* 1995; **48**: 129–32.

79. Nakamura T, Nekarda H, Hoelscher AH *et al.* Prognostic value of DNA ploidy and c-*erbB-2* oncoprotein overexpression in adenocarcinoma of Barrett's esophagus. *Cancer* 1994; **73**: 1785–94.

80. Jankowski J, McMenemin R, Yu C, Hopwood D & Wormsley KG. Proliferating cell nuclear antigen in oesophageal diseases; correlating with transforming growth factor alpha expression. *Gut* 1992; **33**: 587–91.

81. Reid BJ, Blount PL, Rubin CE *et al.* Flow-cytometry and histological progression to malignancy in Barrett's esophagus: prospective endoscopic surveillance of cohort. *Gastroenterology* 1992; **102**: 1212.

82. Galipeau PC, Cowan DS, Sanchez CA *et al.* 17p (p53) allelic losses, 4N (G2/tetraploid) populations, and progression to aneuploidy in Barrett's esophagus. *Proc Natl Acad Sci USA* 1996; **93**: 7081–4.

83. Menke-Pluyners MBE, Mulder AH, Hop WJC & Tilanus HW. The Rotterdam Oesophageal Tumour Study Group. Dysplasia and aneuploidy as markers of malignant degeneration in Barrett's esophagus. *Gut* 1994; **35**: 1348–51.

84. Garewal HS, Sampliner RE & Fennerty MB. Flow cytometry in Barrett's esophagus: what have we learned so far? *Dig Dis Sci* 1991; **36**: 548.

85. Neshat K, Sanchez CA, Gallipeau PC *et al.* p53 mutations on Barrett's metaplasia and high-grade dysplasia. *Gastroenterology* 1994; **106**: 1589–95.

86. Younes M, Lebovitz RM, Lechago LV & Lechago J. p53 protein accumulation in Barrett's metaplasia, dysplasia and carcinoma: follow-up study. *Gastroenterology* 1993; **105**: 1637–42.

87. Blount BL, Galipeau PC, Sanchez CA *et al.* 17p allelic losses in diploid cells of patients with Barrett's esophagus who develop aneuploidy. *Cancer Res* 1994; **54**: 2292–5.

88. Ramel S, Reid BJ, Sanchez CA *et al.* Evaluation of p53 protein expression in Barrett's esophagus by two-parameter flow cytometry. *Gastroenterology* 1992; **102**: 1220–8.

89. Coggi G, Bosari S, Roncalli M, Graziaini D *et al..* P53 accumulation and *p53* gene mutation in esophageal carcinoma. *Cancer* 1997; **79**: 425–32.

90. Cameron AJ. Barrett's esophagus and adenocarcinoma: from the family to the gene. *Gastroenterology* 1992; **102**: 1421–4.

91. Romero Y, Cameron AJ, Locke GR, III *et al.* Familial aggregation of gastroesophageal reflux in patients with Barrett's esophagus and esophageal adenocarcinoma. *Gastroenterology* 1997; **113**: 1449–56.

92. Thompson JJ, Zeinsser KR & Enterline HT. Barrett's metaplasia and adenocarcinoma of the esophagus and esophago-gastric junction. *Hum Pathol* 1983; **14**: 42–60.

93. Mendes de Almeida JC, Chaves P, Pereira AD & Altorki NK. Is Barrett's esophagus the precursor of most adenocarcinomas of the esophagus and cardia? A biochemical study. *Ann Surg* 1997; **226**: 725–35.

94. Provenzale D, Kemp JA, Arora S & Wong JB. A guide for surveillance of patients with Barrett's oesophagus. *Am J Gastroenterol* 1994; **89**: 670–80.

95. Streitz JM, Jr, Andrews CW, Jr & Ellis FH, Jr. Endoscopic surveillance of Barrett's oesophagus. Does it help? *J Thorac Cardiovasc Surg* 1993; **105**: 383–8.

96. Cameron AJ, Zinsmeister AR, Ballard DJ & Carney JA. Prevalence of columnar-lines (Barrett's) oesophagus. Comparison of population-based clinical and autopsy findings. *Gastroenterology* 1990; **99**: 918–22.

97. Falk GW, Chittajalu R, Goldblum JR *et al.* Surveillance of patients with Barrett's esophagus for dysplasia and cancer with balloon cytology. *Gastroenterology* 1997; **112**: 1787–97.

98. van der Burgh A, Dees J, Hop WCJ & van Blankenstein M. Oesophageal cancer is an uncommon cause of death in patients with Barrett's oesophagus. *Gut* 1996; **39**: 5–8.

99. Spechler SJ. Endoscopic surveillance for patients with Barrett's oesophagus: does the cancer risk justify the practice? *Ann Intern Med* 1987; **106**: 902–4.

100. Riddell RH, Goldman H, Ransohoff DF *et al.* Dysplasia in inflammatory bowel disease: standardized classification with provisional clinical implications. *Hum Pathol* 1983; **14**: 931–68.

101. Cameron AJ & Carpenter HA. Barrett's esophagus, high-grade dysplasia and early adenocarcinoma: a pathological study. *Am J Gastroenterol* 1997; **92**: 586–91.

102. Levine DS, Haggitt RC, Blount PL *et al.* An endoscopic biopsy protocol can differentiate high-grade dysplasia from early adenocarcinoma in Barrett's esophagus. *Gastroenterology* 1993; **105**: 40–50.

103. Levine HS, Haggitt RC, Irvine S *et al.* Natural history of high-grade dysplasia in Barrett's esophagus. *Gastroenterology* 1996; **110**: A590.

104. Schnell T, Sontag SJ, Chejfec G *et al.* High-grade dysplasia is not an indication for surgery in patients with Barrett's esophagus. *Gastroenterology* 1996; **110**: A548.

105. Reid BJ, Weinstein WM & Lewin KJ. An endoscopic protocol can differentiate high-grade dysplasia or early adenocarcinoma in Barrett's esophagus without grossly recognizable neoplastic lesions. *Gastroenterology* 1988; **94**: 81–90.

106. Reid BJ, Haggitt RC & Ruben CE. Observer variation in the diagnosis of dysplasia in Barrett's esophagus. *Hum Pathol* 1988; **19**: 166–78.

107. Panjehpour M, Overholt BF, Vo-Dinh T *et al.* Endoscopic fluorescence detection of high-grade dysplasia in Barrett's esophagus. *Gastroenterology* 1996; **111**: 93–101.

108. Dent J, Bremner CG, Collen MJ *et al.* Working party report to the World Congress of Gastroenterology, Sydney 1990. *J Gastroenterol Hepatol* 1991; **6**: 1–22.

109. Fennerty MB. Barrett's esophagus: What do we really know about this disease? *Am J Gastroenterol* 1997; **92**: 1–3.

110. Winters C, Jr, Spurling TJ, Chobanian SJ *et al.* Barrett's esophagus: a prevalent, occult complication of gastroesophageal reflux disease. *Gastroenterology* 1987; **92**: 118–24.

111. Richter JE & Falk GW. Barrett's esophagus and adenocarcinoma. The need for a consensus conference. *J Clin Gastroenterol* 1996; **23**: 88–90.

112. Edwards MJ, Gable DR, Lentsch AB & Richardson JD. The rationale for esophagectomy as the optimal therapy for Barrett's oesophagus with high-grade dysplasia. *Ann Surg* 1996; **223**: 585–91.

113. Rice TW, Falk GW, Acker E & Petras RE. Surgical management of high-grade dysplasia in Barrett's esophagus. *Am J Gastroenterol* 1993; **88**: 1832–6.

114. Pera M, Trastek VF, Carpenter HA *et al.* Barrett's esophagus with high-grade dysplasia: an indication for esophagectomy? *Ann Thorac Surg* 1992; **54**: 199–203.

115. Tygat GNJ & Hameeteman W. The neoplastic potential of columnar-lined (Barrett's) esophagus. *World J Surg* 1992; **16**: 308–12.

116. Robertson CS, Mayberry JF, Nicholson DA *et al.* Value of endoscopic surveillance in the detection of neoplastic change in Barrett's esophagus. *Br J Surg* 1988; **75**: 760–3.

117. Cameron AJ, Carpenter HC, Laukka MA & Trastek VF. Barrett's esophagus: pathologic findings following resection for high-grade dysplasia. *Am J Gastroenterol* 1993; **88**: 1483.

118. Heitmiller RF, Redmond M & Hamilton SR. Barrett's oesophagus with high-grade dysplasia. An indication for prophylactic oesophagectomy. *Ann Surg* 1996; **224**: 66–71.

119. Falk GW, Cataloano MF, Sivak MV, Jr *et al.* Endosonography in the evaluation of patients with Barrett's esophagus and high-grade dysplasia. *Gastrointest Endosc* 1994; **40**: 207–12.

120. Boset JF & Lightdale C. Endoscopic ultrasonography of the upper gastrointestinal tract. *Radiol Clin North Am* 1992; **39**: 1067–83.

121. Rusch VW, Levine DS, Haggitt R & Reid BJ. The management of high-grade dysplasia and early cancer in Barrett's oesophagus. A multidisciplinary problem. *Cancer* 1994; **74**: 1225–9.

122. Siewert JR, Hoelscher AH & Bollscweiler E. Surgical therapy of cancer in Barrett's esophagus. *Dis Esoph* 1992; **5**: 57–62.

123. Bonavina L. Early esophageal cancer: results of a European multicenter survey. *Br J Surg* 1995; **82**: 98–101.

124. Streup WD, de Leyn P, Deniffe G, Van Raemdonck D, Coosemans W & Lerut T. Tumours of the oesophagogastric junction. *J Thorac Cardiovasc Surg* 1996; **111**: 85–9.

125. Menke-Pluymers MB, Schoute NW, Mulder AH, Hop WC, van Blankenstein M & Tilanus HW. Outcome of surgical treatment of adenocarcinoma in Barrett's oesophagus. *Gut* 1992; **33**: 1454–8.

126. Kauer WH, Peters JH, DeMeester TR, Ireland AP, Bremner CG & Hagen JA. Mixed reflux of acid and duodenal juices is more harmful to the oesophagus than gastric juice alone. The need for surgical therapy re-emphasised. *Ann Surg* 1995; **222**: 525–31.

127. Marshall REK, Anggiansah A, Owen WA & Owen WJ. The relationship between acid and bile reflux and symptoms in gastro-oesophageal reflux disease. *Gut* 1997; **40**: 182–7.

128. Sharma P, Samplimer RE & Camargo E. Normalization of esophageal pH with high-dose proton pump inhibitor therapy does not result in regression of Barrett's esophagus. *Am J Gastroenterol* 1997; **92**: 582–5.

129. Sampliner RE. Effect of up to three years of high dose lansoprazole on Barrett's. *Am J Gastroenterol* 1994; **89**: 1844–8.

130. Neumann CS, Iqbal TH & Cooper BT. Long term continuous omeprazole treatment of patients

with Barrett's oesophagus. *Aliment Pharmacol Ther* 1995; **9**: 451–4.

131. Malesci A, Savarino V, Zenith P *et al.* Partial regression of Barrett's oesophagus by long term therapy with high dose omeprazole. *Gastrointest Endosc* 1996; **44**: 700–5.

132. Gore S, Healy CJ, Sutton R *et al.* Regression of columnar lined (Barrett's) oesophagus with continuous omeprazole therapy. *Aliment Pharmacol Ther* 1993; **7**: 622–8.

133. Ireland AP, Peters JH, Smyrk TC *et al.* Gastric juice protects against the development of adenocarcinoma in the rat. *Ann Surg* 1996; **224**: 358–71.

134. Klingenberg-Knol EC, Festen HPN, Jansen JBMJ *et al.* Long-term treatment with omeprazole for refractory reflux esophagitis: efficacy and safety *Ann Intern Med* 1994; **121**: 161–7.

135. Kuipers EJ, Uyterlinde AM, Pena AS *et al.* Long-term sequelae of *Helicobacter pylori* gastritis. *Lancet* 1995; **345**: 1525–8.

136. Kuipers EJ, Uyterlinde AM, Pena AS *et al.* Increase of *Helicobacter pylori*-associated corpus gastritis during acid suppressive therapy: implications for long-term safety. *Am J Gastroenterol* 1995; **90**: 1401–6.

137. Kuypers EJ, Lundell L, Klinkerberg-Knol EC *et al.* Atrophic gastritis and *Helicobacter pylori* infection in patients with reflux esophagitis treated with omeprazole or fundoplication. *N Engl J Med* 1996; **334**: 1018–22.

138. DeMeester TR, Bonavina L & Albertucci. Nissen fundoplication for gastroesophageal reflux diseases: evaluation of primary repair in 100 consecutive patients. *Ann Surg* 1986; **204**: 9–20.

139. Luosterian M, Isolauri J, Laitmen J *et al.* Fate of Nissen fundoplication after 20 years: a clinical, endoscopical and functional analysis. *Gut* 1993; **34**: 1015–20.

140. Wellinger J, Ollyo JB, Savary M *et al.* Le traitment chirurgical de l'endobrachy-oesophage. *Helv Chir Acta* 1988; **55**: 695–8.

141. Attwood SEA, Barlow AP, Norris TL & Watson A. Barrett's oesophagus: effect of anti-reflux surgery on symptom control and development of complications. *Br J Surg* 1992; **79**: 1050–3.

142. McDonald ML, Trastek VF, Allen MS, Deschamps C & Pairolero PC. Barrett's oesophagus: does an anti-reflux procedure reduce the need for endoscopic surveillance? *J Thorac Cardiovasc Surg* 1996; **111**: 1135–40.

143. Martinez deHaro LF, Ortiz A, Parilla P *et al.* Long term results of Nissen fundoplication in reflux oesophagitis without strictures. *Dig Dis Sci* 1992; **37**: 523–7.

144. Trus TL, Laycock WS, Branun G *et al.* Intermediate follow-up of laparoscopic anti-reflux surgery. *Am J Surg* 1996; **171**: 32–5.

145. Spechler SJ. The Veteran Affairs Gastro-esophageal Reflux Study Group. A prospective trial of medical and surgical therapies for gastro-esophageal reflux disease. *N Engl J Med* 1992; **326**: 786–92.

146. Brand DL, Ylvisaker JT, Gelfand M *et al.* Regression of columnar esophageal (Barrett's) epithelium after anti-reflux surgery. *N Engl J Med* 1980; **302**: 844–8.

147. Williamson WA, Ellis FH, Jr, Gibb SB, Shahian DM & Aretz HT. Effect of anti-reflux operation on Barrett's mucosa. *Ann Thorac Surg* 1990; **49**: 537–42.

148. Skinner DB, Walther BC, Riddell RH, Schmidt H, Iascone C & De Mester TR. Barrett's esophagus: comparison of benign and malignant cases. *Ann Surg* 1983; **198**: 554–65.

149. Sagar PM, Ackroyd R, Hosie KB, Patterson JE, Stoddard CJ & Kingsnorth AN. Regression and progression of Barrett's oesophagus after anti-reflux surgery. *Br J Surg* 1995; **82**: 806–10.

150. Ortiz A, Martinez de Haro LF, Parrilla P *et al.* Conservative treatment versus anti-reflux surgery in Barrett's oesophagus: long-term results of a prospective study. *Br J Surg* 1996; **83**: 274–8.

151. Chow WH, Finkle WD, McLaughlin JK, Frankl H, Ziel HK & Fraumeni JF, Jr. The relationship of gastroesophageal reflux disease and its treatment to adenocarcinomas of the oesophagus and gastric cardia. *JAMA* 1995; **274**: 474–7.

152. Hamilton SR, Hutcheon DF, Ravitch WJ *et al.* Adenocarcinoma in Barrett's esophagus after elimination of gastroesophageal reflux. *Gastroenterology* 1984; **86**: 356.

153. McCallum RW, Polepalle S, Davenport K, Frierson H & Boyd S. Role of anti-reflux surgery against dysplasia in Barrett's esophagus. *Gastroenterology* 1991; **100**: A121.

154. Streitz JM, Ellis FH, Gibb SP *et al.* Adenocarcinoma in Barrett's esophagus: a clinicopathologic study of 65 cases. *Ann Surg* 1991; **213**: 122.

155. Crookes PF & DeMeester TR. The diagnosis and management of gastroesophageal reflux disease in a managed care environment. *Arch Surg* 1996; **131**: 1021–3.

156. Berenson MM, Johnson TD, Markowitz NR, Buchi KN & Samowitz WS. Restoration of squamous mucosa after ablation of Barrett's oesophageal epithelium. *Gastroenterology* 1993; **104**: 1686–91.

157. Brandt LJ & Kauvar DR. Laser-induced regression of Barrett's epithelium. *Gastrointest Endosc* 1992; **38**: 619–22.

158. Ertan A, Zimmerman M & Younes M. Esophageal adenocarcinoma associated with Barrett's esophagus: long-term management with laser ablation. *Am J Gastroenterol* 1995; **90**: 2201–3.

159. Sampliner RE, Hixson LJ, Fennerty B *et al.* Regression of Barrett's esophagus by laser ablation in an acid environment. *Dig Dis Sci* 1993; **38**: 365–8.

160. Overholt BF & Panjehpour M. Photodynamic therapy for Barrett's oesophagus: clinical update. *Am J Gastroenterol* 1995; **91**: 1719–23.

161. Barr H, Shepherd NA, Roberts DJH *et al.* Eradication of high-grade dysplasia in columnar lined (Barrett's) oesophagus by photodynamic therapy with endogenously generated protoporphyrin IX. *Lancet* 1996; **348**: 584–5.

162. Overholt BF & Panjehpour M. Barrett's esophagus: photodynamic therapy for ablation of dysplasia, reduction of specialised mucosa, and the treatment of superficial esophageal cancer. *Gastrointest Endosc* 1995; **42**: 64–70.

163. Sampliner RE, Fennerty MB & Garewal MD. Reversal of Barrett's oesophagus with acid suppression and multipolar electrocoagulation: preliminary resuts. *Gastrointest Endosc* 1996; **44**: 523–5.

3

QUALITY OF LIFE

JANE M. BLAZEBY
DEREK ALDERSON

INTRODUCTION

The outcome of treatment of esophageal and gastric cancer, on patient health and general well-being, is of the greatest concern to patients, and a major criterion for measuring the effectiveness of surgical care. This traditionally has been assessed by end-points such as mortality and morbidity rates, as well as symptom control and length of disease-free survival time. In the past, most clinicians found that these measures, together with informal feedback on functional results according to the doctor–patient encounter in the outpatient clinic, provided all the data needed with which to audit their practice. Over the past few decades, the demand for more information about the broader effects of treatment and illness on patients' lives, has required formal definitions and measures of "quality of life" which hitherto have not existed. For patients with cancer of the upper gastrointestinal tract, who often have a poor prognosis and many debilitating symptoms, there is a great need to address quality of life issues alongside more conventional measures of outcome. In this chapter, a summary of quality of life assessment is presented together with a brief critique of some of the frequently cited, but not necessarily more appropriate, measures that have been used in this area. How the treatment of esophageal and gastric cancer impacts on quality of life is also reviewed.

DEFINITION OF QUALITY OF LIFE

The phrase "quality of life" is misleading because within general vocabulary its definition varies widely between individuals. A layman's definition of quality of life may depend on material affluence, emotional satisfaction, personal achievements, or freedom from pain and other health concerns. This spectrum of private definitions has led to the misuse of the term in the scientific literature and although it is a widely used phrase, explicit definitions are rare. Some claim to alter quality of life without any formal attempt either to define the term or to measure it accurately. Others have tended to believe that clinical indicators (e.g., dysphagia grade) adequately reflect patients' quality of life. There is also the view that symptom checklists are sufficient quality of life tools. Psychosocial researchers strongly emphasize the importance of meanings attached by patients to their experiences. Within a medical context, a precise definition of quality if life is required to allow appropriate methodology to produce clinically meaningful data. In medical research it is now generally accepted that quality of life is not a unitary concept, but rather a complex amalgam of the patient's perception of their functioning in at least three core or primary domains.[1] The dimensions of interest vary between studies, but should always include physical, psychologic, and social functioning and may include other specific quality of life issues relevant to the patient and their treatment.

QUALITY OF LIFE ASSESSMENT

Questionnaire structure

Quality of life questionnaires consist of a variable number of domains, each addressing particular aspects of quality of life. Each domain is assessed by items, which are individual questions. Groups of items addressing one domain form a scale. The response to each item may be a yes/no answer (dichotomous), categorical (e.g., not at all, a little, quite a bit, or very much), or in the form of a continuous scale (e.g., a visual analog scale). There is no evidence that a visual analog scale is superior or inferior to a categoric scale, although the latter may be favored for simplicity.[2] The arrival of a final score depends on the format of the instrument. Scores for individual items are aggregated to produce a score for that scale. Some measures use a weighting system, so that a positive response for each item is multiplied by a factor before aggregation into a score for that domain. Aggregation of the scores from separate domains may produce an overall quality of life score, although not many questionnaires are computed in that way. The time frame of a quality of life instrument is the period in which the patient is asked to consider when formulating a response. Many leave the time frame undefined; others make reference to the previous day, week, or month.

Classification of quality of life instruments

Quality of life instruments may be placed on a continuum reflecting their intended spectrum of application: (i) generic instruments; (ii) disease specific measures; (iii) diagnosis-specific measures; and (iv) *ad hoc* instruments.[3] Generic instruments cover a broad range of dimensions and are designed for use in general populations or in patients with chronic diseases. This approach allows for comparisons between patient populations, which is of concern to health policy makers and those interested in resource allocation. The main disadvantage of generic measures of quality of life is that because they are so general, they fail to detect small but clinically significant changes in quality of life. Disease-specific measures are designed to use in homogenous groups of patients, such as those with cancer. They have similar advantages to generic measures of health in that they allow comparisons between different groups of

patients with the same general diagnosis. Like generic measures of quality of life, disease-specific measures are often too broad in their scope to detect changes in symptoms which may be relevant to subgroups of patients. Diagnosis- or treatment-specific questionnaires are assessments for particular disease sites or treatment regimens which focus upon quality of life issues relevant for that patient group. These seem ideal for most patients, but the main obstacle to their use at present is the shortage of reliable and valid tools. The data from diagnosis-specific questionnaires are so specific that comparisons between different patient populations may be difficult. The fourth type of quality of life measure – that formed the bulk of assessments in the past – may be referred to as *ad hoc* quality of life questionnaires. *Ad hoc* measures contain questions that have been chosen without formal development. This approach is quick and easy, but because of lack of methodologic details of questionnaire construction it is not known if the data obtained from these are valid. Thus, this approach to quality of life assessment is not recommended.

Another approach to quality of life assessment which avoids forcing a choice between the two strategies of generic versus disease-specific measures is a compromise which incorporates positive features of both. This is referred to as a modular approach to quality of life assessment.[4] Formalized originally by the European Organization for Research and Treatment of Cancer Quality of Life Study Group, this method uses a core instrument plus a diagnosis- or treatment-specific module.[5] The modular approach reconciles the two requirements of quality of life assessment by providing a sufficient degree of generalizability to allow for cross-study comparisons, and a level of specificity adequate for addressing research questions of particular relevance to a given group of patients.

Criteria of quality of life instruments

Important criteria of quality of life questionnaires are summarized in **Table 3.1**.[6] The instrument should contain relevant quality of life questions which are brief, clearly set out, and easily understood. The coding and scoring system for each instrument may affect the final presentation of the results and needs to be considered. Population norms may be available for some quality of life instruments and help to interpret results. The

Table 3.1   Quality of life instruments

CRITERIA FOR A GOOD QUALITY OF LIFE INSTRUMENT

Function	Contain relevant quality of life domains
Administration	Easily understood Completed within 15 minutes
Format	Clear legible layout Appropriate response categories Specific time frame
Scoring	Easy-to-output scores Appropriate scores for scales in questionnaire Population norms available Easy-to-analyze scores
Clinical use	Designed and tested for particular patients Sensitive to change over time
Reliability	Reproducible scores Lower inter-observer variation High internal consistency
Validity	Content complete and accurate Scores correlate with other outcomes Discriminates between patient subgroups
Translation	Correct guidelines Quality control measures

psychometric (reliability and validity) properties of the questionnaire need to be good. Reliability and validity testing of quality of life instruments ensures the questionnaire is free from measurement error.[7,8] There are many approaches and terms to assess reliability and validity, although it is complex because no "gold standard" quality of life measure exists against which new measures may be validated. Questionnaires which have originated from a different country need to be carefully translated in order to account for differences between cultures in concepts of health and illness, literacy, and socially acceptable questions. Guidelines for cross-cultural adaptation of questionnaires are available.[9] This is important in international multicenter cancer clinical trials in which, nowadays, quality of life assessment is often mandatory.

Data collection

Standardized methods of quality of life assessment have been developed in order to minimize random and systematic measurement errors. The assessments can be based on observations, interviews, or patients' self-report questionnaires. Observations may have to be used if patients suffering from disseminated malignancy are too frail to complete a questionnaire, but this can create difficulties with observer bias and interobserver variation. Many studies have found that observer-rated quality of life scores do not agree with those reported by the patients themselves, and thus observer ratings need to be interpreted with caution.[10-12] Quality of life data may be collected in a standardized interview by a trained researcher, but patients have been shown sometimes to have difficulties revealing their true feelings in a face-to-face situation.[13] It is therefore generally recommended that, wherever possible, questionnaires should be completed by the patient themselves. Ideally, a trained interviewer should be available to clarify the question formatting and if necessary help the patient to complete the questionnaire.

HOW QUALITY OF LIFE DATA CAN HELP IN UPPER GASTROINTESTINAL CANCER

The monitoring of quality of life in patients with esophageal and gastric cancer can be used in a number of clinical and research settings. These are summarized in **Table 3.2**.

Screening

Many patients with cancer suffer significant psychiatric morbidity, especially during the early months of treatment.[14] Quality of life questionnaires can be used as screening tools to identify problems that are not always discovered in the out-patient clinic, especially psychologic

Table 3.2   Applications of quality of life assessment in upper gastrointestinal cancer

APPLICATION

Screening tool	Identify patients who might benefit from additional interventions
Outcome measures	Detailed evaluation of the wide effects of cancer therapy
Decision making	Aid patients and clinicians choose the most appropriate treatment
Economic measure	Data for cost-benefit studies to aid resource allocation decisions

morbidity which might have passed undetected. Questionnaires may act as a prompt for the disclosure of information concerning anxiety and fears. If appropriate support or treatment can be directed to any issues identified by quality of life assessment, it is hoped that it would improve the overall outcome.

Clinical trials

Quality of life information should substantially augment other more conventional outcome measures by providing a detailed appraisal of the patients' perspective of the benefits or harms of treatment. The data can assist clinical decision making, which may be of paramount importance in trials of palliative therapies. Some patients demand every small chance of longevity despite increased side effects, others choose a dignified death with minimal intervention, and some do not want to be involved in decision making. Decisions considering patient preferences should be made with the patient and their family having as much access to good information about general quality of life considerations and survival data as they require. Inclusion of quality of life measurement requires circumspect planning, costing, and analysis. Instruments must be carefully chosen. Assessment points need to be kept to the minimum to reduce statistical difficulties, and resources need to be allocated to aid data collection. This type of scientific approach to quality of life research will improve its quality and produce accurate clinically meaningful results.

Health policy and resource allocation

In the UK, the recent health service reforms now offer the opportunity for district health authorities in their role as purchasing agents to assess the health care requirements of their local populations, and to purchase the most appropriate health care to meet those needs. This means that all types of surgery are undergoing economic evaluation, the aim of which is to compare alternative uses of resources by relating the benefits which result from one particular project to the associated costs in terms of real resource use. There are different levels of economic evaluation appropriate for answering different questions raised in health care, either setting priorities within interventions or between interventions.[15] One common approach is the cost–utility analysis. The only measure of outcome is utility,

a combination of quality and quantity of life, the quality-adjusted life year (QALY). For each intervention, the resulting "cost per QALY gained" can be measured. The disability index developed by Rosser et al.[16] and more recently the Euroqol,[17] which produces a single score, have been used to make these calculations. Such instruments are mostly very crude, however, and not always completed by the patients themselves.[15] Accurate, well-validated self-completion quality of life measures must be used for these types of studies. Few papers have reported cost considerations in the treatment of upper gastrointestinal cancer, although because of expensive new developments there is a growing literature. At present, economic evaluations are still in their infancy and until quality of life tools are standardized, results must be interpreted with caution.

QUALITY OF LIFE MEASURES USED IN ESOPHAGEAL AND GASTRIC CANCER

English language measures commonly used in patients with esophageal and gastric cancer are listed in **Table 3.3**. There are an increasing number of generic quality of life instruments available, as yet none of which is entirely appropriate for patients with gastric or esophageal cancer. Cancer- or domain-specific questionnaires should be used.

Esophageal cancer

Many studies have discussed quality of life in patients with esophageal cancer, but few have made formal attempts to measure it. Success or failure of treatment is judged by survival rates and morbidity data. Some early work itemizes crude outcomes such as fistula formation and the necessity to perform a gastrostomy as attempts to objectively evaluate quality of life, but these simple morbidity measures are not really considered as valid techniques for quality of life assessment.[18] One of the earliest attempts to assess patients' general well-being was in 1968.[19] An index to quantify subjective data based on two independent opinions of post-therapy palliation was designed, though no specific details of what was understood by palliation were recorded. The authors concluded that while cure should continue to be the goal in selected patients, an index of palliation would be a more realistic outcome measure for

Table 3.3 Quality of life measures used in esophageal and gastric cancer

TYPE OF MEASURE	QUESTIONNAIRE
Generic	Sickness Impact Profile (SIP)[70]
Cancer-specific	Rotterdam Symptom Checklist (RSCL)[71]
	Functional Assessment of Cancer Therapy (FACT)[72]
	EORTC Quality of Life Questionnaire (EORTC QLQ-C30)[5]
	Linear Analog Self Assessment Scale (LASA)[78]
	Spitzer Quality of Life Index (QLI)[11]
Gastrointestinal-specific	Visick classification[51]
	Gastrointestinal Quality of Life Index (GIQLI)[81]
Domain-specific	
Psychological function	Hospital Anxiety and Depression Scale (HAD)[82]
Physical function	Karnofsky Performance Scale (KPS)[83]
	World Health Organization Performance Scale (WHO)[84]
	Eastern Cancer Oncology Group Scale (ECOG)[85]
Disease-specific	
Esophageal cancer	Stoller Esophageal Grading System[24]
	EORTC Esophageal Cancer Module (QLQ-OES24)[87]
Gastric cancer	Troidl Gastric Cancer Questionnaire[55]

comparing methods of treatment. Others recognized that satisfactory palliation was not just relief of symptoms, but in their reports no further details were recorded.[20–22] Ong, in his 1975 Moynihan lecture on surgery of resectable esophageal cancer, noted that weight gain and early return to work were important indicators of quality of life.[23] In 1977, Stoller et al.[24] published a new proposal for the evaluation of treatment for carcinoma of the esophagus. Four domains of quality of life were defined: swallowing ability, work habits, the enjoyment of leisure, and sleeping habits. Information on dysphagia was considered of paramount importance, with failure to sleep comfortably ranking secondary to dysphagia grade. Others have sought to evaluate quality of life with a measure of performance status, as well as dysphagia grade.[25–38] This gives more general information about patients' well-being, but most performance measures are based on simple observer scores of physical function. Other questionnaires which lack formal reliability and validity testing have been designed to use in specific studies. Collard and coworkers[39] used a seven-item questionnaire in patients surviving 3 or more years after esophagectomy. Questions covered gastrointestinal symptoms, but no information was collected about patients' emotional or social well-being. Many others consider dysphagia as an important indicator of quality of life in esophageal

cancer, using a multitude of scales with unknown psychometric properties.[40–43] In 1980, Earlam and Cunha-Melo[44] stated "that since the original symptom is dysphagia, it is presumed that removal of this should produce a good quality of life, but there is really no objective evidence available." Few studies have examined this assumption by simultaneously measuring dysphagia grade and quality of life. In those that have, the findings have been mixed, but they generally indicate that dysphagia is by no means the dominant determinant of quality of life. Van Knippenberg et al.[45] adapted the Rotterdam Symptom Checklist to assess quality of life in 83 patients undergoing surgery for early neoplastic lesions. A poor correlation was found between swallowing score and global quality of life (Spearman's rank correlation 0.36 preoperatively and 0.16 at 4 months postoperatively). Loizou et al.[46] studied 38 patients with locally invasive or metastatic disease and found higher correlations (Spearman's rank correlation = 0.51). In another study, Barr et al.[47] randomized 46 patients with advanced disease to receive laser treatment alone, or laser followed by intubation. Spearman's rank correlations between the quality of life scores and the results of a daily dysphagia diary kept by the patients were significant at the 0.005 level, but modest in magnitude (0.27–0.43). Overall, these studies indicated that the proportion of the variance in quality of life that could be accounted for by dysphagia is relatively low at 15–20% or less. A more recent survey of quality of life in patients following esophagectomy or intubation correlated dysphagia score assessed by an observer with quality of life scores using the European Organization for Research and Treatment of Cancer core Quality of Life Questionnaire, the EORTC QLQ-C30.[48] No significant correlations were found with any of the quality of life scales or items at the 1% level. Others claim that relief of pain as well as dysphagia is essential to improvement of quality of life.[42] Studies in terminally ill patients show that factors which determine quality of life include psychosocial components and satisfaction with supportive care.[43,49,50] Clearly, a combination of dysphagia, nutrition, performance status, and other symptoms as well as social and psychologic well-being constitute quality of life for patients with esophageal cancer, and any one aspect such as dysphagia does not predominate.

Gastric cancer

Early work in patients with gastric cancer equated quality of life with nutritional status, weight loss, or the presence of metastases. It then began to emerge that the adverse physical effects of gastrectomy had inevitable consequences on social and psychologic function. Visick was one of the first surgeons to demonstrate this in patients with peptic ulcer disease.[51] In his Hunterian lecture, he stated that satisfactory "surgical" outcomes do not always correlate with patients' functional and emotional well-being. Visick also emphasized the need for outcomes to be assessed by an independent observer, as it was impossible for the surgeon to avoid the bias of enthusiasm. Goligher used the Visick classification to assess the outcome of surgery for duodenal ulcer disease.[52] At this time, Goligher acknowledged that surgeons often adopt too simplistic an approach to the outcome of their handiwork, and they are too frequently content to judge the results in terms of operative mortality, immediate operative morbidity and, in the case of operation of malignant disease, the length of survival.[53] Goligher advocated operation-specific tools to assess functional results of surgery. Troidl et al.[54] further emphasized the need for better techniques to measure quality of life in patients with gastrointestinal cancer, and developed a questionnaire for evaluating the outcome of total gastrectomy.

Eleven items, including disease-specific and sociopersonal variables, were assessed. Questions partly based on the Visick classification and partly on work done in Cologne were included. Each item was scored individually, producing a disease-specific subtotal score and a sociopersonal subtotal score which together yielded a total quality of life score. One general inquiry was also asked – "What is disturbing you most?" To this open-ended question patients reported a combination of upper gastrointestinal symptoms, physical, and psychologic complaints. Kusche et al.[55] compared the standardized Troidl questionnaire with the Spitzer Index of Quality of Life and the original Visick Scale. Results from a cohort of 30 patients indicated that the Visick Scale produced similar results to that of the Troidl instrument, but that the Spitzer Quality of Life Index did not discriminate between extremes of well-being. Although the Troidl Index appears to be promising, it is difficult to assume from this small study that it is an appropriate instrument to use in patients with gastric cancer. Modified versions of the Visick classification have since been used in both esophageal and gastric cancer.[55–61] More recently, Svedlund et al.[62] published detailed quality of life data collected after a 60-minute interview with a psychiatrist, and completion of a battery of questionnaires including the Sickness Impact Profile. Results were compared with data from the normal population, as well as from patients with irritable bowel syndrome, peptic ulcer disease, and a group of unselected cancer survivors. Overall functional quality of life scores from the Sickness Impact Profile were similar to those scored by the general population and cancer survivors. Some 25% of patients with gastric cancer reported significant eating difficulties – figures which probably indicate that the Sickness Impact Profile is not sensitive to detect important quality of life problems in patients with gastric cancer. Others have suggested that quality of life measurement in patients with gastric cancer might include an assessment of the patients' expectations of treatment, of the degree of family understanding and cooperation, and even a measure of spirituality.[63,64] Siegrist and Siegrist[65] undertook a large observational study of 1444 gastric cancer patients to consider how the disease was influenced by social support and education. No information was given about data collection, but it was presumed that a postal questionnaire was used. Most patients reported a good outlook on life with good daily support. The main psychologic problem resulting from their diagnosis was anxiety about possible disease progression. Performance scores such as those described by Karnofsky, the World Health Organization and the Eastern Cooperative Oncology Group have been used with nutritional outcomes in several studies.[66–68] Koster et al.[69] collected data from 1081 German patients with gastric cancer to try and validate the Karnofsky Performance Score and the Spitzer Quality of Life index, a surgeon completing the instruments while interviewing the patient. Among this mixed group of patients, resections were performed in 81%. More than 80% of patients had the highest values on the Spitzer Quality of Life Index and the Karnofsky Scale. Median scores obtained in these gastric cancer patients were in the same range as healthy Australian individuals. These results may be interpreted differently: the authors suggest that only a performance measure is needed to assess quality of life in patients with gastric cancer because the psychosocial scales in the Spitzer Scale did not greatly influence the overall score. Alternatively, the results may indicate that both observer-rated scales are unable to detect quality of life problems in patients with gastric cancer, and a more sensitive disease specific instrument is needed. Until a reliable and valid questionnaire for patients with gastric cancer is produced, such questions will remain unanswered.

Generic quality of life measures
The Sickness Impact Profile

The Sickness Impact Profile (SIP) was developed in the United States as a measure of perceived health status.[70] It was designed for a wide range of health problems, the questionnaire containing 136 items which addressed 12 areas: work, recreation, emotion, affect, home life, sleep, rest, eating, ambulation, mobility, communication, and social interaction. It may be self- or interview-administered and it takes 20–30 minutes to complete. Extensive reliability and validity testing has produced good results. It is a long questionnaire, which limits its use in patients with advanced disease, but is probably not specific enough to detect important quality of life issues in patients with esophageal or gastric cancer.[62]

Cancer-specific quality of life measures
The Rotterdam Symptom Checklist

The Rotterdam Symptom Checklist was originally designed to measure the toxicity and impact that treatment for cancer had on psychosocial functioning.[71] The list contains 30 items which can be divided into two primary scales measuring physical and psychosocial disability. The questionnaire is easy to complete within 5–10 minutes. Population norms are available and there is work to demonstrate good sensitivity and specificity. An adapted version for patients with esophageal cancer has been developed in The Netherlands (not available in English).[45]

The Functional Assessment of Cancer Therapy (FACT) Scale

This 34-item questionnaire has been developed and tested in an American population.[72] It contains four scales addressing physical, social, emotional, and functional well-being, as well as containing a scale which considers the doctor–patient relationship. At the end of each set of items assessing a quality of life dimension, a single item asks patients to rate how much that dimension affects his/her quality of life. The FACT is completed within 5–10 minutes, usually without help. Data show that it is responsive to clinical changes in health, reliable, and valid. Specific modules are available for some disease sites.

The European Organization for Research and Treatment of Cancer (EORTC) Core Questionnaire

The EORTC QLQ-C30 incorporates five functional quality of life scales, a global health scale, and three symptom scales. Six single items assess symptoms and problems commonly found in patients with cancer.[5] It was developed with a modular approach so that disease-specific questionnaires can be added to the core instrument.[73] Reliability and validity testing has been extensively performed in several groups of patients, including those with esophageal cancer.[48,74–77] It is currently available in over 20 languages, and is a useful tool for international oncology trials.

The Linear Analog Self-Assessment (LASA) Scale

The linear analog self-assessment scale was developed for patients with advanced breast cancer.[78] It has 25 items, 10 of which are related to disease symptoms, while five examine psychologic disabilities and five measure other physical indices. The scale has been validated and tested for reliability, but many patients find it difficult to accustom themselves to representing their feelings on a continuum. It has been used in patients with gastric and esophageal cancer, although it lacks items relating to eating and dysphagia.

The Spitzer Quality of Life Index

This brief measure of quality of life was developed for use by physicians in patients with cancer or chronic illnesses.[11] It consists of five items assessing activity, daily life, overall health, support, and outlook. Each question is scored on a three-point scale (0 to 2) which is summated to produce an overall score ranging between 0 and 10. The average completion time is 1 minute. The observer can also rate their confidence of the accuracy of the scores. Psychometric testing of the questionnaire has been carried out in various populations of patients, although some recent studies have questioned its reliability, validity, and sensitivity.[10,79,80]

Gastrointestinal-specific measures
The Visick classification

The Visick classification was designed to assess the outcome of surgery for peptic ulcer disease.[51] It is an observer-rated scale which addresses nutrition, weight loss, dysphagia, and regurgitation as well as the ability to enjoy leisure and the ability to work. This produces five grades: Grade I, patients with no complaints; Grade II, patients are well but interrogation reveals light symptoms; Grade III, patients require regular doctor's help and cannot work; Grade IV, patients with troublesome symptoms who cannot leave the house; and Grade V, patients who are in bed with repeated hospital visits. Many have used the Visick classification in patients with gastric and esophageal cancer.[55–61] Some reliability data have been published, but there is a lack of strict validation testing. This scale mainly assesses symptoms without considering the psychosocial impact of ill health.

The Gastrointestinal Quality of Life Index

The Gastrointestinal Quality of Life Index (GIQLI) was carefully developed in patients with a wide range of benign and malignant gastrointestinal disorders.[81] Some reliability and validity data are available, although it is not known if the instrument is sensitive to changes in quality of life in patients with gastric and esophageal cancer. It is available in German and English.

Domain-specific measures

Domain-specific measures are subdivisible into scales monitoring psychologic morbidity and physical function.

The Hospital Anxiety and Depression Scale

The Hospital Anxiety and Depression Scale is a brief assessment of psychologic well-being, consisting of 14 items divided into two subscales for anxiety and depression.[82] It does not address physical symptoms even related to psychologic dysfunction. The questionnaire is easy and quick to administer, complete, and score. Good reliability and validity data have been published and it is available in several different languages.

The Karnofsky Performance Scale

The Karnofsky Performance Scale is frequently referred to as proxy measure of quality of life in clinical trials, because it only measures physical function.[83] Despite its inadequacy as a quality of life measure it is often used to make clinical judgements and to influence decision making. The scale comprises of 11 categories ranging from normal performance (100%) to death (0%). It is particularly weak at accurately measuring quality of life in patients who are immobile due to poor physical health. Such patients may score very low on a physical scale but may also be emotionally and socially strong (which it will fail to detect). Other disadvantages, apart from being crude and limited in content, is that it is an observer-rated scale.

The World Health Organization Performance Scale

The WHO five-point scale is physician-rated.[84] Patients who are fully active and well score zero, while those completely disabled score four. This old instrument has the same disadvantages already listed for the Karnofsky Performance Scale.

The Eastern Cancer Oncology Group (ECOG) Scale

The ECOG scale is another simple scale which examines performance status.[85] It is graded on a five-point scale by an observer: grade zero, able to carry out all normal activity without restriction; grade one, restricted in physically strenuous activity but ambulatory and able to do light work; grade two, ambulatory and capable of all self care but unable to carry out any work; grade three, capable of only limited self care, confined to bed or chair for more than 50% of waking hours; and grade four, completely disabled. Like the Karnofsky and WHO Scales, this measure does not address social and psychologic issues and is generally considered to be outdated.

Disease-specific measures
Esophageal Grading System

In 1977, Stoller *et al.*[24] published a new proposal for the evaluation of treatment for carcinoma of the esophagus which considered five domains of quality of life: swallowing ability, pain, work habits, the enjoyment of leisure, and sleeping habits. The questionnaire is completed by an independent observer. It has been used by several groups in a variety of clinical situations, but no formal reliability or validity data exist.[25,35,86] This questionnaire has probably been superseded by instruments that patients are able to complete themselves.

The EORTC Oesophageal Cancer Module

The EORTC QLQ-OES24 is designed to supplement the EORTC QLQ-C30 core questionnaire.[87] It is designed for patients with esophageal cancer, irrespective of disease stage. The questionnaire was developed in patients undergoing esophagectomy with or without neoadjuvant or adjuvant chemoradiation, patients undergoing primary radiotherapy or chemoradiation, and patients being intubated or undergoing endoscopic tumor ablation with laser, diathermy, or alcohol injection. It has 24 items, hypothesized to contain six scales and five individual symptoms items. The scales include: dysphagia, deglutition, eating, upper gastrointestinal symptoms, pain, and emotional problems relating to esophageal cancer. The five

symptoms are: coughing, alopecia, dry mouth, trouble with talking, and taste problems. It is a self-completion questionnaire which takes less than 10 minutes to complete. No reliability or validity data have been published, although it is currently undergoing an international validation study.[88]

The Troidl Gastric Cancer Questionnaire

This standardized quality of life questionnaire has been developed in Germany for patients undergoing gastrectomy.[55] It contains 13 items addressing disease-specific variables related to the side effects of surgery and sociopersonal variables including: fatigue, sleep, pain, ability to work, ability to walk, and immobility. Troidl and colleagues have used the instrument in several studies with promising results, though no psychometric data have been published.

THE EFFECT OF TREATMENT FOR ESOPHAGEAL CANCER ON QUALITY OF LIFE

Physical problems, especially eating difficulties, associated with the diagnosis and treatment of esophageal cancer have been well documented in the literature. Less is known about the psychosocial distress suffered with the disease and its treatment. This section discusses the effects of esophagectomy and radiotherapy on patients' physical, social and psychologic function, as well as considering how purely palliative treatments (endoscopic relief of dysphagia and palliative chemoradiation) impact on quality of life.

Esophagectomy

The effect of esophagectomy on dysphagia and other eating-related symptoms has been extensively recorded. Early work using the Visick classification and simple questionnaires have measured problems with nutrition and weight loss which are common sequelae of esophageal cancer. Following esophagectomy, most patients have some difficulty in consuming foods and many experience a degree of heartburn. In a personal series of 49 patients who had undergone thoracoabdominal resection, Watson found that 90% were Visick grade I, with normal swallowing.[61] Patients report that meals take a long time to eat, and that they have lost their appetite, though five-year survivors claim that appetite eventually returns.[28] Early satiety is another common residual symptom which leads patients to eat small, but frequent, meals. Whether transhiatal or thoracoabdominal esophagectomy affects functional eating ability has been frequently questioned. Roder et al.[89] found no significant correlations between quality of life scores from three validated instruments and the type of resection or histology of the tumor. Significant correlations were found, however, between quality of life scores and relative body weight. Weight loss following esophagectomy may reflect difficulties eating, recurrence of disease, or psychologic problems. Patients who have relatively low body weight or a sudden decrease in weight more than 6 months after esophagectomy require an intense physical and psychologic examination. Others have compared the outcome after esophagectomy with an intrathoracic anastomosis with the outcome of a retrosternal bypass.[90] Patients with an intrathoracic anastomosis had less problems with dysphagia than those with the other reconstruction. No significant differences were observed between other parameters of quality of life. The effect of esophagectomy with lymphadenectomy on quality of life and survival has been studied.[91] No differences were observed between three- or two-field dissection in terms of mortality, morbidity, and postoperative quality of life, although patients undergoing three-field dissection survived for longer. Problems with pain control after surgery for esophageal cancer are not commonly reported. Following thoracotomy, less than one-third of patients report residual scar pain.[92] Other authors have reported 80% of patients to be pain-free after surgery, which has a major influence on quality of survival.[42,45] The effect of esophagectomy on performance status and physical well-being has been well documented. In the postoperative period, patients suffer a clear decrease in general performance and severe fatigue usually lasting for at least 6 months after surgery.[29,36,45,77,93] This gradually returns to normal in those who remain free from recurrence. This profound effect on physical function dramatically influences patients' ability to return to work. Sugimachi et al.[28] interviewed patients surviving one or more years after esophagectomy and found that only one-fifth of those working before surgery were able to continue. Collard et al.[39] achieved a 100% response rate to a questionnaire mailed to patients surviving 3 years

or more; three-fourths of these patients were able to resume some sort of occupational activity. Another study using the EORTC QLQ-C30 questionnaire indicated that, following esophagectomy, 67% of patients reported a partial or complete incapacity in their jobs or household tasks.[77]

Little is known about psychologic distress and social problems following esophageal surgery for cancer. Roder et al.[89] compared quality of life data from patients following esophagectomy with a representative random group of the normal population, healthy persons, and a group of patients with varying types of malignancies. They found that the loss of ability to socialize caused much anxiety. A prospective study using a modified version of the Rotterdam Symptom Checklist obtained completed sets of data from 62 to 83 patients before and 3 months after esophagectomy;[45] psychologic function was seen to improve following surgery. Zieren et al.[77] evaluated quality of life by asking patients to complete the EORTC QLQ-C30. At the same time, a psychologist completed the Spitzer Quality of Life Index, studying 119 patients one year after esophagectomy and 30 patients before and after treatment. Patients with recurrence and those who died within the study period were excluded ($n = 18$). Only 33% reported emotional disturbances, while social function decreased in the early postoperative period. Further work is needed in this area such that appropriate psychosocial support may enhance the quality of patients' lives.

Neoadjuvant treatment

The effect of neoadjuvant chemotherapy or radiotherapy on the quality of life of patients is still undergoing investigation, although a few early studies have reported results using simple measures. One prospective study compared preoperative radiotherapy and surgery with surgery alone on patients' quality of life.[45] Those who had received neoadjuvant treatment had lower mean dysphagia scores postoperatively, but no other differences were seen in other aspects of quality of life. Further studies using disease-specific measures are needed.

Palliative surgery

The increasing numbers of safe endoscopic methods of relieving the obstructed esophageal lumen have led many to feel there is little place for palliative surgery in the management of esophageal cancer. Better staging techniques have also improved patient selection. Others, however, continue to believe that dysphagia is most effectively relieved by surgery, despite its associated costs in terms of morbidity and mortality. In the pooled patient study published by Muller et al.,[94] palliative resection resulted in 3- and 5-year survival rates of 6% and 2%, respectively. Hospital mortality rates were about 10%, and 46% of patients had significant postoperative complications. The results of bypass surgery were even worse, with mortality rates of 20–35%.[95,96] The only notable exception was the series reported by Mannell et al.,[97] where the hospital mortality was 11%, with 82% of patients experiencing complete relief of dysphagia. In 1980, Stoller evaluated the results of palliative bypass surgery in 14 patients with unresectable esophageal tumors.[98] Using an in-house outcome classification, Stoller demonstrated that a reasonable quality of life was obtained in 11 of the surviving patients. Welvaart and De Jong[41] prospectively studied quality of life in 40 patients undergoing palliative esophagogastrectomy, quality of life being calculated using a score based on ability to eat and survival time. Nine patients died in hospital, though of the 28 who recovered, quality of life scores were high. The authors concluded that palliative resection is a worthwhile procedure. Sawant and Moghissi[99] reported the results of 70 patients who underwent substernal bypass with stomach or transverse colon for unresectable esophageal tumors. The hospital mortality rate was 22%, but the quality of life of the survivors was graded as moderate to good because the operation allowed patients to eat almost normal food for a mean duration of 10 months. Although palliative resection can relieve dysphagia and prevent problems such as haemorrhage, aspiration, and the risk of aerodigestive fistula, all of these can usually be addressed by other approaches. Accurate quality of life data are needed to help patients and clinicians make informed decisions. Controlled studies with multidimensional quality of life measures should be prospectively performed. Dysphagia may be effectively relieved by surgery, but more information about other physical, social, and psychologic effects of palliative surgery are required.

Radiotherapy

Many clinicians have felt that external-beam radiotherapy alone or in combination with intracavity radiation has less deleterious effects on the patients' overall well-being, and similar outcomes in terms of survival and symptom relief as esophagectomy. Although this hypothesis remains to be proven in controlled clinical trials, several longitudinal studies have been performed. Between 1985 and 1988, Flores treated 211 patients with a combination of intracavity and external-beam irradiation.[32] Performance, measured with the Eastern Cooperative Oncology Group system, improved in patients who had started with reasonable pretreatment scores. Swallowing ability, odonyphagia, and body weight improved in most patients. In a larger study, Flores et al. reported the effect of combined external-beam radiotherapy and intracavity radiation on patients' performance scores, swallowing, and weight loss.[31] When quality of life was assessed 6 months after treatment, 56% of patients had improved swallowing with less pain and performance scores improved in most patients. Albertsson et al.[33] reported the effect of radiotherapy on the Karnofsky Performance Status of 149 patients and found that high pretreatment scores correlated well with good outcome. A non-randomized prospective study reported in 1984 compared the results of surgery with primary radiotherapy in 88 patients using the Stoller Esophageal Questionnaire.[86] Survival was similar in the two groups, although patients treated with primary radiotherapy suffered less morbidity than those who underwent surgery. Esophageal palliation scores were similar at each follow-up appointment in the two groups. The authors concluded that since palliation levels were as good following radiotherapy as after operation, it may be the better treatment. Sawant and Moghissi assessed quality of life after palliative radiotherapy in three categories: poor; moderate; and good.[99] The authors admitted that lack of standard quality of life tools made it difficult to assess, but concluded that most patients had poor relief of dysphagia and morbidity rates were high. O'Rourke et al. compared palliative radiotherapy with intubation in a non-randomized study;[36] no significant differences in performance status, swallowing, or pain relief were observed. Further studies which include assessment of the burden of repeated treatments and hospitalization are required in order to fully evaluate the effect of radiotherapy on patients' quality of life.

Intubation

Patients who present with metastatic disease or who are unfit for radical treatment may be palliated by a number of methods, the aim of which is to relieve dysphagia with minimum morbidity and mortality and maximum quality of life. Measuring quality of life in patients who are terminally ill can be difficult because they are frail, frequently confused, and often not receptive to repeated interviews or questionnaires. It is generally recommended that patients complete the questionnaires themselves wherever possible, although it is recognized that data collected by proxy may be required.

Intubation, which is the main stay of palliative treatment for malignant dysphagia, continues to have a considerable morbidity and mortality. Morbidity from the insertion of a plastic prosthesis is about 30–40% and procedure-related mortality rates are between 3% and 16%.[61,100]

It is still unknown if expanding metal stents reduce these figures. The relevance of quality of life data in these patients has been emphasized by many, but there is still a lack of studies using validated cancer-specific measures. Chest pain lasting for several days is not uncommon, although it is important to ensure that it does not represent a small perforation. Other immediate symptoms include respiratory problems resulting from aspiration pneumonia, gastroesophageal reflux if the tube crosses the lower esophageal sphincter, and eating-related difficulties as the patient adjusts to a soft diet. Late complications mainly related to recurrent dysphagia greatly impinge on patients' quality of life by requiring repeated hospital admissions. Most plastic tubes allow 10–15% of patients to eat virtually normally, 50–60% to eat a semi-solid diet, and the remainder only to drink liquids.[100] Metal stents theoretically produce a better relief of dysphagia because the fully expanded stent lumen is 18–25 mm compared with lumens of between 12–18 mm provided by plastic tubes. Most studies have only assessed dysphagia as an indicator of quality of life. They generally report that esophageal prostheses improve quality of life because of relief of dysphagia.[27,40] O'Hanlon et al.[93] used the Rotterdam Symptom Checklist to assess quality of life in patients either undergoing radiation treatment or intubation, and found that although dysphagia initially improved following intubation, it remained static until death. At 4 months after palliative treatment, several other parameters of quality of life were significantly worse and no improvements were seen.

Laser treatment

The immediate morbidity associated with endoscopic laser treatment is generally less than that following intubation with a plastic prosthesis. Tumor recurrence causing dysphagia, however, is much more common, which requires the patient to remain closely tied to the hospital for repeated endoscopic follow-up. This is perceived by some (clinicians and patients) as burdensome and disruptive.[101] Few studies, however, have objectively measured patients' views about this matter. Some pilot work performed in the mid-1980s assessed dysphagia and performance status, using the Eastern Cooperative Oncology Group Scale before and after laser treatment.[34] Overall performance status improved, as did dysphagia grade. At about the same time, Mellow and Pinkas[26] investigated the role of laser treatment for junctional tumors. In an attempt to assess the impact of the treatment on patients' quality of life, their dysphagia, eating ability, and performance status (Eastern Cooperative Oncology Group) were assessed. Laser treatment achieved luminal patency in 29 of the 30 patients. Technical success in establishing luminal patency usually correlated well with improvement in dysphagia, although eating ability was not always improved. Performance status improved in just over 50% of patients. The authors concluded that, despite the attractive aspects of laser therapy, many other factors had an impact on the functional outcome besides simply establishing a patent lumen. Rutgeerts et al.[30] performed a similar study of 31 patients with advanced disease. Among these, 63% of patients had immediate relief of dysphagia, but this was short lasting (1 month) and such improvement was not reflected in general performance status. Gasparri et al.[56] studied the short- and long-term results of 248 prostheses (a combination of Nottingham, Celestin and Medoc tubes) in inoperable carcinoma of the esophagus. Patients were sent a questionnaire which addressed feeding problems using the Visick classification, but the authors obtained only a 55% response rate. Some 50% of patients reported normal swallowing (Visick grade I), 36% dysphagia to solids, and 10% dysphagia for semi-solids. These results are not in accordance with most reports but, based on only a 55% response rate, they may be invalid. Loizou et al.[46] evaluated the effect of laser therapy and intubation on quality of life using the Linear Analog Self Assessment questionnaire and the Spitzer Quality of Life Index. Dysphagia grade improved in all patients after treatment, as did quality of life scores, though these changes were transient and patients gradually deteriorated until death.

The effect of photodynamic therapy on quality of life has also been investigated. McCaughan et al.[25] examined the Karnofsky Performance Status and the Stoller Esophageal Questionnaire in a pilot study of 16 patients. Photodynamic therapy was delivered a few days after an intravenous injection of a photosensitizer. Patients required between one and five treatments approximately every 3 months. At 1 month after initial treatment, the Karnofsky Performance Status improved in four patients and 15 had an overall improvement in Esophageal grade. The authors stated that this improvement was mostly due to increased swallowing ability.

Chemotherapy for advanced esophageal cancer

Few quality of life studies after palliative chemotherapy for esophageal cancer have been published. Bamias et al.[102] used the EORTC QLQ-C30 to assess the effect of epirubicin, cisplatin, and 5-flurouracil on quality of life in patients ($n = 235$) with esophagogastric adenocarcinoma. A complete or partial response was seen in 66% of patients, and toxicity scores were reported as generally mild, although there were six treatment-related deaths. Complete quality of life data were collected from only 55 patients. No signifcant negative impact on emotional function was demonstrated in this small subset of patients, and symptoms were reported as low. Global quality of life scores significantly improved at the follow-up appointment, although no difference was detected between the responders and non-responders. Thus, it is difficult to draw meaningful conclusions from this incomplete data set.

Randomized trials with quality of life as an outcome measure

Despite the growing interest in quality of life assessment, there are still very few randomized

trials which have included a quality of life assessment in patients with esophageal cancer (**Table 3.4**). Often, only a performance measure and dysphagia grade are assessed which fail to reflect the patients' true perspective. Barr et al.[47] randomized 40 patients to laser therapy alone, or to laser therapy followed by intubation. Quality of life was assessed with the Linear Analog Self Assessment scale and the Spitzer Quality of Life Index. No significant differences in dysphagia grade or quality of life scores were found, and morbidity was significantly higher in intubated patients, though these required fewer endoscopic procedures. In a small trial, Reed et al.[35] randomized 27 patients to intubation alone, intubation and palliative radiotherapy, or endoscopic laser therapy and radiotherapy. Quality of life was assessed by the Stoller Esophageal Questionnaire and Karnofsky Performance Status. They found that the overall Stoller Esophageal Score was most affected by the change in swallowing, which improved in all three groups. The average Karnofsky score improved modestly in the intubation group and in the group receiving laser therapy and radiotherapy. Patients receiving laser and radiotherapy required significantly more time in hospital than those undergoing intubation alone, despite intubation producing a significantly greater morbidity. The authors concluded that radiotherapy in addition to intubation did not produce any advantages, and therefore either intubation alone or laser plus radiotherapy were good palliative treatments for malignant dysphagia. Fuchs et al.[58] randomized 40 patients to laser therapy or endoscopic intubation; quality of life was evaluated using the Visick classification. No significant differences were seen between the two treatment arms, and the authors concluded that the choice of procedure should depend on the technical facilities available and the personal experience of the surgeon. Low and Pagliero[38] randomized 43 patients to either laser photoablation or brachytherapy, and assessed dysphagia and performance scores. Dysphagia and performance status showed a similar improvement in both groups. Retreatments were three times more common with laser therapy, but both groups had similar morbidity rates. There is one published randomized trial comparing a metal Wallstent with plastic endoprostheses.[37] Quality of life was crudely measured with the Karnofsky Performance Scale and a dysphagia score. In this small study, a lower rate of

Table 3.4 Randomized studies with quality of life as an outcome measure – esophageal cancer

REFERENCE	YEAR	GROUP 1	GROUP 2	GROUP 3	QUALITY OF LIFE TOOL	OUTCOME
Barr et al.[47]	1990	Intubation	Laser	–	LASA, Spitzer Index	No significant differences in quality of life. Morbidity lower in laser group
Reed et al.[35]	1991	Intubation and radiotherapy	Intubation	Laser and radiotherapy	Stoller, Karnofsky	No significant differences in quality of life data. In-patient stay longer in laser group
Fuchs et al.[58]	1991	Laser therapy	Intubation	–	Visick classification	No significant differences
Low and Pagliero[38]	1992	Laser	Brachytherapy	–	Performance score	No significant differences
Knyrim et al.[37]	1993	Plastic prostheses	Metal stents	–	Performance score	No significant differences

DXT, radiotherapy.
LASA, linear analog self-assessment scale.

immediate complications was reported in the metal stent group, although no difference was seen in the 30-day mortality. The Wallstents were uncovered and a number of design problems occurred. Patients receiving conventional tubes were treated under general anesthetic, whereas those receiving metal stents had only intravenous sedation. Technical complications encountered with the plastic tube were substantial, but most esophageal surgeons consider it unnecessarily aggressive to use a 20-mm balloon dilator before inserting a prosthesis. Recurrent dysphagia was equally common in both groups and most frequently resulted from tumor ingrowth in the group treated with metal stents and tube migration in the plastic endoprosthesis group. No significant differences were seen in performance status between the two groups. Despite their higher costs, the metal stents proved cost-effective because of the decreased complication rate and shorter hospital stay.

There is a great need to define outcomes for patients with inoperable esophageal cancer. Dysphagia scores should be standardized and future palliative trials should include an objective assessment of quality of life of patients, as well as cost-effectiveness during the follow-up period. Every effort to improve the quality of the remaining life of these patients is required. A short hospital stay, adequate pain relief, supportive social care, and appropriate help from oncologists, palliative care physicians, and nurses should be arranged in addition to effective management of dysphagia.

THE EFFECT OF TREATMENT FOR GASTRIC CANCER ON QUALITY OF LIFE

Surgery for gastric cancer is the mainstay of treatment, even for patients with advanced disease. The functional consequences of total or subtotal resection are controversial and many have searched for the best method of reconstructing the gastrointestinal tract to improve patients' quality of life. This section discusses the physical, emotional, and social outcomes of surgery as well as reviewing how palliative chemotherapy impacts on patients' quality of life.

Total or subtotal gastrectomy?

For patients with carcinoma of the distal stomach, opinions are divided as to the most appropriate operation. The choice between distal or total gas-

trectomy does not only rely on surgical and oncologic factors such as postoperative morbidity and mortality and disease-free survival time, but also on the quality of life of patients with the two procedures. This should be taken into consideration, particularly if differences in other outcomes are marginal. There is an extensive knowledge of the nutritional consequences of total gastrectomy and the mode of gastrointestinal reconstruction. There is also growing evidence that malnutrition, even if only slight, affects patients more after total gastrectomy than subtotal gastrectomy and this may impair patients' quality of life. Bozzetti et al.[103] investigated the variation of nutritional indexes, food intake, the degree of anorexia and problems with dumping syndrome in 44 (23 total gastrectomy, 21 subtotal) disease-free patients a mean of 3 years after surgery. Both groups progressively lost weight for 15 months after the operation, though weight loss and general status was worse in patients after total gastrectomy. In general, almost all patients complain of some symptoms following total gastrectomy; these vary from minor disorders of esophagitis and dumping syndrome to very disabling difficulties with swallowing, postprandial discomfort, abdominal pain, and diarrhoea.[60,67] Anderson and Macintyre studied 57 patients undergoing esophagogastrectomy, total gastrectomy with or without reconstruction, or partial gastrectomy.[104] Symptomatic outcome was recorded in a standard proforma, including whether the patient thought the operation was successful. Resection relieved abdominal pain, nausea, and vomiting in all patients. Less symptoms were experienced following partial gastrectomy and esophagogastrectomy than after total gastrectomy. New symptoms developed most frequently after total gastrectomy. In all groups, about 70% were able to enjoy their food and about 80% considered their operation successful. Although the study by Korenaga et al.[67] received several criticisms, it did attempt to assess quality of life variables after R2 gastrectomy.[105] Performance scores were seen to gradually increase following surgery, but a significant difference in food tolerance and body weight was seen between patients who had undergone total or partial gastrectomy. Total gastrectomy was more disabling. More recently, Braga et al.[106] investigated the results of total versus subtotal gastrectomy for patients with adenocarcinoma of the lower two-thirds of the stomach. Postoperative mortality and morbidity were higher in the total gastrectomy group, but the extent of gastric resection did not influence 5-year survival. Patients in the subtotal gastrectomy group increased their body weight significantly more quickly than those undergoing total gastrectomy. The present authors recommend distal gastrectomy when a cancer-free proximal resection margin can be guaranteed. A literature review by Haglund et al.[107] noted that patient selection into different groups tends to bias results, as patients with more advanced tumors are more likely to be subjected to total rather than subtotal gastrectomy. This should be considered when interpreting non-randomized studies. Furthermore, although patients suffer nutritional problems after total gastrectomy, it is still not really known if these impinge on other aspects of quality of life.

There is extensive discussion in the literature as to whether a gastric substitute helps totally gastrectomized patients and improves quality of life. Buhl et al.[68] evaluated functional results and quality of life in patients a minimum of 12 months postoperatively. Patients underwent total gastrectomy and Hunt–Lawrence–Rodino pouch reconstruction ($n = 59$), an esophagojejunostomy ($n = 24$), or a distal gastrectomy ($n = 21$). Quality of life was assessed with the Visick Scale, the Karnofsky Performance Index, the Troidl gastric cancer questionnaire, the Spitzer Quality of Life index as well as three German questionnaires for complaints, depression, and impact of events on the patients. No significant differences were seen between total gastrectomy with pouch reconstruction and distal gastrectomy with respect to dumping syndrome or heartburn. Patients after total gastrectomy and esophagojejunostomy suffered from both, in addition to a reduced nutritional status. Buhl et al. concluded that total gastrectomy with pouch reconstruction was the treatment of choice, with no threat to postoperative quality of life. Moreover, distal gastrectomy should be reserved for surgery performed with purely palliative intent. Other randomized studies are discussed below.

Palliative surgery

The benefit of palliative surgery for gastric cancer is controversial. Partial gastrectomy is commonly performed, but total gastrectomy is not universally accepted for palliation because of its high attendant morbidity and mortality and the question of adverse long-term side effects.[108] Many patients with proximal tumors still require total gastrectomy to excise gross tumor if intubation or laser treatment are not appropriate. Few studies have properly examined quality of life in these groups of patients. Monson et al.[109] reviewed 53 consecutive patients undergoing total gastrectomy for advanced disease. Patients' quality of life was based on the following criteria: the ability to maintain adequate oral intake; the ability to do normal activities; the presence of dysphagia; and the ability to maintain a constant body weight. If patients satisfied all these criteria and did not require further hospital admissions, they were thought to have a good quality of life. Using this classification, 59% were considered to have a good outcome and a poor quality of life was only observed in 13%. In 1983, Meijer et al.[110] presented the results of 51 patients undergoing total or subtotal gastrectomy or gastroenterostomy for advanced carcinoma of the stomach, using a similar observer-rated crude scoring system. Only 13 patients had good results, seven were considered moderate, and 22 poor; patients with a gastroenterostomy generally had poor results.

To summarize, further quality of life research is urgently needed using appropriate validated disease-specific instruments. Indeed, until more is known about the patients' perception of outcome it is difficult to draw meaningful conclusions about the role of gastrectomy in patients with metastases or locally advanced disease.

Chemotherapy

The extent to which chemotherapy in advanced gastric cancer relieves symptoms, improves quality of life, and influences survival is incompletely known. The Japanese Research Society evaluated quality of life using a self-completion linear analog scale in patients with inoperable disease undergoing chemotherapy with a prodrug of 5-fluorouracil and cisplatin in different doses and regimens.[63] Quality of life, in particular, appetite, general well-being and fatigue, was significantly better in patients receiving the higher-frequency drug combination. Response rates were similar in both groups. Jager et al.[111] reported the results of a Phase II study of 5-fluorouracil, folinic acid, and alpha-interferon 2B in advanced gastric cancer. Quality of life was measured with the Karnofsky Performance Status and an unspecified questionnaire. The authors concluded that this regimen had a low toxicity profile and a positive impact on quality of life.

The use of chemotherapy in advanced gastric cancer requires further study. A more recent trial randomized patients to 5-fluorouracil, doxorubicin, and methotrexate or best supportive care.[112] Survival was significantly better in the treatment group and chemotherapy was well tolerated. However, similar trials using disease-specific quality of life measures are needed to determine how palliative chemotherapy affects quality as well as quantity of life.

Randomized trials with quality of life as an outcome measure

The randomized trials in patients with gastric cancer including a quality of life measure are listed in **Table 3.5**. Results of a trial comparing reconstruction after total gastrectomy by the Hunt–Lawrence–Rodino pouch method or esophagojejunostomy have been reported in various formats.[54,55,113] Sixty patients were evaluated with the Visick classification, the Spitzer Quality of Life Index, and a local instrument constructed in Cologne. In general, quality of life decreased in the early postoperative period and then improved until death occurred. Following esophagojejunostomy, more patients complained of inability to eat normal meals and subsequent weight loss. The sociopersonal results from the quality of life questionnaire tended to remain constant, with little variability. This may reflect inaccurate, unsuitable instruments or it may reflect that patients mainly suffer nutritional problems which do not affect other aspects of health. Fuchs *et al.*[59] randomized 120 patients to either a jejunal interposition with pouch or a Roux-en-Y reconstruction with a pouch. The Visick classification and Spitzer index were used to assess postoperative quality of life in patients surviving 3 or more years ($n = 46$). Complications, mortality, and operation times were similar in both groups, and no significant differences were seen in all quality of life scores or body weight. Based on these figures, the authors recommended using the less technically difficult procedure. More recently, the quality of life results from 60 patients randomized to an Ulm pouch, a Hunt–Lawrence–Rodino pouch reconstruction or a Roux-en-Y reconstruction without a pouch were published.[114] Quality of life was assessed by means of a standardized questionnaire which the authors claimed was validated and highly specific, though no validation data were included. At 6 months after surgery, patients with an Ulm pouch were found to have a significantly better quality of life, higher body weight, and better physiologic regulation of gastrointestinal hormones (in contrast to other methods of reconstruction). This study was heavily criticized by Troidl and Eypasch,[115] who questioned the validity of the quality of life measure and results obtained.

Many attempts to palliate unresectable gastric cancer have included chemotherapy.[116] A double-blind, randomized trial compared 5-fluorouracil and methyl CCNU with a placebo group in 193 patients. Quality of life was assessed by an observer looking at the patients' sense of well-being and activity levels, and their need for analgesia. No statistical differences were observed between the treatment arms and placebo group in terms of overall survival, performance (ECOG), or quality of life; indeed, many patients who were particularly frail found chemotherapy detrimental. Another early randomized trial of chemoradiation treatment for gastric cancer found no differences between several combinations of treatment and a control group in terms of survival and quality of life assessed with the Visick classification.[117] Glimelius *et al.*[66] reported a small trial of palliative chemotherapy (leucovorin and 5-fluorouracil ± etoposide) or best supportive care. The Karnofsky Performance Status and a questionnaire designed for colorectal cancer patients was used to assess quality of life. A significant overall survival advantage was seen in the group randomized to chemotherapy, while quality of life also improved in the treatment group, though this did not reach statistical significance. The authors claimed that, on the whole the drug regimen was tolerable except for complete alopecia in all patients. The use of cancer-specific quality of life instruments in trials will allow for cross-study comparisons of results, and these are urgently needed in studies of new treatment for gastric cancer.

CONCLUSIONS

The importance of broadening outcome measures in surgery and oncology to include quality of life parameters is increasingly recognized. There are now good psychometrically robust cancer specific measures available which, when used correctly, can produce reliable data about patients' general

Table 3.5 Randomized studies with quality of life as an outcome measure – gastric cancer

REFERENCE	YEAR	GROUP 1	GROUP 2	GROUP 3	QUALITY OF LIFE TOOL	OUTCOME
Kingston et al.[116]	1978	5-Fluorouracil and methyl CCNU	Placebo	–	Performance score and observer scale	No significant differences
Dent et al.[117]	1979	5-Fluorouracil and radiation	Thiopeta	Control	Observer Visick score	No significant differences
Kusche et al.[55]	1987	Hunt–Lawrence pouch (TG)	Esophagogastrectomy (TG)	–	Visick, Spitzer and Troidl questionnaire	More eating problems after esophagogastrectomy
Glimelius et al.[66]	1994	Leucovorin 5-fluorouracil ± etoposide	Best supportive care	–	Karnofsky Score and colorectal tool	No significant differences
Fuchs et al.[59]	1995	Jejunal interposition and pouch (TG)	Roux-en-Y and pouch (TG)	–	Visick and Spitzer	No significant differences
Schwarz et al.[114]	1996	Ulm pouch (TG)	Hunt–Lawrence pouch (TG)	Roux-en-Y without pouch (TG)	Standardized local questionnaire	Significantly better quality of life with Ulm pouch

TG, total gastrectomy.

quality of life. Instruments designed especially for patients with esophageal and gastric cancer are being developed. It is hoped that these tumor-specific modules will provide additional specificity to address questions of particular relevance in a given clinical trial. The use of these tools in controlled trials requires thoughtful administration and statistical analysis. The mode of administering the questionnaires carries large resource implications for multicenter studies, particularly in patients receiving treatment of palliative intent. Whether telephone interviews or data collected by an interviewer are appropriate remains unclear. Nonetheless, whatever the method of administration used, problems with incomplete data sets occur and new models of analysing quality of life data are currently being elucidated.

As yet, relatively little is known about the psychosocial distress caused by the diagnosis and treatment of upper gastrointestinal cancer. Whether psychiatric and social difficulties simply correlate with physical problems is uncertain, and to what extent these issues can be successfully treated is at present unpredictable. Until results from well-designed studies using appropriate quality of life instruments are available, the full extent of how different treatments for esophageal and gastric cancer diminish or enhance patients' quality of life remains unknown. Current research, however, into the best ways of measuring the patients' view of their own quality of life is continuing, and many trial organizations advocate greater use of these outcome measures. It is hoped, therefore, that clinical decision-making in the selection of patients for major surgery, adjuvant chemoradiation, or palliative treatment alone will be based on morbidity, mortality, and survival data and on valid information regarding the likely effect on the patients' short- and long-term quality of life.

REFERENCES

1. Fallowfield LJ. *The Quality of Life: The Missing Measurement in Health Care.* London: Souvenir Press Ltd, 1990.

2. McQuay HJ. Assessment of pain and effectiveness of treatment. In: Hopkins A & Costain D (eds) *Measuring Outcomes of Medical Care.* London: Royal College of Physicians, 1990: 43–57.

3. Aaronson NK, Cull A, Kaasa S & Sprangers MAG. The EORTC modular approach to quality of life assessment in oncology. *Int J Ment Health* 1994; **23**: 75–96.

4. Aaronson NK, Bullinger M & Ahmedzai S. A modular approach to quality-of-life assessment in cancer clinical trials. *Recent Res Cancer Res* 1988; **111**: 231–49.

5. Aaronson NK, Ahmedzai S, Bergman B *et al.* The European Organization for Research and Treatment of Cancer QLQ-C30: a quality of life instrument for use in international clinical trials in oncology. *J Natl Cancer Inst* 1993; **85**: 365–76.

6. Maguire P & Selby P. Assessing quality of life in cancer patients. *Br J Cancer* 1989; **60**: 437–40.

7. Carmines E & Zeller R. *Reliability and Validity Assessment.* Beverly Hills: Sage, 1979.

8. Nunnally JC. *Psychometric Theory.* New York: McGraw-Hill, 1978.

9. Guillemin F, Bombardier C & Beaton D. Cross-cultural adaptation of health related quality of life measures: literature review and proposed guidelines. *J Clin Epidemiol* 1993; **46**: 1417–32.

10. Slevin ML, Plant H, Lynch D, Drinkwater J & Gregory WM. Who should measure quality of life, the doctor or the patient? *Br J Cancer* 1988; **57**: 109–12.

11. Spitzer WO, Dobson AJ, Hall J *et al.* Measuring the quality of life of cancer patients. A concise QL-index for use by physicians. *J Chron Dis* 1981; **34**: 585–97.

12. Blazeby JM, Williams MH, Alderson D & Farndon JR. Observer variation in assessment of quality of life in patients with oesophageal cancer. *Br J Surgery* 1995; **82**: 1200–3.

13. Bremer BA & McCauley CR. Quality of life measures: hospital interview versus home questionnaire. *Health Psychol* 1986; **5**: 171–7.

14. Ford S, Lewis S & Fallowfield L. Psychological morbidity in newly referred patients with cancer. *J Psychosom Res* 1995; **39**: 193–202.

15. Coast J. The role of economic evaluation in setting priorities for elective surgery. *Health Policy* 1993; **24**: 243–57.

16. Rosser R & Kind P. A scale for valuations of states of illness: is there a consensus? *Int J Epidemiol* 1978; **7**: 347–57.

17. The Euroqol group. Euroqol – a facility for the measurement of health related quality of life. *Health Policy* 1990; **16**: 199–228.

18. Hankins JR, Cole FN, Ward A, Carter EA, Weiner S & McLaughlin JS. Carcinoma of the oesophagus: the philosophy of palliation. *Ann Thorac Surg* 1972; **14**: 189–97.

19. Clark RL & Lott S. Comparative study of symptom relief in oesophageal cancer with the development of a useful index of palliation. *Radiology* 1968; **90**: 971–4.

20. Carey JS & Plested WG. Oesophago-gastrectomy: superiority of the combined abdominal-right thoracic approach. *Ann Thorac Surg* 1972; **14**: 59–68.

21. Ward AS & Collis JL. Late results of oesophageal and oesophagogastric resection in the treatment of oesophageal cancer. *Thorax* 1971; **26**: 1–5.

22. Pearson JG. The value of radiotherapy in the management of squamous oesophageal cancer. *Br J Surg* 1971; **58**: 794–8.

23. Ong GB. Unresectable carcinoma of the oesophagus. *Ann R Coll Surg Engl* 1975; **56**: 3–14.

24. Stoller JL, Samer KJ, Toppin DI & Flores AD. Carcinoma of the oesophagus. A new proposal for the evaluation of treatment. *Can J Surg* 1977; **20**: 454–9.

25. McCaughan JS, Jr, Williams TE, Jr & Bethel BH. Palliation of oesophageal malignancy with photodynamic therapy. *Ann Thorac Surg* 1985; **40**: 113–20.

26. Mellow MH & Pinkas H. Endoscopic laser therapy for malignancies affecting the oesophagus and gastroesophageal junction. *Arch Intern Med* 1985; **145**: 1443–6.

27. Chavy AL, Rougier M, Pieddeloup SA *et al.* Oesophageal prosthesis for neoplastic stenosis. A prognostic study of 77 cases. *Cancer* 1986; **57**: 1426–31.

28. Sugimachi K, Maekawa S, Koga Y, Ueo H & Inokuchi K. The quality of life is sustained after operation for carcinoma of the oesophagus. *Surg Gynecol Obstet* 1986; **162**: 544–7.

29. Mahoney JL & Condon RE. Adenocarcinoma of the oesophagus. *Ann Surg* 1987; **205**: 557–62.

30. Rutgeerts P. Vantrappen G, Broeckaert L *et al.* Palliative Nd:YAG laser therapy for cancer of the oesophagus and gastroesophageal junction: impact on the quality of remaining life. *Gastrointest Endosc* 1988; **34**: 87–9.

31. Flores AD, Nelems B, Evans K, Hay JH, Stoller J & Jackson SM. Impact of new radiotherapy modalities on the surgical management of cancer of the oesophagus and cardia. *Int J Radiat Oncol Biol Phys* 1989; **17**: 937–44.

32. Flores AD. Cancer of the oesophagus and cardia: overview of radiotherapy. *Can J Surg* 1989; **32**: 404–9.

33. Albertsson M, Ewers SB, Widmark H, Hambraeus G, Lillo-Gil R & Ranstam J. Evaluation of the palliative effect of radiotherapy for oesophageal carcinoma. *Acta Oncol* 1989; **28**: 267–70.

34. Eckhauser MI. Palliative therapy of upper gastrointestinal malignancies using the Nd-Yag laser. *Am Surg* 1990; **56**: 158–62.

35. Reed CE, Marsh WH, Carlson LS, Seymore CH & Kratz JM. Prospective, randomized trial of palliative treatment for unresectable cancer of the oesophagus. *Ann Thorac Surg* 1991; **51**: 552–6.

36. O'Rourke IC, McNeil RJ, Walker PJ & Bull CA. Objective evaluation of the quality of palliation in patients with oesophageal cancer comparing surgery, radiotherapy and intubation. *Aust NZ J Surg* 1992; **62**: 922–30.

37. Knyrim K, Wagner HJ, Bethge N, Keymling M & Vakil N. A controlled trial of an expansile metal stent for palliation of oesophageal obstruction due to inoperable cancer. *N Engl J Med* 1993; **329**: 1302–7.

38. Low DE & Pagliero KM. Prospective randomized clinical trial comparing brachytherapy and laser photoablation for palliation of oesophageal cancer. *J Thorac Cardiovasc Surg* 1992; **104**: 173–9.

39. Collard JM, Otte JB, Reynaert M & Kestens J. Quality of life three years or more after oesophagectomy for cancer. *J Thorac Cardiovasc Surg* 1992; **104**: 391–4.

40. Diamantes T & Mannell A. Oesophageal intubation for advanced oesophageal cancer: the Baragwanath experience 1977–1981. *Br J Surg* 1983; **70**: 555–7.

41. Welvaart K & De Jong PL. Palliation of patients with carcinoma of the lower oesophagus and cardia: the question of quality of life. *J Surg Oncol* 1986; **32**: 197–9.

42. Bluett MK, Sawyers JL & Healy D. Oesophageal carcinoma. Improved quality of survival with resection. *Am Surg* 1987; **53**: 126–32.

43. Neal TJ & Krasner N. Is the endoscopic view too narrow? *J Med Ethics* 1992; **18**: 186–8.

44. Earlam R & Cunha-Melo JR. Oesophageal squamous cell carcinoma: 1. A critical review of surgery. *Br J Surg* 1980; **67**: 381–90.

45. van Knippenberg FCE, Out JJ, Tilanus HW, Mud HJ, Hop WCJ & Verhage F. Quality of life in patients with resected oesophageal cancer. *Soc Sci Med* 1992; **35**: 139–45.

46. Loizou LA, Rampton D, Atkinson M, Robertson C & Bown SG. A prospective assessment of quality of life after endoscopic intubation and laser therapy for malignant dysphagia. *Cancer* 1992; **70**: 386–91.

47. Barr H, Krasner N, Raouf A & Walker RJ. Prospective randomized trial of laser therapy

only and laser therapy followed by endoscopic intubation for the palliation of malignant dysphagia. *Gut* 1990; **31**: 252–8.

48. Blazeby JM, Williams MH, Brookes ST, Alderson D & Farndon JR. Quality of life measurement in patients with oesophageal cancer. *Gut* 1995; **37**: 505–8.

49. Payne SA. A study of quality of life in cancer patients receiving palliative chemotherapy. *Soc Sci Med* 1992; **35**: 1505–9.

50. Higginson I, Wade A & McCarthy M. Palliative care: views of patients and their families. *Br Med J* 1990; **301**: 277–81.

51. Visick AH. A study of the failures after gastrectomy. *Ann R Coll Surg Engl* 1948; **3**: 266–84.

52. Goligher JC, Pulvertaft CN, de Dombal FT *et al.* Five- to eight year results of Leeds/York controlled trial of elective surgery for duodenal ulcer. *Br Med J* 1968; **2**: 781–7.

53. Goligher JC. Judging the quality of life after surgical operations. *J Chron Dis* 1987; **40**: 631–3.

54. Troidl H, Kusche J, Vestweber K, Eypasch E, Koeppen L & Bouillon B. Quality of life: an important endpoint both in surgical practice and research. *J Chron Dis* 1987; **40**: 523–8.

55. Kusche J, Vestweber KH & Troidl H. Quality of life after total gastrectomy for stomach cancer. *Scand J Gastroenterol* 1987; **22** (Suppl 133): 96–101.

56. Gasparri G, Casalegno PA, Camandona M *et al.* Endoscopic insertion of 248 prostheses in inoperable carcinoma of the oesophagus and cardia: short-term and long-term results. *Gastrointest Endosc* 1987; **33**: 354–6.

57. Barbier PA, Luder PJ, Schupfer G, Becker CD & Wagner HE. Quality of life and patterns of recurrence following transhiatal oesophagectomy for cancer: results of a prospective follow-up in 50 patients. *World J Surg* 1988; **12**: 270–6.

58. Fuchs KH, Freys SM, Schaube H, Eckstein AK, Selch A & Hamelmann H. Randomized comparison of endoscopic palliation of malignant oesophageal stenoses. *Surg Endosc* 1991; **5**: 63–7.

59. Fuchs KH, Thiede A, Engemann R, Deltz E, Stemme O & Hamelmann H. Reconstruction of the food passage after total gastrectomy: randomised trial. *World J Surg* 1995; **19**: 698–706.

60. Sue-Ling HM, Martin I, Griffith J *et al.* Early gastric cancer: 46 cases treated in one surgical department. *Gut* 1992; **33**: 1318–22.

61. Watson A. A study of the quality and duration of survival following resection, endoscopic intubation and surgical intubation in oesophageal carcinoma. *Br J Surg* 1982; **69**: 585–8.

62. Svedlund J, Sullivan M, Sjodin I, Liedman B & Lundell L. Quality of life in gastric cancer prior to gastrectomy. *Qual Life Res* 1996; **5**: 255–64.

63. Kurihara M & Matsukawa M. Recent advances in inoperable gastric cancer chemotherapy. *Int Med* 1995; **34**: 296–8.

64. Rau E. Tumour biology and quality of life in patients with gastric cancer. In: Sugarbaker P (ed.) *Management of Gastric Cancer.* Boston: Kluwer Academic Publishers, 1991: 325–38.

65. Siegrist K & Siegrist J. Psychological factors in the course of gastric cancer. *Scand J Gastroenterol* 1987; **22** (suppl 133): 90–2.

66. Glimelius B, Hoffman K, Haglund U, Nyren O & Sjoden PO. Initial or delayed chemotherapy with best supportive care in advanced gastric cancer. *Ann Oncol* 1994; **5**: 189–90.

67. Korenaga D, Orita H, Okuyama T, Moriguche T, Maehara S & Sugimachi K. Quality of life after gastrectomy in patients with carcinoma of the stomach. *Br J Surg* 1992; **79**: 248–50.

68. Buhl K, Lehnert T & Herfarth C. Reconstruction after gastrectomy and quality of life. *World J Surg* 1995; **19**: 558–64.

69. Koster R, Gebbensleben B, Stutzer H, Salzberger B, Ahrens P & Rohde H. Quality of life in gastric cancer. *Scand J Gastroenterol* 1987; **22** (suppl 133): 102–6.

70. Bergner M, Bobbit RA, Carter WB & Gilson BS. The Sickness Impact Profile: development and final revision of a health status measure. *Med Care* 1981; **19**: 787–805.

71. de Haes JCJM, van Knippenberg FCE & Neijt JP. Measuring psychological and physical distress in cancer patients: structure and application of the Rotterdam Symptom Checklist. *Br J Cancer* 1990; **62**: 1034–8.

72. Cella DF, Tulsky DS, Gray G *et al.* The Functional Assessment of Cancer Therapy Scale: development and validation of the general measure. *J Clin Oncol* 1993; **11**: 570–9.

73. Sprangers MAG, Cull A, Bjordal K, Groenvold M & Aaronson NK. The European Organisation for Research and Treatment of Cancer approach to quality of life assessment: guidelines for developing questionnaire modules. *Qual Life Res* 1993; **2**: 287–95.

74. Osoba D, Zee B, Pater J, Warr D, Kaizer L & Latreille J. Psychometric properties and responsiveness of the EORTC Quality of Life Questionnaire (QLQ-C30) in patients with breast, ovarian and lung cancer. *Qual Life Res* 1994; **3**: 353–64.

75. Osoba D, Aaronson NK, Muller M *et al.* The development and psychometric validation of a brain cancer quality of life questionnaire for use in combination with general and cancer-specific questionnaires. *Qual Life Res* 1996; **5**: 139–50.

76. Ringdal GI & Ringdal K. Testing the EORTC Quality of Life Questionnaire on cancer patients with heterogeneous diagnoses. *Qual Life Res* 1993; **2**: 129–40.

77. Zieren HU, Jacobi CA, Zieren J & Muller JM. Quality of life following resection of oesophageal carcinoma. *Br J Surg* 1996; **83**: 1772–5.

78. Priestman TJ & Baum M. Evaluation of quality of life in patients receiving treatment for advanced breast cancer. *Lancet* 1976; **i**: 899–900.

79. Morris JN, Suissa S, Sherwood S, Wright SA & Greer D. Last days: a study of the quality of life of terminally ill cancer patients. *J Chron Dis* 1986; **39**: 47–62.

80. Morris JN & Sherwood S. Quality of life of cancer patients at different stages in the disease trajectory. *J Chron Dis* 1987; **40**: 545–53.

81. Eypasch E, Williams JI, Wood-Dauphinee S *et al.* Gastrointestinal quality of life index: development, validation and application of a new instrument. *Br J Surg* 1995; **82**: 216–22.

82. Zigmond AS & Snaith RP. The hospital anxiety and depression scale. *Acta Psychiatr Scand* 1983; **67**: 361–70.

83. Karnofsky DA & Burchenal JH. The clinical evaluation of chemotherapeutic agents in cancer. In: Macleod CM (ed.) *Experimental Cancer Therapy.* New York: Columbia University Press, 1949: 191–205.

84. World Health Organization. *World Health Organization Handbook for Reporting Results of Cancer Treatment.* Geneva: WHO, 1979.

85. Zubrod CG, Schneiderman M, Frei E *et al.* Appraisal of methods for the study of chemotherapy of cancer in man: comparative therapeutic trial of nitrogen mustard and triethylene thiophosphoramide. *J Chron Dis* 1960; **11**: 7–33.

86. Stoller JL & Brumwell ML. Palliation after operation and after radiotherapy for cancer of the oesophagus. *Can J Surg* 1984; **27**: 491–5.

87. Blazeby JM, Alderson D, Winstone K *et al.* Development of a EORTC questionnaire module to be used in quality of life assessment for patients with oesophageal cancer. *Eur J Cancer* 1996; **32**: 1912–17.

88. Blazeby JM, Alderson D & Farndon JR. An international field study to test the EORTC QLQ-C30 and oesophageal cancer module (EORCT QLQ-OES24) among patients with oesophageal cancer. EORTC Protocol No 15961, 1997.

89. Roder JD, Herschbach P, Sellschopp A & Siewert JR. Quality-of-life assessment following oesophagectomy. *Theor Surg* 1991; **6**: 206–10.

90. Kuwano H, Ikebe M, Baba K *et al.* Operative procedures of reconstruction after resection of oesophageal cancer and the post operative quality of life. *World J Surg* 1993; **17**: 773–6.

91. Fujita H, Kakegawa T, Yamana H *et al.* Mortality and morbidity rates, postoperative course, quality of life, and prognosis after extended radical lymphadenectomy for oesophageal cancer. *Ann Surg* 1995; **222**: 654–62.

92. Orel JJ, Erzen JJ & Hrabar BA. Results of resection of carcinoma of the oesophagus and cardia in 196 patients. *World J Surg* 1981; **5**: 259–67.

93. O'Hanlon D, Harkin M, Daya K, Sergeant T, Hayes N & Griffin SM. Quality of life assessment in patients undergoing treatment for oesophageal carcinoma. *Br J Surg* 1995; **82**: 1682–5.

94. Muller JM, Erasmi H, Stelzner M, Zieren U & Pichlmaier H. Surgical therapy of oesophageal carcinoma. *Br J Surg* 1990; **77**: 845–57.

95. Abe S, Tachibana M, Shimokawa T, Shiraishi M & Nakamura T. Surgical treatment of advanced carcinoma of the oesophagus. *Surg Gynecol Obstet* 1989; **168**: 115–20.

96. Orringer MB. Sub-sternal bypass of the excluded oesophagus – Results of an ill advised operation. *Surgery* 1984; **96**: 467–71.

97. Mannell A, Becker PJ & Nissenbaum M. Bypass surgery for unresectable oesophageal cancer: early and late results in 124 cases. *Br J Surg* 1988; **75**: 283–6.

98. Stoller JL. Preliminary results of bypass surgery for unresectable strictures of the oesophagus. *Am J Surg* 1980; **139**: 654–6.

99. Sawant D & Moghissi K. Management of unresectable oesophageal cancer: a review of 537 patients. *Eur J Cardiothorac Surg* 1994; **8**: 113–17.

100. Ogilvie AL, Dronfield MW, Ferguson R & Atkinson M. Palliative intubation of oesophago-gastric neoplasms at fibreoptic endoscopy. *Gut* 1982; **23**: 1060–7.

101. Mathus-Vliegen EMH & Tytgat GNJ. Palliation by laser photoablation: a multidisciplinary quality assessment. *Gastrointest Endosc* 1992; **38**: 365–8.

102. Bamias A, Hill ME, Cunningham D *et al.* Epirubicin, cisplatin, and protracted venous infusion of 5-fluorouracil for oesophagogastric adenocarcinoma. *Cancer* 1996; **77**: 1978–85.

103. Bozzetti F, Ravera E, Dossena G *et al.* Comparing the nutritional status after total or subtotal gastrectomy. *Nutrition* 1990; **6**: 371–5.

104. Anderson ID & Macintyre IMC. Symptomatic outcome following resection of gastric cancer. *Surg Oncol* 1995; **4**: 35–40.

105. Eypasch E & Troidl H. Quality of life after gastrectomy in patients with carcinoma of the stomach. *Br J Surg* 1992; **79**: 974–5.

106. Braga M, Molinari M, Zuliani W *et al.* Surgical treatment of gastric adenocarcinoma: Impact on survival and quality of life. A prospective ten year study. *Hepatogastroenterology* 1996; **43**: 187–93.

107. Haglund U, Wollert S & Gustavsson S. Gastric cancer. *Acta Chir Scand* 1990; **156**: 99–104.

108. Lawrence WJ & McNeer G. The effectiveness of surgery for palliation of incurable gastric cancer. *Cancer* 1958; **11**: 28–32.

109. Monson JRT, Donohue JH, McIlrath DC, Farnell MB & Ilstrup DM. Total gastrectomy for advanced cancer. A worthwhile palliative procedure. *Cancer* 1991; **68**: 1863–8.

110. Meijer S, DeBakker OJGB & Hoitsma HFW. Palliative resection in gastric cancer. *J Surg Oncol* 1983; **23**: 77–80.

111. Jager E, Bernhard H, Klein O *et al.* Combination 5-fluorouracil (FU), folinic acid (FA) and α-interferon 2B in advanced gastric cancer: results of a phase II trial. *Ann Oncol* 1995; **6**: 153–6.

112. Murad AM, Santiago FF, Petroianou A, Rocha PRS, Rodrigues MAG & Rausch M. Modified therapy with 5-fluorouracil, doxorubicin, and methotrexate in advanced gastric cancer. *Cancer* 1993; **72**: 37–41.

113. Troidl H, Kusche J, Vestweber KH, Eypasch E & Maul U. Pouch versus oesophagojejunostomy after total gastrectomy: a randomized clinical trial. *World J Surg* 1987; **11**: 699–712.

114. Schwarz A, Buchler M, Usinger K *et al.* Importance of the duodenal passage and pouch volume after total gastrectomy and reconstruction with the Ulm pouch: prospective randomized clinical study. *World J Surg* 1996; **20**: 60–7.

115. Troidl H & Eypasch E. Invited commentary. *World J Surg* 1996; **20**: 67–8.

116. Kingston RD, Ellis DJ, Powell J *et al.* The West Midlands gastric carcinoma chemotherapy trial: planning and results. *Clin Oncol* 1978; **4**: 55–69.

117. Dent DM, Werner ID, Novis B, Cheverton P & Brice P. Prospective randomized trial of combined oncological therapy for gastric carcinoma. *Cancer* 1979; **44**: 385–91.

PART
2

Gastric cancer

4

SURGICAL MANAGEMENT OF GASTRIC CANCER: THE WESTERN EXPERIENCE

RODERICH E. SCHWARZ
MARTIN S. KARPEH
MURRAY F. BRENNAN

INTRODUCTION

In contradistinction to Japanese and Korean centers with vast experience in gastric cancer screening and treatment, a lower incidence and advanced stage presentation in the United States and Western Europe has prohibited many centers from developing a specialized approach to this disease. Inferior outcome after surgical treatment of gastric cancer reported from European and American centers have led to speculations that the natural history of this disease is different than in the countries of East Asia. Nevertheless, adoption of "Japanese" treatment principles with regard to surgical staging and radicality of resection have led to a significant improvement in "Western" treatment results in several larger European and American series. The evaluation of prospectively collected clinical data on gastric cancer patients at Memorial Sloan-Kettering Cancer Center (MSKCC) in New York City since 1985 has enabled us to answer several relevant questions regarding diagnostic and therapeutic decision making. When we report on this clinical experience, it does not reflect a widely practiced "Western" standard of gastric cancer treatment in the Western world; it does emphasize what treatment outcome is possible with the use of certain staging and therapeutic standards in a large tertiary

care cancer center within the United States, a country with low incidence of gastric carcinoma and no active screening programs. In this respect, our approach to the surgical management of gastric cancer may show more similarities to the "Japanese" experience, as outlined in Chapter 5 by Sasako, than to the commonly practiced approach to this disease within the United States.

Since separate chapters within this book are dedicated to combined modality therapy, early gastric cancer, and gastric lymphoma, we will adhere closely to our analysis of surgical implications for the treatment of gastric adenocarcinoma.

GASTRIC CANCER INCIDENCE, MORTALITY AND TREATMENT OUTCOME IN THE UNITED STATES

Within much of the Western world, gastric adenocarcinoma represented the leading cause of cancer death 50 years ago.[1] While this phenomenon continues in many countries of the Third World, the incidence and mortality of gastric cancer have experienced a drastic decline in the United States over the past 40 years, and estimated deaths from gastric cancer in this country now represent 2.5% of all cancer-related deaths in 1997.[2] Despite an increase in the incidence of adenocarcinoma of the gastroesophageal junction over the past 10 years,[3] the projected total number of new gastric cancer cases in the U.S. for 1997 was 22 400, with 14 000 estimated deaths from disease.[2] The fall in incidence appears to have plateaued throughout the past 5 years. Of all individual organ sites, stomach cancer ranges eighth in total cancer deaths within the U.S.[2] In comparison with countries with an epidemic incidence of gastric cancer, like Japan, Costa Rica or Chile, or compared with other European countries, the magnitude of gastric cancer incidence and mortality within the United States is significantly smaller (**Figures 4.1** and **4.2**). However, the magnitude of survival difference for gastric cancer between the U.S. and developing countries remains small, reflecting a lack of highly effective treatment options and methods for early detection.[5]

Surgical standards of gastric cancer treatment have been reviewed for representative parts of the United States through the American College of Surgeons[6] and the National Cancer Data Base.[7] Accordingly, two-thirds of patients presenting

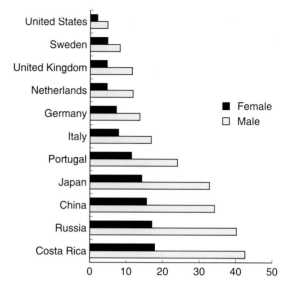

Figure 4.2 Age-adjusted death rates from gastric adenocarcinoma per 100 000 population in various countries, 1990–1993.[1] *Reproduced with permission from Reference 1.*

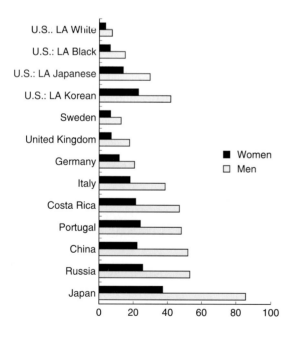

Figure 4.1 Age-standardized incidence of gastric adenocarcinoma in various countries and populations.[4] Incidence (per 100 000 population) in the United States is displayed for various ethnic or racial populations within Los Angeles County (LA).

with newly diagnosed gastric cancer were aged over 65 years, and more than 50% were older than 70. The male:female ratio was 1.6:1. The percentage of patients clinically staged according to the American Joint Committee on Cancer (AJCC) improved from 46% in 1986 to 77% in 1991.[7] Lesions within the upper third of the stomach were as frequent as lower-third cancers (35.6% versus 35.7%).[6] Some 19% of patients belonged to ethnic or racial minorities, with a comparable stage profile at diagnosis, except for a tendency towards earlier stage diagnosis in patients of Asian descent (23.7% stage 1 compared with 16.9% stage 1 in Caucasian patients). Some 72% of patients were treated surgically, of whom three-fourths underwent a form of gastric resection. Only 4.7% of patients with a clear-margin resection had undergone an extended lymphadenectomy. The overall 5-year survival rate after resection was 19%, and the 5-year disease-specific survival rate was 26%.

These U.S. American "standards" in the operative treatment of gastric cancer remain clearly inferior to collectively reviewed Japanese results after surgical treatment.[8,9] Reasons for this discrepancy between East and West have been examined in detail.[10,11] Rather than expecting the presence of a different biologic behavior of gastric cancer in

Japan and the West, it appears that early diagnosis, accuracy of Japanese staging, and a more aggressive approach to surgical treatment may account for the greater part of this difference. Recent changes in the incidence of proximal gastric lesions and in the frequency of signet-cell cancers have also been documented in Japanese centers, indicating similarities in the pathogenesis of gastric cancer in Japan and in Western countries.[12] Although a better survival for patients of Asian descent compared with White American patients has been shown in a recent study,[13] racial factors as the reason between superior Japanese treatment results in gastric cancer have been ruled out by comparing Tokyo Japanese patients with Japanese patients in Honolulu, treated according to common U.S. methods.[14] Adherence to Japanese principles of staging and lymphadenectomy in the treatment of "Western" patients within some European or American centers have indeed produced results more comparable with those previously only achieved in Japan (**Tables 4.1** and **4.2**).[15–17] Whether other comorbid conditions, adiposity, "Western" body habitus, and tobacco abuse present to the surgeon in the U.S. specific "Western" treatment limitations is unproven, but likely.

ANATOMIC AND PATHOLOGIC CONSIDERATIONS

Rich arterial blood supply and extensive lymphatic drainage create organ-specific conditions in the surgical treatment of gastric cancer. Major resections are frequently well tolerated, despite minimal remaining direct arterial blood flow. The complexity of perigastric, second-echelon, and more remote lymph nodes has been put into a useful classification by the Japanese Research Society for Gastric Cancer.[18] While strict adherence to this classification for the pathologic staging may not be feasible for most Western centers, it provides useful guidelines for the surgical approach to extended lymphadenectomy. The ability of the surgeon to predict the presence of a lymph node metastasis is generally poor. In lymph nodes <15 mm in maximum diameter, an accurate prediction by the surgeon about the presence or absence of metastatic cancer was obtained in <20% of cases.[19] In addition, up to 25% of lymph nodes <10 mm in size are involved with metastatic cancer.[9] It therefore appears useful to follow a systematic scheme not only to perigastric, but also to second- or third-echelon lymph node dissection for potentially curative gastrectomy, even if only for the purpose of accurate staging. Based on the location of the primary tumor, the assignment of lymph nodes to D1, D2, or D3 groups varies, which has important implications for performing a D2 dissection. The extent of D2 dissection has been graphically displayed for gastric lesions within the proximal, middle or lower thirds of the stomach.[20,21]

Although only reported in 9% of U.S. gastrectomy specimens,[6] the Lauren classification of intestinal and diffuse histologic types of gastric adenocarcinoma has been shown to provide prognostic information.[22,23] The intestinal type correlates with advanced age and male gender, is more common in areas of high incidence, and has a lesser tendency for submucosal or systemic spread.[24] Although the Borrmann classification can also provide important prognostic information,[25] we have not routinely used this as a criterion for pathologic tumor evaluation.

Table 4.1 Five-year survival rate by stage in selected series from Japan and the United States

		Maruyama[8]	ACS[6]	NCDB[7]	MSKCC[62]	MSKCC[17]
Time interval		1971–1985	1982, 1987	1985–1986, 1991	1955–1975	1985–1994
Patients (n)		3176	18 365	16 992	101	675
5-year survival rate (%)	Stage I	91	50	43	47	84
	Stage II	72	29	37	27	61
	Stage III	44	13	18	0	29
	Stage IV	9	3	10	0	25

ACS, American College of Surgeons; MSKCC, Memorial Sloan-Kettering Cancer Center; NCDB, National Cancer Data Base.
Adapted from Brennan & Karpeh.[17]

Table 4.2 Five-year survival rate by N classification in selected series

		JAPAN[9]	JAPAN[8]	GERMANY[15]	MSKCC[17]
Patients (*n*)		3145	3176	977	675
5-year survival rate (%)	N0	80	85	74	78
	N1	53	61	36	30
	N2	26	31	20	17
	N3	10	10	10	–
	N4	3	2	–	–

Since the pathologic stage based on TNM classifications is the single most important prognostic factor for survival in gastric cancer, exact staging is mandatory. Stage at presentation, clinical or pathologic, may vary more widely among Western centers than those in Japan or Korea. In many centers within the U.S., up to 50% of patients present with stage 4 disease, and have limited treatment options.[26] In our own experience at Memorial Sloan-Kettering Cancer Center (MSKCC), the stage distribution of patients newly diagnosed with gastric cancer over the past 10 years has shifted towards earlier stages and earlier T classification, likely reflecting an increased gastric cancer awareness and the more liberal use of diagnostic endoscopy (**Figure 4.3**). A recent trend towards more frequent proximal gastric cancer has not been observed at MSKCC, where gastroesophageal junction lesions (34%) and fundus lesions (14%) have made up nearly half of all gastric cancer sites for each year during the same time period (**Figure 4.4**).

Whether other pathobiologic parameters such as DNA ploidy,[27,28] signet ring cell features,[29] CD 44 expression,[30] expression of p53,[31–33] erbB-2,[34,35] K-*ras*,[36] E-cadherin,[37] proliferating cell nuclear antigen,[38] sialyl Tn antigen[39] or estrogen receptors,[39a] dendritic cell infiltration,[40] thymidylate synthetase inhibition,[38] or angiogenesis markers[41] have truly independent prognostic relevance is unclear. We have not relied on any of these for clinical therapeutic or monitoring decision making. An interesting approach to better assessing a cancer's ability for systemic spread, even in the presence of "low-risk" T or N classifications, is the investigation of cytokeratin-positive cells in bone marrow.[42] This holds promise to identify a subgroup of patients with presumed early stages of gastric cancer who may benefit from additional therapeutic means.

Infection with *Helicobacter pylori* appears to correlate with the presence of intestinal-type gastric cancer.[24] It is suspected that *H. pylori* acts as a contributing factor to gastric carcinogenesis, and recently has been classified as a class-I carcinogen for gastric cancer.[43] Prevalence of *H. pylori* infection in endemic areas can be as high as 75%, and a prognostic relevance to gastric cancer survival has

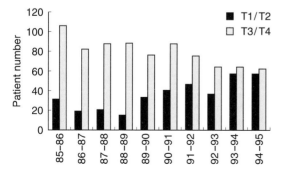

Figure 4.3 Changes in the T classification distribution over time, gastric adenocarcinoma at MSKCC, 1985–1995.

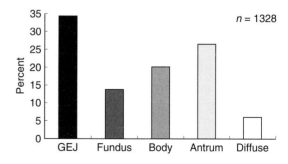

Figure 4.4 Site distribution, gastric adenocarcinoma at MSKCC, 1985–1995. GEJ, gastroesophageal junction.

not been established.[44] If diagnosed preoperatively, we prefer to treat the infection before proceeding with a gastrectomy.

DIAGNOSIS AND STAGING

Diagnostic goals for suspected gastric cancer include the histologic confirmation of the presence of carcinoma, assessment of resectability criteria, identification of patients with advanced tumor stages that may not be adequately served with operative treatment alone, and identification of patients with metastatic disease (M1). Anamnestic patient evaluation can identify symptoms due to metastatic disease. The physical examination should include palpation for supraclavicular lymphadenopathy (Virchow's node), ovarian masses (Krukenberg tumors), periumbilical masses (Sister Mary Joseph's nodule), and pelvic peritoneal implants felt on rectal exam (Blumer's shelf). Comorbid conditions that would preclude the safe performance of operative treament require specialized evaluation, e.g., cardiac stress performance and pulmonary function tests. Although slightly younger than the U.S. average,[6] the majority of patients with gastric cancer seen at MSKCC are aged over 60 years (**Figure 4.5**), and cardiac or pulmonary risk factors are not uncommon.

Upper gastrointestinal endoscopy is the mainstay of diagnosis for adenocarcinoma of the stomach. Histologic analysis of biopsy material is more likely to succeed than cytology of brushings (94% versus 74%).[6] Endoscopy commonly allows description of the tumor location and intragastric extent. In adenocarcinomas of the gastroesophageal junction, endoscopic assessment of the more proximal esophagus with biopsies is helpful to rule out the presence of Barrett's esophageal changes with dysplasia. The use of upper gastrointestinal contrast radiographs has decreased over the past 10 years, secondary to increased use of endoscopy and computed tomography (CT). High-resolution CT of the abdomen and pelvis can identify local extent of the gastric tumor, contiguous organ invasion, or possible parenchymal involvement of liver, adrenal, or ovary. CT evaluation has been helpful to define the depth of gastric wall invasion by the primary tumor.[45] CT scans, however, have limited ability to identify peritoneal serosal metastases or metastatic lymph nodes, unless they are extensive or accompanied by ascites.[46] Nevertheless, we routinely obtain CT scans of the abdomen and pelvis to evaluate gastric and extragastric extent, and, if positive, to avoid an unrewarding operative exploration. CT scans of the chest are obtained for presumably advanced gastric lesions, and if plain chest radiographs were equivocal or suggestive for the presence of pulmonary metastases. Magnetic resonance imaging (MRI) has not found a routine application in the work-up of gastric cancer, although it allows better definition of the gastric mural architecture than CT scans.[47]

Endoscopic ultrasonography (EUS) has been used with increasing frequency to assess the thickness of the primary tumor and the presence of enlarged lymph nodes.[48] Although the concordance for EUS with the pathologic T classification is not higher than 86%, EUS assessment of the tumor thickness is highly predictive of clinical outcome or recurrence.[17,49] Therefore, the preoperative identification of T1/2 versus T3/4 lesions has become a very desirable goal, since the high rate of treatment failure in the latter group strongly suggests a preoperative treatment approach with systemic agents. Over the last years, patients thus staged preoperatively underwent experimental chemotherapy and subsequent restaging before any potentially curative gastrectomy.[50] Our recent experience with laparoscopic staging, including laparoscopic ultrasonography, has been shown to be equally effective in obtaining a useful measure of tumor thickness, in addition to the ability of visualization of peritoneal surfaces and of obtaining biopsies from D3 lymph nodes.[51,52] If preopera-

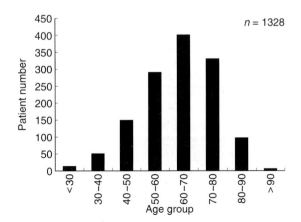

Figure 4.5 Age distribution, gastric adenocarcinoma at MSKCC, 1985–1995.

tive chemotherapy protocols for high-risk patients with curative treatment intent are available, either endoscopic or laparoscopic ultrasonography in addition to endoscopy and CT scanning appear to be useful in determining the tumor thickness. The role for laparoscopy at gastrectomy is discussed in more detail below.

OPERATIVE STRATEGIES IN THE SURGICAL TREATMENT OF GASTRIC CANCER

Since the first successful partial gastrectomy for a pyloric carcinoma by Billroth in 1881,[53] and since the first total gastrectomy by Schlatter in 1897,[54] surgical treatment of gastric cancer has evolved through a century of continued technical and multi-disciplinary refinements. Early challenges to the surgeon performing gastric resections were reconstitution of upper gastrointestinal continuity, control of anastomotic leaks, and control of postoperative infection. Extensive procedures in the absence of antibiotics, blood replacement, and sophisticated anesthesiologic techniques were fraught with a high mortality rate. Operative treatment principles were not different for malignant or benign disorders of the stomach. Total gastrectomy became more feasible after the description of the Roux-en-Y esophagojejunostomy, eliminating reflux esophagitis.[55] An early report from our institution reviewed failure and recurrence patterns after subtotal gastric resection for adenocarcinoma, and found a local recurrence rate of 80%, with involvement of the gastric remnant in as many as 50% of cases.[56] In order to improve on local control, total gastrectomy was proposed as the treatment of choice for any patient with gastric cancer.[57,58] Routine use of "second-look" laparotomies was advocated to salvage patients with early locoregional recurrence after gastrectomy.[59] Recognition of a frequent pattern of failure involving nodal tissues around the celiac plexus and splenic vessels lent support to the inclusion of splenectomy and nodal dissection at the time of gastric resection.[60] McNeer and colleagues, reviewing their experience at MSKCC, provided an anatomic basis and technical description of an extended gastrectomy with routine lymphadenectomy, splenectomy and distal pancreatectomy in order to improve local control.[61] With the decline of gastric cancer incidence in the U.S., poor overall survival, and the recognition that most patients continue to present

with locally advanced disease, many surgeons here had lost enthusiasm for radical surgical approaches. For these reasons, the next definition of the surgical approach to gastric cancer came from Japan. Adherence to strict surgical principles, meticulous pathologic examination of resected specimens, and a large clinical experience allowed Japanese surgeons to set unsurpassed standards for diagnosis, staging and treatment outcome.[8] This observation has been the primary reason that the discussion over the extent of gastric or lymph node resection has been reignited in the United States and other parts of the Western world.

Extent of gastric resection

An earlier retrospective study from MSKCC showed a significant survival benefit of extended total gastrectomy over proximal subtotal gastrectomy for the treatment of cancer of the cardia.[62] Only patients with stage 1 or 2 disease were among long-term survivors. The operative mortality rate, however, was as high as 15%. There was a high incidence of locoregional recurrences, particularly in the subtotal gastrectomy group. It is possible that these recurrences in part were caused by uncontrolled lymphatic metastatic disease. Review of a larger patient cohort by the same authors found development of an anastomotic recurrence in only 23% of patients with positive margins at resection.[63] No positive margin was found with resection of 12 cm or more of esophagus proximal to the macroscopic tumor. Most patients with positive resection margins and more advanced cancer stages died of systemic disease before ever developing an anastomotic recurrence, supporting the importance to consider underlying cancer biology in the assessment of recurrence risk based on the presence of microscopically tumor-positive margins.

The interpretation of a positive resection margin continues to be debated.[15,64–66] It is clear from most studies that the presence of tumor at the resection margin is an adverse prognostic factor, predicting decreased survival, and decreased disease-free survival. This may be supported by multivariate analysis as independent prognostic factor, or simply as univariate phenomenon (own analysis). It is also clear that not all patients with involved margins develop local recurrence.[63,66] The International Union against Cancer (UICC) R classification attempts to reflect the worse prognosis attached to microscopically (R1) or macroscopically (R2) involved margins. The argument whether a positive margin causes increased recurrence or merely reflects (otherwise unmeasured) disease factors that create a greater likelihood for recurrence has not been solved. It is likely, however, that an R1/2 status may have different implications in early stage gastric cancer than in advanced disease,[62] and may carry different meaning based on the histologic type.[15] In our experience, the likelihood for a "palliative" R1 or R2 resection increases significantly with the underlying disease stage, allowing "curative" R0 resections for the vast majority of patients with stages smaller or equal to 3A (**Figure 4.6**). This has been supported by findings from the German multicenter trial, where extended lymphadenectomy allowed for more R0 resections of tumors with T1–4 and N0–2 classifications.[67] Furthermore, the presence of positive margins in our analysis correlated significantly with diffuse gastric involvement, poorly differentiated histologic grade, and performance of a total gastrectomy.

In an attempt to define a possible survival advantage of total gastrectomy prospectively, two prospective randomized trials have examined the role of gastric resections of lesser extent. A French multicenter trial with 169 patients compared total with subtotal gastrectomies for primary antral adenocarcinoma.[68] Both procedures had a low morbidity and mortality rate, and there was no appreciable 5-year survival difference (**Table 4.3**). The conclusion was that total gastrectomy did not confer a benefit in the treatment of distal gastric cancer. A second study comparing subtotal D1 gastrectomy with total D3 gastrectomy enrolled 55 patients.[69] Although total gastrectomy was performed with minimal mortality, there was significant morbidity from the splenectomy and distal pancreatectomy included in this aggressive

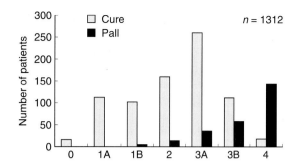

Figure 4.6 Cancer stage in curative versus non-curative resections, gastric adenocarcinoma at MSKCC, 1985–1995. Cure, Curative (R0) resections; Pall, Palliative (R1 or R2) resections.

approach, and survival was significantly better in the group undergoing limited resections without splenectomy or distal pancreatectomy. Based on these experiences and our own analysis, we perform a subtotal gastrectomy for gastric carcinomas of the middle or distal third whenever possible with an approximate 5 cm proximal margin clearance. We attempt to generate negative proximal margins on every patient undergoing curative gastrectomy. However, we do not attempt to generate negative margins with extended resections in the presence of advanced nodal metastasis, since this is not supported by the data presented above.

The approach to proximal stomach lesions has been debated. While some surgeons prefer a thoracoabdominal approach or a two-cavity procedure according to Lewis-Tanner, it appears that for most proximal gastric neoplasms, especially those of intestinal type, a transabdominal approach with transhiatal resection of the distal esophagus is sufficient.[70,70a] For proximal-third gastric cancer, our data show no morbidity or survival benefit of a total gastrectomy compared

Table 4.3 Total versus limited gastrectomy for antral adenocarcinoma

	TOTAL GASTRECTOMY	LIMITED (SUBTOTAL) GASTRECTOMY
Patients (*n*)	93	76
Postoperative mortality rate (%)	1.3	3.2
Postoperative morbidity rate (%)	32	34
5-year survival rate (%)	48	48

Data from a prospective French multicenter study.[68]

with proximal subtotal gastrectomy (**Table 4.4**). The functional side effects of proximal gastrectomy, in particular reflux esophagitis, have not apparently been a major deterrent in our patients. In summary, we prefer a subtotal gastric resection, proximal or distal, over a total gastrectomy, if this does not compromise adequacy of resection of potentially curable gastric carcinomas.

Extent of lymphadenectomy

The extent of lymphadenectomy in "Western" countries is an ongoing debate. Interest in extended lymphadenectomy has increased in European and American centers as a result of the superior outcome seen in Japan in association with a systematic approach to lymph node metastasis.[8,9] Several Western publications, based on retrospective observations, have supported a survival benefit for extended lymphadenectomy.[71–74] It remains unclear, however, if extended lymph node dissection can be carried out in Western patients with acceptable morbidity, and whether the apparent benefits in survival could be primarily based on a stage migration phenomenon. The prospective German gastric carcinoma study, although not based on randomized comparison, found evidence for a survival benefit in patients undergoing D2 lymphadenectomy over D1 dissection.[67] Patients with N0 or N1 classifications appeared to have the greatest benefit. As histologic negative lymph nodes may carry individual tumor cells only identifiable on immunohistochemistry,[75] and as systemic disease frequently accompanies N2 disease, these observations appear appropriate.

Four prospective randomized trials have compared extended with limited lymph node resections. The Cape Town trial compared small numbers of patients (D1: $n = 22$; D2: $n = 21$),

and found an increase in blood transfusion rate and hospital stay in the D2 dissection group.[76] There was no appreciable survival difference at 3 years. It is however likely that the sample size is inadequate to support this notion with the appropriate statistical power. The second study from Hong Kong was discussed earlier.[69] Comparison of D1 subtotal gastrectomy and D3 total gastrectomy showed a significantly increased morbidity in the D3 group, likely due to the effect of splenectomy and pancreatectomy performed. Survival was significantly worse in this group, although postoperative mortality remained low.

Two European prospective multicenter trials have attempted to examine the benefits of D2 lymphadenectomy compared with limited D1 dissection. The Dutch multicenter trial studied 711 patients undergoing curative resections in terms of morbidity and mortality.[77] Although well designed and controlled, a significant number of protocol violations occurred, leading to non-compliance (in 84%) and contamination (in 48%) effects between the two groups to be studied.[78] In addition, the D2 dissection group had a significantly higher number of splenectomies and pancreatectomies performed (**Table 4.5**). There were a higher incidence of postoperative complications, a longer hospital stay, and more fatal complications in the D2 dissection group. A survival benefit has not been found at early follow-up based on the perioperative events.

The Medical Research Council Trial in the United Kingdom compared 200 patients in each lymphadenectomy group,[79] and came to similar conclusions (**Table 4.5**). Patients undergoing D2 dissection had more complications, higher mortality, a somewhat extended hospital stay, but also a greater likelihood of splenectomy or

Table 4.4   Total versus proximal gastrectomy for adenocarcinoma of the proximal stomach

	TOTAL GASTRECTOMY	PROXIMAL (SUBTOTAL) GASTRECTOMY
Patients (*n*)	33	65
Postoperative mortality rate (%)	3	6
Length of stay: median (days)	18	16.5
Length of stay: range (days)	8–48	8–55
5-year survival rate (%)	41	43

Data from Harrison *et al.*[70a]

Table 4.5 Comparison of morbidity and mortality after D1 and D2 lymphadenectomies in two large prospective multicenter trials

	PARAMETER OF ANALYSIS	UNIT	D1	D2	*P*-VALUE
Dutch Multicenter Trial[77]	Patients analyzed (curative resections)	*n*	380	331	
	Postoperative deaths	%	4	10	0.004
	Non-fatal complications	%	25	43	<0.001
	Reoperations	%	8	18	<0.001
	Mean hospital stay (range)	days	18 (7–143)	25 (7–277)	<0.001
	Splenectomy	%	11	38	<0.0001[†]
	Distal pancreatectomy	%	3	30	<0.0001[†]
Medical Research Council Trial[79]	Patients analyzed (curative resections)	*n*	200	200	
	Postoperative deaths	%	6.5	13	0.04
	Non-fatal complications	%	21	33	0.001*
	Median hospital stay (range)	days	14 (6–101)	14 (10–147)	0.01
	Splenectomy	%	31	65.5	<0.0001[†]
	Pancreatosplenectomy	%	4	56.5	<0.0001[†]

*P-value reflects comparison of overall complications, including postoperative deaths.
[†] P-value reflects Fisher's exact test/chi-square re-analysis based on the original data displayed.

pancreatectomy. A comparison of survival between these groups has not been reported.

Our own observations, based on a retrospective analysis of prospectively collected data over 10 years, do not support these findings. In an earlier report from MSKCC, extended lymphadenectomies did not lead to an increase in morbidity, mortality or hospital stay when compared with D1 lymph node resections.[20] The only significant difference occurred in the amount of postoperative drainage, which did not have any significant impact on clinical outcome. Mortality and reoperation rate were lower than in the European trials (**Table 4.6**), and it is our impression that extended lymphadenectomies can be performed without increased mor-

bidity or mortality. For the purpose of accurate staging and for an observed survival benefit in our patient group (see outcome analysis), we are biased towards performing extended (D2) lymphadenectomies in all patients with gastric cancer undergoing potentially curative gastric resections.

Resection of extragastric organs

Resection of other organs in case of direct tumor extension in the absence of systemic spread can lead to long-term control or cure.[80] However, resection of extragastric organs, whether directly involved with tumor or not, is accompanied by a significant increase in morbidity and hospital stay. An earlier analysis from MSKCC examined the role

Table 4.6 Morbidity and mortality associated with lymphadenectomy, gastric adenocarcinoma at MSKCC, 1985–1995

	D1	D1–2	D2	D3	TOTAL
n	80	95	479	37	691
Postoperative deaths: *n* (%)	3 (4)	2 (2)	16 (3)	0	21 (3)
LOS: median (days)	13	15	14	13	14
LOS: range (days)	6–81	9–182	5–88	8–108	5–182
Reoperation: *n* (%)	9 (11)	7 (7)	27 (6)	4 (11)	47 (7)

LOS, length of stay.
The total number of 691 excluded patients for whom the lymphadenectomy extent was not clearly defined. Adapted from Brennan & Karpeh.[17]

of splenectomy at the time of gastrectomy for gastric cancer,[81] and found a significant increase in the overall complication rate when splenectomy was performed, primarily based on an increase in postoperative infections (**Table 4.7**). Others have confirmed these observations.[26,82–84] Distal pancreatectomy is equally correlated with increased morbidity, primarily through pancreatic leaks.[69,77] A splenectomy *per se* is not required to perform an adequate lymphadenectomy,[82] although a splenectomy may be necessary to clear bulky nodal involvement at the splenic artery and hilus (levels 10 and 11). Extended lymphadenectomy should be performed without distal pancreatectomy, unless there is T4 involvement of the pancreas.[85] We make attempts to avoid a splenectomy or pancreatectomy, unless local factors of tumor extension or nodal involvement dictate otherwise. Surgical resection of liver metastases from gastric carcinoma has been shown to be of benefit in some highly selected patients, limited to those with T1/2 disease or late metachronous recurrences.[86] We do not consider that resection of bulky discontiguous disease or peritoneal or hepatic metastases at the time of gastrectomy under curative intent is indicated. In these situations, cancer of the stomach is not considered curable, and a limited gastric resection should be performed if indicated for palliative purposes. More radical procedures that include resection of celiac vascular structures in order to enhance the potential benefit of extended lymphadenectomy[87] have not been widely accepted in the West,

although it appears that they can be performed safely in highly experienced units.

Use of laparoscopy

Laparoscopic staging as an extent of the preoperative staging work-up has recently become commonplace as part of the surgical management of gastric cancer.[52,65,88–90] In the series quoted, laparoscopy at the beginning of an operation for gastric cancer was able to prevent a subsequent laparotomy based on identification of contraindications for resection in 23% to 42%. It has become our routine practice to start every operative exploration in patients qualifying for potentially curative procedures with laparoscopy. Examination of peritoneal surfaces, parenchymal organs, and D3 lymph node stations is performed to identify presence of metastases that would preclude a resection with curative potential. Cytology samples from peritoneal washings are obtained, and suspicious areas are biopsied. If advanced disease precludes a curative procedure, and the patient has no indication for palliative resection, we treat the patient with experimental preoperative chemotherapy.[50] Patients not undergoing resections based on laparoscopic findings had a significantly decreased hospital stay compared with those undergoing laparotomy without gastrectomy (**Table 4.8**).[91] This is expected to result in significant cost savings.

Laparoscopic ultrasound has been suggested as an additional option for operative staging, and was shown to be useful in a subset of patients with proximal gastric cancer.[92] Should the patient have

Table 4.7 Complications associated with splenectomy in the operative treatment of gastric cancer, curative resections at MSKCC, 1960–1984[81]

	SPLENECTOMY	NO SPLENECTOMY
NO. OF PATIENTS	163	229
Pneumonia (%)	14.1	5.7
Intra-abdominal abscess (%)	8.6	1.3
Wound infection (%)	6.7	2.2
Fistula (%)	6.1	5.2
Cardiac complications (%)	1.2	3.5
Bleeding (%)	1.2	1.3
Thromboembolism (%)	2.5	0
Fever of unknown origin (%)	1.8	0
Complications: total (%)	45	21

The numbers reflect percentages of afflicted patients within each treatment group.

Table 4.8 Laparoscopy compared with exploratory laparotomy in patients not undergoing gastric resection

	LAPAROSCOPY	LAPAROSCOPY / LAPAROTOMY	LAPAROTOMY
Patients (*n*)	24	4	60
Mean age (years)	58	75	60
Mean length of stay (days)	1.4	6.5	6.8
Postoperative complications (%)	4	0	13.3
Mean operative time (min)	74	138	83

Data from MSKCC.[91]

had a preoperative endoscopic ultrasound with unequivocal T1 or T2 readings, we do not advocate laparoscopic ultrasound. With less clear preoperative findings or a larger primary tumor classification on EUS, we have made attempts to identify or confirm the presence of T3 or T4 lesions with laparoscopic ultrasound.[52] Our initial experience suggests that laparoscopic ultrasonography is useful for intraoperative confirmation of T3/4 primary lesions of the stomach.

Although the laparoscopic approach to gastrectomy for cancer treatment has been described and applied,[93] we do not see an obvious advantage to this strategy, and fear compromise in an area where extended local resections may yield a therapeutic benefit. Our use of laparoscopy in gastric cancer has been diagnostic.

Implications of perioperative transfusions

The effect of blood transfusions on the long-term outcome of surgical treatment of gastric cancer is controversial. Several reports suggest that use of blood transfusions during gastrectomy has an adverse effect on survival, but that this effect may not be an independent mechanism, since subgroup comparison of stage-matched patients with and without transfusions appear to have similar outcomes.[94,95] In both studies, need for blood transfusions was greater with larger tumor size and a more advanced stage. Others have found that extended lymphadenectomy causes higher transfusion requirements,[69,76] but in one retrospective series this phenomenon did not negatively impact on survival.[72] An earlier analysis from our institution reviewed 232 patients undergoing curative gastrectomy for gastric cancer between 1985 and

1992.[96] As many as 58% of patients received perioperative blood transfusions, the need for which correlated with cancer stage, T classification, and the extent of gastrectomy. Need for transfusion was an independent prognostic factor influencing long-term survival. Whether this finding was reflective of a direct deleterious effect of the transfused blood, or a measure of other associated mechanisms (e.g., associated complications, splenectomy, etc.) remains unclear. We attempt to avoid the use of blood transfusions in the operative treatment of gastric cancer whenever the patients general condition permits, and encourage the use of autologous blood donation in cases of anticipated large blood loss.

Implications of positive peritoneal cytology

Positive cytologic examination of washings obtained from the peritoneal cavity before gastrectomy have shown some correlation to tumor thickness (positive in 12% of T3/4 lesions) and nodal metastases (positive in 7.5% of N+ cancers) in a large prospective trial.[97] Survival of patients with positive cytology was significantly lower, irrespective of whether a curative or palliative resection had been performed. The pattern of recurrence in patients with positive cytology, however, may not necessarily be intraperitoneal, as many patients develop visceral metastases or local recurrence.[98] This may be an important factor for the design of adjuvant treatment strategies favoring systemic rather than intraperitoneal chemotherapy.[99] In addition, many patients with subsequent peritoneal carcinomatosis did not have a positive cytology at the time of their operation.[98] Attempts to enhance the predictive value of peritoneal washings by measuring carcinoembryonic antigen (CEA) levels in the peritoneal fluid have not found wide acceptance.[100] We are currently evaluating the predictive role of information obtained from peritoneal cytology, and it appears that the incidence of positive cytology in patients with M0 disease is low. Patients with T1/2 M0 disease had no positive peritoneal cytology, patients with T3/4 M0 disease had a 10% incidence of positive cytology, and patients with M1 disease had a 50% rate of positive cytology.[91] Nevertheless, all patients with peritoneal washings positive for gastric carcinoma and T3/4 M0 disease have experienced early postoperative peritoneal recurrences and have died of their disease. Until more complete information is obtained from this analysis, our selection of high-risk patients for the purpose of additional systemic and/or intraperitoneal treatment remains based on the ultrasonographic T classification during EUS or laparoscopy.

Postgastrectomy reconstruction

Various methods of reconstruction after gastrectomy have been described and have been reviewed elsewhere.[101] These include Roux-en-Y esophago-jejunostomy, jejunal interposition, Braun esophagojejunostomy with enteroenterostomy, and various pouch reconstructions. The main area of concern after gastrectomy includes rapid intestinal transit time, malabsorption (especially fat absorption), dumping, afferent or efferent limb syndrome, and possibly Roux stasis. Comparisons between patients undergoing distal gastrectomy (Billroth I) and those undergoing total gastrectomy with pouch reconstruction have failed to show a significant nutritional difference in these groups.[102–104] When Billroth I procedures were compared with Billroth II reconstructions after distal gastrectomy for adenocarcinoma of the antrum, digestive parameters and survival were not different, although fistula formation and local recurrence were observed more frequently in the Billroth 1 group.[105] The preservation of duodenal passage at the time of pouch reconstruction has not been superior to Roux-en-Y reconstructions with pouch in two studies,[106,107] but was considered superior in another.[108] Answers to the fundamental question whether a pouch should be used for postgastrectomy reconstruction at all have been attempted. The strongest evidence in favor of a pouch comes from two randomized studies, in which the Hunt–

Lawrence pouch and Roux-en-Y esophagojejunostomy were components.[102,107] Decreased incidence of dumping and pyrosis, slowed emptying time, and some improved nutritional parameters were considered to render the pouch reconstruction superior to a plain Roux-en-Y technique. In contradistinction, the use of a pouch failed to improve nutritional adaptation in other trials.[103,109] In our own experience, the benefits of a pouch have not been considered significant enough to warrant their routine use.

Palliative resections

Despite the common advanced stage presentation of patients with gastric cancer in Europe or the U.S.,[26,110] little has been published on the technical aspects and clinical outcome of palliative resections. While UICC R1 and R2 resections are considered "palliative," since they lead to a high failure rate, up to 13% of these may have been performed with the intent to cure the patient.[64] Indications for procedures with truly palliative intent are primarily obstruction and bleeding, less frequently perforation. Operations of this category have a high complication rate, especially when performed under emergent conditions.[111] When the indication for a palliative operation is given, gastrectomy appears to be linked to a better outcome than simple bypass procedures.[112,113] We do not advocate an extended lymphadenectomy at the time of palliative resection, although this issue has been debated recently.[114] Palliative resection in the presence of liver metastases is rarely effective and should be offered only to highly selected patients.[115] For unresectable, symptomatic tumors at the gastroesophageal junction, a side-to-side gastroesophagostomy using a mobilized fundus may be useful,[116] but is technically difficult, and therefore rarely performed. An alternative method of palliation for this lesion may exist through the use of endoscopic YAG laser application or a wall stent placement.[117] The ability of chemoradiation therapy to relieve obstruction in these patients obviates the need for most such procedures.

Perioperative nutrition

Many patients with gastric cancer have experienced some mild to moderate weight loss before operative treatment is performed. Attempts nutritionally to replete these patients with parenteral hyperalimentation have not been very successful.

In a prospective multicenter trial, Buzby et al.[118] have demonstrated that only patients with severe nutritional deficits benefit from preoperative repletion with parenteral nutrition, and that this method correlates with a higher rate of infectious complications. Our own experience with perioperative parenteral nutrition in patients with pancreatic cancer has also shown no significant advantage.[119] A recent prospective study evaluated the role for postoperative enteral nutrition in patients with upper gastrointestinal cancer, and found a significant benefit to this method compared with patients taking an oral diet only.[120] Improved nutritional parameters, postoperative complications, re-hospitalization rate, and completion rate of adjuvant treatment were seen after enteral feeding. In a comparable prospective trial of postoperative enteral nutrition in patients with upper gastrointestinal cancer at MSKCC, we were unable to demonstrate a significant benefit of this technique over no postoperative feeding.[121] The complication rate between the two study groups were not different, due to low overall complications and a few complications related to the feeding tube placement itself. Consequently, we do not advocate routine early postoperative enteral or parenteral feeding in patients after gastrectomy. Placement of a feeding tube at the time of gastric resection is only performed, if a prolonged postoperative intestinal dysmotility can be anticipated.

Prolonged postoperative paralytic ileus and intestinal dysmotility are common after upper gastrointestinal surgical procedures.[122] Although intravenous erythromycin has been shown to improve postoperative gastric emptying after esophagogastrectomy,[123] and may also be of benefit after limited gastrectomy for gastric cancer, we have not applied motility-enhancing agents routinely after gastrectomy for lack of evidence that they improve postoperative recovery.

SURGICAL TREATMENT OUTCOME ANALYSIS

Survival

Survival is the ultimate outcome measure after operative treatment for gastric cancer; treatment administered with curative intent should significantly prolong survival from the time of diagnosis. The main predictor of survival after resections of

gastric cancer is the stage of the disease.[23,25] Stage by stage, survival from gastric cancer appears to be worse in Western countries compared with Japan (**Table 4.1**), although in specialized centers within the Western world this stage-specific survival appears to approach Japanese results. The result for this phenomenon may partly reside in a more compatible approach to staging based on extended lymphadenectomy.

Our results in terms of survival after resection of primary gastric cancer with curative intent based on stage group are displayed in **Figure 4.7**. The median survival of all patients undergoing resection for primary gastric cancer at MSKCC between 1985 and 1995 was 23.6 months (range 0.2 to 148 months). Survival based on univariate comparison of T classification or N status is displayed in **Figures 4.8** and **4.9**. Factors that influence survival independently have been analyzed in a Cox multiple regression model (**Table 4.9**). They include T classification, N classification, presence of complications, histologic grade, and performance of an extended lymphadenectomy. Other patient-, disease-, or treatment-related factors that showed a significant influence on survival on univariate analysis, but failed to qualify as independent prognostic variables on multivariate analysis, are displayed in the same table. The results are only valid for patients undergoing resection of a primary adenocarcinoma of the stomach with curative intent,

Table 4.9 Results of a multivariate analysis for survival, gastric adenocarcinoma at MSKCC (1985–1995)

COVARIATE FACTOR	P-VALUE
T classification	<0.0001
N classification	<0.0001
Presence of complications	0.0001
Histologic grade	0.016
Lymphadenectomy: D2 or greater	0.019
M classification	NS
Gender	NS
Location of primary tumor	NS
Amount of tumor left (R status)	NS
Resection of other organs	NS
Margin status	NS

NS, not significant ($P > 0.05$).
Only covariates that had shown a statistically significant effect on overall and disease-specific survival in a univariate analysis were entered into this proportional hazards model.

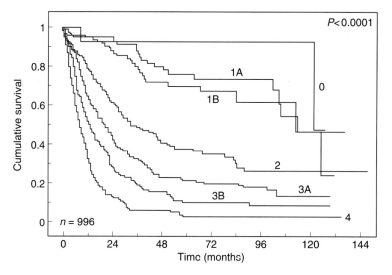

Figure 4.7 Survival by pathologic stage, resections for primary gastric adenocarcinoma at MSKCC, 1985–1995.

hence the lack of multivariate significance for the M classification. The impact of complications on survival is discussed in one of the following sections within this chapter.

Recurrences and disease-free survival

Detection of gastric cancer recurrences depends on many factors, including onset of symptoms, clinical follow-up schedules, the use of tumor markers, or routine imaging. Since most local recurrences are harbingers of impending systemic failure, and since no effective systemic treatment for metastatic gastric cancer is available at the current time, most recurrences are not effectively approachable with operative or non-operative treatment. For these reasons, we have not made efforts to measure disease-free survival in our patients with gastric

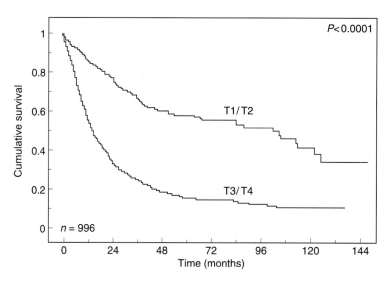

Figure 4.8 Survival by T classification, resections for primary gastric adenocarcinoma at MSKCC, 1985–1995.

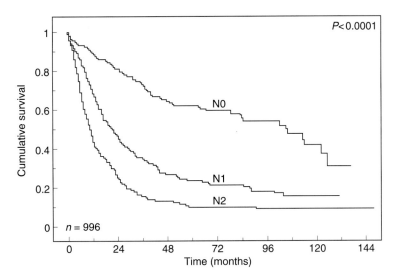

Figure 4.9 Survival by N classification, resections for primary gastric adenocarcinoma at MSKCC, 1985–1995.

cancer. Data on gastric cancer recurrence from the American College of Surgeons survey are shown in **Figure 4.10**.[6] For all different locations of the primary tumors within the stomach, systemic recurrences limit disease-free survival in over 50%. Local recurrences appear to be more common for lesions within the upper third of the stomach, and regional recurrence rates are highest for distal gastric cancers. The problem of local recurrence has been addressed with various additional treatment modalities, designed to improve locoregional control at the time of primary treatment. These include intra-

operative radiation therapy to high-risk sites and intraperitoneal perfusion with cytotoxic agents.[124] While the incidence of local recurrences appears to benefit from these modalities, an obvious survival advantage rarely exists, leading to the conclusion that more aggressive locoregional treatment approaches may just affect the pattern of disease failure, but rarely overall survival. In selected patients, particularly those with symptomatic, isolated recurrences, an aggressive operative approach can be justified.[125] Based on these retrospective data, the 2-year survival after combination treatment of recurrent gastric cancer with reresection and chemotherapy can be as high as 66%, although this is at least in part expected to be a function of patient selection as well. We currently employ phase I/II investigational regimens, the FAMTX regimen, or symptomatic care in such patients.

Complications and hospital stay

Length of hospital stay has become an important outcome measure for any operative treatment. Since the duration of hospitalization is the major factor contributing to the overall treatment costs, analyzing factors that influence the length of stay has an important economic impact. We have shown in an analysis of elderly patients with gastric cancer that the most significant predictor of

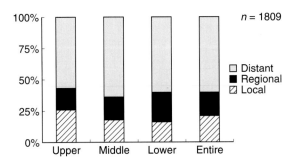

Figure 4.10 Type of first recurrence of gastric cancer after operative therapy, by location of the primary stomach lesion (American College of Surgeons, data from 1982 to 1987).[6] *Reproduced with permission from Reference 6.*

increased hospital stay is the presence of any complication.[126] Patients with infectious complications had a longer hospital stay than those with non-infectious complications. In elderly patients, stage of disease and extent of the surgical procedure were other prognostic variables. Results of an analysis of hospital stay data for patients of all age groups undergoing resections of primary gastric cancers at MSKCC between 1985 and 1995 are displayed in **Figure 4.11**. The median hospital stay after gastric resection was 15 days (range 5 to 182 days). Results of a multivariate analysis of all covariates that had shown significant effects on univariate testing are listed in **Table 4.10**. Besides complications, only increased age and higher T classification were predictive of increased length of stay. The performance of procedures commonly associated with development of postoperative complications, e.g., splenectomy or pancreatectomy, had no independent impact on length of admission in this analysis. This can in part be explained by the relatively low rate of splenectomies or pancreatectomies, since only 14.4% of our patients undergoing gastrectomy for primary gastric cancer underwent splenectomy or partial pancreatectomy at the same time. The hospital stay of patients not undergoing gastrectomy depended strongly on the mode of abdominal exploration (**Figure 4.8**). Those patients undergoing laparoscopy only had a mean hospital stay

Table 4.10 Results of a multivariate analysis for length of hospital stay, gastric adenocarcinoma at MSKCC (1985–1995)

COVARIATE FACTOR	P-VALUE
Presence of any complication	<0.0001
Age	0.015
T classification	0.023
Pancreatectomy	NS
Splenectomy	NS
Resection of other extragastric organs	NS
Type of gastrectomy	NS
Primary tumor site	NS

NS, not significant ($P > 0.05$).
Only covariates that had shown a statistically significant effect on length of hospital stay in a univariate analysis were entered into this proportional hazards model.

of 1.4 days, those undergoing laparotomy had an average stay of 6.8 days.[91] This difference in outcome for unresected patients provides the main rationale to employ laparoscopy as the initial step of operative evaluation in every patient who is to undergo potentially curative gastrectomy.

Association of disease- or treatment-related factors with the occurrence of complications was analyzed for those patients undergoing gastrectomy with curative intent at MSKCC. Factors positively correlated with postoperative complications included resection of additional organs including

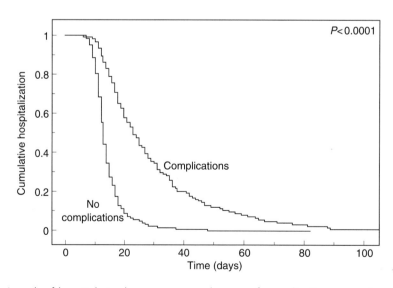

Figure 4.11 Length of hospital stay by presence or absence of complications, resections for primary gastric adenocarcinoma at MSKCC, 1985–1995.

splenectomy or pancreatectomy, primary tumors at the gastroesophageal junction, proximal gastrectomy, stage 3A (but not stage 4) disease, age, and the use of parenteral nutrition. No significant correlation with complications was seen for extended lymphadenectomies. No measurable patient-related parameter except age showed any correlation to complications.

Our postoperative mortality rate was 4.2%. In contradistinction to the findings of a German multicenter analysis on in-hospital mortality,[127] postoperative lethal events in our series were associated with the occurrence of complications and with advanced age, but not with tumor stage, tumor location, or type of gastrectomy. The extent of lymphadenectomy was not a predictor of postoperative death, unlike in the prospective trials of extended versus limited lymphadenectomy.[77,79] Palliative procedures did not have a higher rate of subsequent lethal complications. There was no statistically significant difference in the mortality rate between patients with infectious and non-infectious complications, although the latter group had a slightly higher occurrence (14.5 versus 11.1%).

The overall complication rate in our series was 34%. While this may appear high, it reflects prospective data collection and accurate recording of 30-day overall or longer than 30-day in-hospital postsurgical morbidity and mortality events. In addition, 72% of patients did undergo a D2 or more extensive lymphadenectomy. Complication rates in the two recent multicenter prospective trials randomizing patients to limited versus extended lymphadenectomy were 32.6%[77] and 36.8%,[79] with postoperative mortality figures of 6.6% and 9.8%, respectively. These numbers give some representation of outcome results for morbidity and mortality in Western tertiary care centers with a programmatic approach to the operative treatment of gastric cancer, using prospective data recording.

Quality of life assessment

The analysis of quality of life after operative treatment of gastric cancer is a complex task. Categories influencing quality of life can be highly subjective and difficult to measure. Yet, assessing the activity level, general health, self-image, and dependency on support structures besides survival after gastrectomy is a worthwhile effort to evaluate treatment outcome. Attempts have been made to compare several methods for quality of life analysis after operative treatment of gastric cancer, and the most useful test appears to be the Spitzer index.[128,129] Although most of the quality of life studies have focused on outcome after different type of gastric reconstructions,[102,104] it is apparent that patients with gastric cancer may have special limitations in quality of life or support structures even before any treatment.[130] In this respect, elderly patients with gastric cancer represent a patient subset with increased needs for supportive care and special challenges to the treating surgeon. Poor overall condition limits treatment options in elderly patients more than in younger patients.[110] Although the relative survival after gastrectomy is similar between all age groups,[131] complication rate, postoperative mortality, and length of hospital stay are all increased in elderly patients.[126] This frequently leads to the need for more intensive outpatient support, more frequent readmissions, increased treatment costs, and the resulting limitation in quality of life for elderly patients after surgical treatment of gastric cancer.

SPECIAL CONSIDERATIONS RELEVANT TO THE SURGICAL MANAGEMENT OF GASTRIC CANCER

Adjuvant approaches affecting surgical treatment

Postoperative adjuvant therapy approaches to gastric cancer have been studied extensively, but to date, for the most part, have failed to demonstrate a convincing survival benefit.[132] Among the few exceptions to this general observation is a recent randomized multicenter study from Italy, which demonstrated an increased survival after postoperative triple chemotherapy in patients with nodal-positive gastric carcinoma.[133] Given the general lack of evidence of a survival benefit after postoperative chemotherapy, a rationale for preoperative chemotherapy has been formulated.[134] So far, there is no convincing evidence suggesting a significant benefit to this approach.[135] We nevertheless have attempted to identify patients with T3/4, N3, or M1 disease limited to the peritoneum, based on EUS and/or laparoscopy, for enrollment in trials of preoperative systemic treatment. In these cases, the gastrectomy was deferred, the patient then re-evaluated after chemotherapy administration, and a gastrectomy with curative intent performed in those patients who showed evidence for treatment response and were considered to have potentially curable disease at re-evaluation. In our experience with patients undergoing gastrectomy, preoperative chemotherapy was not an independent prognostic factor associated with increased complications, longer hospital stay, or altered postoperative outcome. Therefore, preoperative systemic treatment does not seem to have an obvious detrimental effect on conduct or outcome of gastric cancer resections.

Intraperitoneal adjuvant chemotherapy has been studied in patients with tumors at high risk for peritoneal failure, e.g., T3/4 lesions or advanced lymph node metastasis. Preoperative intraperitoneal chemotherapy has shown significant early and delayed local complications, mainly related to the formation of adhesions.[136] Postoperative intraperitoneal treatment has been studied more extensively,[99,124,137] but without convincing beneficial effect on survival. In our own experience, intraperitoneal chemotherapy was administered through a port system placed at the time of gastrectomy.[50] There were very few device-related complications, and intraperitoneal treatment was generally well tolerated. The commencement of intraperitoneal treatment within five days from the operation was noted to allow for a better peritoneal distribution. Initial limitations due to peritoneal fibrosis were successfully addressed by lowering the pH of the perfusate. At a median follow-up of 29 months, the peritoneal failure rate was only 16%.

The initial Japanese experience with intraoperative hyperthermic chemotherapy perfusion for selected patients with gastric cancer and high potential for peritoneal failure or established peritoneal metastasis has shown acceptable toxicity and a relatively good outcome with low intraperitoneal recurrence rates.[138–140] Since the complexity of technical set-up and the potential for enhanced toxicity are major limitations, more evidence is required before this approach can be widely accepted.

The impact of postoperative radiation therapy as part of adjuvant multimodality treatment for gastric cancer is equally poorly defined.[141] Intraoperative radiation (IORT) to the area of gastrectomy dissection has been linked to an improved local control rate compared with postoperative external beam radiation therapy in a prospective trial at the National Cancer Institute.[142] There was no obvious benefit, however, to overall survival. A tendency towards survival benefit to IORT compared with resection alone has been seen for patients with stage 2 through 4 gastric cancer in a large Japanese series.[143] This benefit was most evident in patients with N2–3 classifications or serosal involvement by the primary tumor. We have no extensive experience in the use of IORT for gastric cancer at our institution, and do not apply this method routinely. A detailed discussion of adjuvant treatment options for adenocarcinoma of the stomach and the current clinical results is provided by Kelsen in Chapter 6.

The problem of gastric remnant cancer

The possibility of gastric cancer to occur after prior partial gastrectomy for non-malignant diseases of the stomach or duodenum had been described as early as 1922.[144] Although the exact etiologic mechanism remains unclear, two meta-analyses support the notion that there is an increased risk for the development of gastric cancer after prior subtotal gastrectomy.[145,146] Cancer of the gastric remnant appears to present with a higher rate of lymphatic and hematogenous metastases, but fewer instances of peritoneal serosal involvement.[147,148] The rationale to detect these lesions early to facilitate curative treatment is clear.[149] So far, however, specific attempts to perform endoscopic surveillance and screening for patients at risk for the development of gastric remnant cancer have not convincingly shown any clinical benefit.[150] The treatment should consist of reresection or completion gastrectomy for disease limited to the stomach whenever possible, regardless of the underlying disease that led to the prior gastrectomy.[151] A benefit to extended lymphadenectomy for gastric stump carcinoma appears to be limited to T2 lesions or smaller.[148]

Postoperative follow-up

A generally accepted schedule for postoperative follow-up after curative gastrectomy for gastric cancer does not exist. The goal of regular follow-up is identification of clinically silent recurrent or *de novo* disease that is treatable and can lead to a survival benefit. Failure patterns after operative treatment of gastric cancer in the United States indicate the presence of hematogenous metastatic disease in the majority of patients (**Figure 4.10**).[6] Since this problem cannot be considered curable, the focus of follow-up efforts should lie on the identification of local or regional recurrences, as well as secondary cancers. Since locoregional recurrence in the absence of systemic disease is more likely to occur after gastrectomy for early stage disease, and since long-term survival in this patient group can be as high as 60–85% (**Table 4.1**), the patient group that would likely benefit from regular postoperative screening tests is expected to be quite small. Furthermore, the benefit of detecting clinically asymptomatic versus symptomatic recurrences remains unclear. In a recent review, the combination of radiologic imaging and CEA serum tests for gastric cancer follow-up yielded a lead time of at least 2 months prior to symptomatic presentation in only 33% of patients developing a recurrence.[152] Only 17% of patients with recurrence were able to undergo further treatment, and no benefit in survival was detected. The high costs of routine follow-up testing, an increased economic awareness, and the lack of clear clinical advantage prevent us from recommending a tightly regimented follow-up scheme after curative resections for gastric cancer. Regular clinical evaluations, with radiographic imaging or endoscopic examinations directed by clinical symptoms, appear to be most useful and cost-effective. Patients' anxiety over indeterminate test results is avoided. We see no benefit to the routine evaluation of any tumor marker for gastric cancer. Detection of isolated recurrences, including metachronous liver metastases, has been approached with resection attempts.[86,125] Non-isolated recurrences may be effectively treated with systemic chemotherapy, even if not symptomatic. This has been shown to be survival-enhancing and cost-effective.[153] It is hoped that the development of specific markers will allow for a concentration of follow-up efforts in patients who are at high risk for local recurrence, but have a higher likelihood for successful salvage treatment.

REFERENCES

1. Parker SL, Tong T, Bolden S & Wingo PA. Cancer statistics, 1996 (see comments). *Cancer J Clin* 1996; **46**: 5–27.

2. Parker SL, Tong T, Bolden S & Wingo PA. Cancer statistics, 1997. *Cancer J Clin* 1997; **47**: 5–27.

3. Salvon-Harman JC, Cady B, Nikulasson S et al. Shifting proportions of gastric adenocarcinomas. *Arch Surg* 1994; **129**: 381–8.

4. Parkin DM, Muir CS, Whelan SL et al. *Cancer Incidence in Five Continents*. International Agency for Research on Cancer, Lyon, 1992.

5. Sankaranarayanan R, Swaminathan R & Black RJ. Global variations in cancer survival. Study group on cancer survival in developing countries. *Cancer* 1996; **78**: 2461–4.

6. Wanebo HJ, Kennedy BJ, Chmiel J et al. Cancer of the stomach. A patient care study by the American College of Surgeons. *Ann Surg* 1993; **218**: 583–92.

7. Lawrence W, Jr., Menck HR, Steele G, Jr. & Winchester DP. The National Cancer Data Base report on gastric cancer. *Cancer* 1995; **75**: 1734–44.

8. Maruyama K, Okabayashi K & Kinoshita T. Progress in gastric cancer surgery in Japan and its limits of radicality. *World J Surg* 1987; **11**: 418–25.

9. Noguchi Y, Imada T, Matsumoto A et al. Radical surgery for gastric cancer. A review of the Japanese experience. *Cancer* 1989; **64**: 2053–62.

10. Brennan MF. Radical surgery for gastric cancer. A review of the Japanese experience (editorial). *Cancer* 1989; **64**: 2063.

11. Fielding JW. Gastric cancer: different diseases. *Br J Surg* 1989; **76**: 1227.

12. Kampschoer GH, Nakajima T & van de Velde CJ. Changing patterns in gastric adenocarcinoma. *Br J Surg* 1989; **76**: 914–16.

13. Fortner JG, Lauwers GY, Thaler HT et al. Nativity, complications, and pathology are determinants of surgical results for gastric cancer. *Cancer* 1994; **73**: 8–14.

14. Hundahl SA, Stemmermann GN & Oishi A. Racial factors cannot explain superior Japanese outcomes in stomach cancer. *Arch Surg* 1996; **131**: 170–5.

15. Hermanek P. Prognostic factors in stomach cancer surgery. *Eur J Surg Oncol* 1986; **12**: 241–6.

16. Bollschweiler E, Boettcher K, Hoelscher AH et al. Is the prognosis for Japanese and German patients with gastric cancer really different? *Cancer* 1993; **71**: 2918–25.

17. Brennan MF & Karpeh M, Jr. Surgery for gastric cancer: the American view. *Semin Oncol* 1996; **23**: 352–9.

18. Nishi M, Omori Y & Miwa K. *Japanese Research Society for Gastric Cancer: Japanese Classification of Gastric Carcinoma.* Tokyo, Kanehara & Co, Ltd, 1995.

19. Okamura T, Tsujitani S, Korenaga D *et al.* Lymphadenectomy for cure in patients with early gastric cancer and lymph node metastasis. *Am J Surg* 1988; **155**: 476–80.

20. Smith JW, Shiu MH, Kelsey L & Brennan MF. Morbidity of radical lymphadenectomy in the curative resection of gastric carcinoma. *Arch Surg* 1991; **126**: 1469–73.

21. Lawrence W, Jr. & Horsley Jr. "Extended" lymph node dissections for gastric cancer – is more better? (editorial). *J Surg Oncol* 1996; **61**: 85–9.

22. Lauren P. The two histological main types of gastric carcinoma: diffuse and so-called intestinal-type carcinoma: an attempt at a histoclinical classification. *Acta Pathol Microbiol Scand* 1965; **64**: 31–49.

23. Maruyama K. The most important prognostic factors for gastric cancer patients. *Scand J Gastroenterol* 1987; **22**(suppl. 133): 63–8.

24. Neugut AI, Hayek M & Howe G. Epidemiology of gastric cancer. *Semin Oncol* 1996; **23**: 281–91.

25. Roder JD, Bonenkamp JJ, Craven J *et al.* Lymphadenectomy for gastric cancer in clinical trials: update. *World J Surg* 1995; **19**: 546–53.

26. Crookes PF, Incarbone R, Peters JH *et al.* A selective therapeutic approach to gastric cancer in a large public hospital. *Am J Surg* 1995; **170**: 602–5.

27. Nanus DM, Kelsen DP, Niedzwiecki D *et al.* Flow cytometry as a predictive indicator in patients with operable gastric cancer. *J Clin Oncol* 1989; **7**: 1105-12.

28. Sakusabe M, Kodama M, Sato Y *et al.* Clinical significance of DNA ploidy pattern in stage III gastric cancer. *World J Surg* 1996; **20**: 27–31.

29. Maehara Y, Watanabe A, Kakeji Y *et al.* Prognosis for surgically treated gastric cancer patients is poorer for women than men in all patients under age 50. *Br J Cancer* 1992; **65**: 417–20.

30. Mayer B, Jauch KW, Gunthert U *et al.* De-novo expression of CD44 and survival in gastric cancer. *Lancet* 1993; **342**: 1019–22.

31. Martin HM, Filipe MI, Morris RW *et al.* p53 expression and prognosis in gastric carcinoma. *Int J Cancer* 1992; **50**: 859–62.

32. Joypaul BV, Hopwood D, Newman EL *et al.* The prognostic significance of the accumulation of p53 tumour-suppressor gene protein in gastric adenocarcinoma. *Br J Cancer* 1994; **69**: 943–6.

33. Victorzon M, Nordling S, Haglund C *et al.* Expression of p53 protein as a prognostic factor in patients with gastric cancer. *Eur J Cancer* 1996; **2**: 215–20.

34. Oda N, Tsujino T, Tsuda T *et al.* DNA ploidy pattern and amplification of ERBB and ERBB2 genes in human gastric carcinomas. *Virchows Arch B [Cell Pathol Incl Mol Pathol]* 1990; **58**: 273–7.

35. Lee HR, Kim JH, Uhm HD *et al.* Overexpression of c-ErbB-2 protein in gastric cancer by immunohistochemical stain. *Oncology* 1996; **53**: 192–7.

36. Motojima K, Furui J, Kohara N *et al.* Expression of Kirsten-ras p21 in gastric cancer correlates with tumor progression and is prognostic. *Diagn Mol Pathol* 1994; **3**: 184–91.

37. Yonemura Y, Ninomiya I, Kaji M *et al.* Decreased E-cadherin expression correlates with poor survival in patients with gastric cancer. *Anal Cell Pathol* 1995; **8**: 177–90.

38. Nakano H, Namatame K, Suzuki T *et al.* Prognostic evaluation of curatively resected locally advanced gastric cancer patients with preoperative downstaging chemotherapy assessed by histochemical and pharmacologic means. *Oncology* 1995; **52**: 474–82.

39. Victorzon M, Nordling S, Nilsson O *et al.* Sialyl Tn antigen is an independent predictor of outcome in patients with gastric cancer. *Int J Cancer* 1996; **65**: 295–300.

39a. Maehara Y, Sakaguchi Y, Moriguchi S *et al.* Signet ring cell carcinoma of the stomach. *Cancer* 1992; **69**: 1645–50.

40. Tsujitani S, Kakeji Y, Maehara Y *et al.* Dendritic cells prevent lymph node metastasis in patients with gastric cancer. *In Vivo* 1993; **7**: 233–7.

41. Maeda K, Chung YS, Ogawa Y *et al.* Prognostic value of vascular endothelial growth factor expression in gastric carcinoma. *Cancer* 1996; **77**: 858–63.

42. Maehara Y, Yamamoto M, Oda S *et al.* Cytokeratin-positive cells in bone marrow for identifying distant micrometastasis of gastric cancer. *Br J Cancer* 1996; **73**: 83–7.

43. Forman D. *Helicobacter pylori* and gastric cancer. *Scand J Gastroenterol Suppl* 1996; **215**: 48–51.

44. Lee WJ, Lin JT, Shun CT *et al.* Comparison between resectable gastric adenocarcinomas seropositive and seronegative for *Helicobacter pylori*. *Br J Surg* 1995; **82**: 802–5.

45. Minami M, Kawauchi N, Itai Y *et al.* Gastric tumors: radiologic-pathologic correlation and

accuracy of T staging with dynamic CT. *Radiology* 1992; **185**: 173–8.

46. Halvorsen R, Jr., Yee J & McCormick VD. Diagnosis and staging of gastric cancer. *Semin Oncol* 1996; **23**: 325–35.

47. Matsushita M, Oi H, Murakami T *et al.* Extraserosal invasion in advanced gastric cancer: evaluation with MR imaging. *Radiology* 1994; **192**: 87–91.

48. Botet JF, Lightdale CJ, Zauber AG *et al.* Preoperative staging of gastric cancer: comparison of endoscopic US and dynamic CT [see comments]. *Radiology* 1991; **181**: 426–32.

49. Smith JW, Brennan MF, Botet JF *et al.* Preoperative endoscopic ultrasound can predict the risk of recurrence after operation for gastric carcinoma. *J Clin Oncol* 1993; **11**: 2380–5.

50. Kelsen D, Karpeh M, Schwartz G *et al.* Neoadjuvant therapy of high-risk gastric cancer: a phase II trial of preoperative FAMTX and postoperative intraperitoneal fluorouracil-cisplatin plus intravenous fluorouracil. *J Clin Oncol* 1996; **14**: 1818–28.

51. Bartlett DL, Conlon KC, Gerdes H & Karpeh M, Jr. Laparoscopic ultrasonography: the best pretreatment staging modality in gastric adenocarcinoma? Case report. *Surgery* 1995; **118**: 562–6.

52. Conlon KC & Karpeh M, Jr. Laparoscopy and laparoscopic ultrasound in the staging of gastric cancer. *Semin Oncol* 1996; **23**: 347–51.

53. Billroth T. Über einen neuen Fall von gelungener Resektion des carcinomatösen Pylorus. *Wien Med Wochenschr* 1881; **31**: 1427–30.

54. Schlatter C. Further observations on a case of total extirpation of the stomach in the human subject. *Lancet* 1898; **2**: 1314.

55. Orr TG. A modified technique for total gastrectomy. *Arch Surg* 1947; **54**: 279–83.

56. McNeer G, Vandenberg H & Donn F. A critical evaluation of subtotal gastrectomy for cure of cancer of the stomach. *Ann Surg* 1951; **134**: 2–7.

57. Longmire WP. Total gastrectomy for carcinoma of the stomach. *Surg Gynecol Obstet* 1947; **84**: 21–5.

58. Lahey FH. Total gastrectomy for all patients with operable gastric cancer of the stomach. *Surg Gynecol Obstet* 1950; **90**: 246–9.

59. Wangensteen OH, Lewis FJ & Arhelger SW. An interim report upon the second-look procedure for cancer of the stomach, colon and rectum and for limited intraperitoneal carcinomatosis. *Surg Gynecol Obstetr* 1954; **99**: 257–67.

60. Arhelger SW, Lober PH & Wangensteen OH. Dissection of the hepatic pedicle and retro-pancreaticoduodenal area for cancer of the stomach. *Surgery* 1955; **38**: 675–8.

61. McNeer G, Sunderland DA, McInnes G *et al.* A more thorough operation for gastric cancer. *Cancer* 1951; **4**: 957–67.

62. Papachristou DN & Fortner JG. Adenocarcinoma of the gastric cardia. The choice of gastrectomy. *Ann Surg* 1980; **192**: 58–64.

63. Papachristou DN, Agnanti N, D'Agostino H & Fortner JG. Histologically positive esophageal margin in the surgical treatment of gastric cancer. *Am J Surg* 1980; **139**: 711–13.

64. Hallissey MT, Jewkes AJ, Dunn JA *et al.* Resection-line involvement in gastric cancer: a continuing problem. *Br J Surg* 1993; **80**: 1418–20.

65. Roder JD, Stein HJ, Bottcher K & Siewert JR. Surgical therapy for gastric cancer. *J Infus Chemother* 1995; **5**: 97–103.

66. Gall CA, Rieger NA & Wattchow DA. Positive proximal resection margins after resection for carcinoma of the oesophagus and stomach: effect on survival and symptom recurrence. *Aust N Z J Surg* 1996; **66**: 734–7.

67. Siewert JR, Bottcher K, Roder JD *et al.* Prognostic relevance of systematic lymph node dissection in gastric carcinoma. German Gastric Carcinoma Study Group (see comments). *Br J Surg* 1993; **80**: 1015–18.

68. Gouzi JL, Huguier M, Fagniez PL *et al.* Total versus subtotal gastrectomy for adenocarcinoma of the gastric antrum. A French prospective controlled study. *Ann Surg* 1989; **209**: 162–6.

69. Robertson CS, Chung SC, Woods SD *et al.* A prospective randomized trial comparing R1 subtotal gastrectomy with R3 total gastrectomy for antral cancer (see comments). *Ann Surg* 1994; **220**: 176–82.

70. Siewert JR, Bottcher K, Stein HJ *et al.* Problem of proximal third gastric carcinoma. *World J Surg* 1995; **19**: 523–31.

70a. Harrison LE, Karpeh MS & Brennan MF. Total gastrectomy is not necessary for proximal gastric cancer. *Surgery* 1998; **123**: 127–30.

71. Shiu MH, Moore E, Sanders M *et al.* Influence of the extent of resection on survival after curative treatment of gastric carcinoma. A retrospective multivariate analysis. *Arch Surg* 1987; **122**: 1347–51.

72. Pacelli F, Doglietto GB, Bellantone R *et al.* Extensive versus limited lymph node dissection for gastric cancer: a comparative study of 320 patients (see comments). *Br J Surg* 1993; **80**: 1153–6.

73. Viste A, Svanes K, Janssen C, Jr. *et al.* Prognostic importance of radical lymphadenectomy in curative resections for gastric cancer. *Eur J Surg* 1994; **160**: 497–502.

74. Volpe CM, Koo J, Miloro SM *et al.* The effect of extended lymphadenectomy on survival in patients with gastric adenocarcinoma. *J Am Coll Surg* 1995; **181**: 56–64.

75. Siewert JR, Kestlmeier R, Busch R *et al.* Benefits of D2 lymph node dissection for patients with gastric cancer and pN0 and pN1 lymph node metastases. *Br J Surg* 1996; **83**: 1144–7.

76. Dent DM, Madden MV & Price SK. Randomized comparison of R1 and R2 gastrectomy for gastric carcinoma. *Br J Surg* 1988; **75**: 110–12.

77. Bonenkamp JJ, Songun I, Hermans J *et al.* Randomised comparison of morbidity after D1 and D2 dissection for gastric cancer in 996 Dutch patients [see comments]. *Lancet* 1995; **345**: 745–8.

78. Bunt AM, Hermans J, Boon MC *et al.* Evaluation of the extent of lymphadenectomy in a randomized trial of Western- versus Japanese-type surgery in gastric cancer. *J Clin Oncol* 1994; **12**: 417–22.

79. Cuschieri A, Fayers P, Fielding J *et al.* Postoperative morbidity and mortality after D1 and D2 resections for gastric cancer: preliminary results of the MRC randomised controlled surgical trial. The Surgical Cooperative Group (see comments). *Lancet* 1996; **347**: 995–9.

80. Kodama I, Takamiya H, Mizutani K *et al.* Gastrectomy with combined resection of other organs for carcinoma of the stomach with invasion to adjacent organs: clinical efficacy in a retrospective study. *J Am Coll Surg* 1997; **184**: 16–22.

81. Brady MS, Rogatko A, Dent LL & Shiu MH. Effect of splenectomy on morbidity and survival following curative gastrectomy for carcinoma. *Arch Surg* 1991; **126**: 359–64.

82. Griffith JP, Sue-Ling HM, Martin I *et al.* Preservation of the spleen improves survival after radical surgery for gastric cancer. *Gut* 1995; **36**: 684–90.

83. Okajima K & Isozaki H. Splenectomy for treatment of gastric cancer: Japanese experience. *World J Surg* 1995; **19**: 537–40.

84. Soreide JA, van Heerden JA, Burgart LJ *et al.* Surgical aspects of patients with adenocarcinoma of the stomach operated on for cure. *Arch Surg* 1996; **131**: 481–6.

85. Maruyama K, Sasako M, Kinoshita T *et al.* Pancreas-preserving total gastrectomy for prox-imal gastric cancer. *World J Surg* 1995; **19**: 532–6.

86. Ochiai T, Sasako M, Mizuno S *et al.* Hepatic resection for metastatic tumours from gastric cancer: analysis of prognostic factors. *Br J Surg* 1994; **81**: 1175–8.

87. Takenaka H, Iwase K, Ohshima S & Hiranaka T. A new technique for the resection of gastric cancer: modified Appleby procedure with reconstruction of hepatic artery. *World J Surg* 1992; **16**: 947–51.

88. Ajani JA, Mansfield PF & Ota DM. Potentially resectable gastric carcinoma: current approaches to staging and preoperative therapy. *World J Surg* 1995; **19**: 216–20.

89. Molloy RG, McCourtney JS & Anderson JR. Laparoscopy in the management of patients with cancer of the gastric cardia and oesophagus. *Br J Surg* 1995; **82**: 352–4.

90. Lowy AM, Mansfield PF, Leach SD & Ajani J. Laparoscopic staging for gastric cancer. *Surgery* 1996; **119**: 611–14.

91. Burke EC, Karpeh MS, Conlon KC & Brennan MF. Laparoscopy in the management of gastric adenocarcinoma. *Ann Surg* 1997; **225**: 262–7.

92. Bemelman WA, van Delden OM, van Lanschot JJ *et al.* Laparoscopy and laparoscopic ultrasonography in staging of carcinoma of the esophagus and gastric cardia. *J Am Coll Surg* 1995; **181**: 421–5.

93. Ballesta-Lopez C, Bastida-Vila X, Catarci M *et al.* Laparoscopic Billroth II distal subtotal gastrectomy with gastric stump suspension for gastric malignancies. *Am J Surg* 1996; **171**: 289–92.

94. Kampschoer GH, Maruyama K, Sasako M *et al.* The effects of blood transfusion on the prognosis of patients with gastric cancer. *World J Surg* 1989; **13**: 637–43.

95. Choi JH, Chung HC, Yoo NC *et al.* Perioperative blood transfusions and prognosis in patients with curatively resected locally advanced gastric cancer. *Oncology* 1995; **52**: 170–5.

96. Fong Y, Karpeh M, Mayer K & Brennan MF. Association of perioperative transfusions with poor outcome in resection of gastric adenocarcinoma (see comments). *Am J Surg* 1994; **167**: 256–60.

97. Bonenkamp JJ, Songun I, Hermans J & van de Velde CJ. Prognostic value of positive cytology findings from abdominal washings in patients with gastric cancer. *Br J Surg* 1996; **83**: 672–4.

98. Abe S, Yoshimura H, Tabara H *et al.* Curative resection of gastric cancer: limitation of peritoneal lavage cytology in predicting the outcome. *J Surg Oncol* 1995; **59**: 226–9.

99. Jones AL, Trott P, Cunningham D *et al.* A pilot study of intraperitoneal cisplatin in the management of gastric cancer. *Ann Oncol* 1994; **5**: 123–6.

100. Nishiyama M, Takashima I, Tanaka T *et al.* Carcinoembryonic antigen levels in the peritoneal cavity: useful guide to peritoneal recurrence and prognosis for gastric cancer. *World J Surg* 1995; **19**: 133–7.

101. Lawrence W, Jr. Reconstruction after total gastrectomy: what is preferred technique? (editorial). *J Surg Oncol* 1996; **63**: 215–20.

102. Buhl K, Lehnert T, Schlag P & Herfarth C. Reconstruction after gastrectomy and quality of life. *World J Surg* 1995; **19**: 558–64.

103. Liedman B, Andersson H, Berglund B *et al.* Food intake after gastrectomy for gastric carcinoma: the role of a gastric reservoir. *Br J Surg* 1996; **83**: 1138–43.

104. Roder JD, Stein HJ, Eckel F *et al.* [Comparison of the quality of life after subtotal and total gastrectomy for stomach carcinoma]. *Dtsch Med Wochenschr* 1996; **121**: 543–9.

105. Chareton B, Landen S, Manganas D *et al.* Prospective randomized trial comparing Billroth I and Billroth II procedures for carcinoma of the gastric antrum (see comments). *J Am Coll Surg* 1996; **183**: 190–4.

106. Fuchs KH, Thiede A, Engemann R *et al.* Reconstruction of the food passage after total gastrectomy: randomized trial. *World J Surg* 1995; **19**: 698–705.

107. Nakane Y, Okumura S, Akehira K *et al.* Jejunal pouch reconstruction after total gastrectomy for cancer. A randomized controlled trial. *Ann Surg* 1995; **222**: 27–35.

108. Schwarz A, Buchler M, Usinger K *et al.* Importance of the duodenal passage and pouch volume after total gastrectomy and reconstruction with the Ulm pouch: prospective randomized clinical study. *World J Surg* 1996; **20**: 60–6.

109. Bozzetti F, Bonfanti G, Castellani R *et al.* Comparing reconstruction with Roux-en-Y to a pouch following total gastrectomy. *J Am Coll Surg* 1996; **183**: 243–8.

110. Allum WH, Powell DJ, McConkey CC & Fielding JW. Gastric cancer: a 25-year review. *Br J Surg* 1989; **76**: 535–40.

111. Alexander HR, Turnbull AD, Salamone J *et al.* Upper abdominal cancer surgery in the very elderly. *J Surg Oncol* 1991; **47**: 82–6.

112. Meijer S, De Bakker OJ & Hoitsma HF. Palliative resection in gastric cancer. *J Surg Oncol* 1983; **23**: 77–80.

113. Cosendey BA & Chapuis G. [Cancer of the esophago-gastric area. Palliative resection and anastomosis by laparotomy alone]. *Helv Chir Acta* 1989; **55**: 703–6.

114. Baba H, Okuyama T, Hiroyuki O *et al.* Prognostic factors for noncurative gastric cancer: univariate and multivariate analyses. *J Surg Oncol* 1992; **51**: 104–8.

115. Chow LW, Lim BH, Leung SY *et al.* Gastric carcinoma with synchronous liver metastases: palliative gastrectomy or not? *Aust N Z J Surg* 1995; **65**: 719–23.

116. Kwun K & Kirschner PA. Palliative side-to-side oesophagogastrostomy for unresectable carcinoma of the oesophagus and cardia. *Thorax* 1981; **36**: 441–5.

117. Tranberg KG, Stael von Holstein C, Ivancev K *et al.* The YAG laser and Wallstent endoprosthesis for palliation of cancer in the esophagus or gastric cardia. *Hepatogastroenterology* 1995; **42**: 139–44.

118. Buzby GP. Perioperative total parenteral nutrition in surgical patients. The Veterans Affairs Total Parenteral Nutrition Cooperative Study Group (see comments). *N Engl J Med* 1991; **325**: 525–32.

119. Brennan MF, Pisters PW, Posner M *et al.* A prospective randomized trial of total parenteral nutrition after major pancreatic resection for malignancy. *Ann Surg* 1994; **220**: 436–41.

120. Daly JM, Weintraub FN, Shou J *et al.* Enteral nutrition during multimodality therapy in upper gastrointestinal cancer patients. *Ann Surg* 1995; **221**: 327–38.

121. Heslin MJ, Latkany L, Leung D *et al.* A prospective, randomized trial of early enteral feeding after resection of upper gastrointestinal malignancy. *Ann Surg* 1997; **226**: 567–77.

122. Summers G, Jr. & Hocking MP. Preoperative and postoperative motility disorders of the stomach. *Surg Clin North Am* 1992; **72**: 467–86.

123. Burt M, Scott A, Williard WC *et al.* Erythromycin stimulates gastric emptying after esophagectomy with gastric replacement: a randomized clinical trial. *J Thorac Cardiovasc Surg* 1996; **111**: 649–54.

124. Averbach AM & Jacquet P. Strategies to decrease the incidence of intra-abdominal recurrence in resectable gastric cancer. *Br J Surg* 1996; **83**: 726–33.

125. Shchepotin I, Evans SR, Shabahang M *et al.* Radical treatment of locally recurrent gastric cancer. *Am Surg* 1995; **61**: 371–6.

126. Schwarz RE, Karpeh MS & Brennan MF. Factors predicting hospitalization after operative

treatment for gastric carcinoma in patients older than 70 years (see comments]). *J Am Coll Surg* 1997; **184**: 9–15.

127. Rohde H, Rau E, Gebbensleben B *et al.* What causes in-hospital mortality of surgical patients with cancer of the stomach? *Scand J Gastroenterol Suppl* 1987; **133**: 76–9.

128. Köster R, Gebbensleben B, Stützer H *et al.* Quality of life in gastric cancer. *Scand J Gastroenterol Suppl* 1987; **133**: 102–6.

129. Kusche J, Vestweber KH & Troidl H. Quality of life after total gastrectomy for stomach cancer. *Scand J Gastroenterol Suppl* 1987; **133**: 96–101.

130. Svedlund J, Sullivan M, Sjodin I *et al.* Quality of life in gastric cancer prior to gastrectomy. *Qual Life Res* 1996; **5**: 255–64.

131. Winslet MC, Mohsen YM, Powell J *et al.* The influence of age on the surgical management of carcinoma of the stomach. *Eur J Surg Oncol* 1996; **22**: 220–4.

132. Kelsen DP. Adjuvant and neoadjuvant therapy for gastric cancer. *Semin Oncol* 1996; **23**: 379–89.

133. Neri B, de Leonardis V, Romano S *et al.* Adjuvant chemotherapy after gastric resection in node-positive cancer patients: a multicentre randomised study. *Br J Cancer* 1996; **73**: 549–52.

134. Leach SD, Lowy AM, Mansfield PF & Ajani JA. Adjuvant therapy for resectable gastric adenocarcinoma: preoperative and postoperative chemotherapy trials. *J Infus Chemother* 1995; **5**: 104–11.

135. Fink U, Stein HJ, Schuhmacher C & Wilke HJ. Neoadjuvant chemotherapy for gastric cancer: update. *World J Surg* 1995; **19**: 509–16.

136. Adachi W, Koike S, Rafique M *et al.* Preoperative intraperitoneal chemotherapy for gastric cancer, with special reference to delayed peritoneal complications. *Surg Today* 1995; **25**: 396–403.

137. Yu W. Intraperitoneal 5-fluorouracil and mitomycin C as adjuvants to resectable gastric cancer: a status report. *Cancer Treat Res* 1996; **81**: 177–83.

138. Yonemura Y, Ninomiya I, Kaji M *et al.* Prophylaxis with intraoperative chemohyperthermia against peritoneal recurrence of serosal invasion-positive gastric cancer. *World J Surg* 1995; **19**: 450–4.

139. Kaibara N. [Prophylaxis and treatment of peritoneal metastasis from gastric cancer]. *Nippon Geka Gakkai Zasshi* 1996; **97**: 308–11.

140. Yonemura Y, Fujimura T, Nishimura G *et al.* Effects of intraoperative chemohyperthermia in patients with gastric cancer with peritoneal dissemination. *Surgery* 1996; **119**: 437–44.

141. Gunderson LL, Burch PA & Donohue JH. The role of irradiation as a component of combined modality treatment for gastric cancer. *J Infus Chemother* 1995; **5**: 117–24.

142. Sindelar WF, Kinsella TJ, Tepper JE *et al.* Randomized trial of intraoperative radiotherapy in carcinoma of the stomach. *Am J Surg* 1993; **165**: 178–86.

143. Abe M, Nishimura Y & Shibamoto Y. Intraoperative radiation therapy for gastric cancer. *World J Surg* 1995; **19**: 544–7.

144. Balfour D. Factors influencing the life expectancy of patients operated on for gastric surgery. *Ann Surg* 1922; **76**: 405–8.

145. Stalnikowicz R & Benbassat J. Risk of gastric cancer after gastric surgery for benign disorders. *Arch Intern Med* 1990; **150**: 2022–6.

146. Tersmette AC, Offerhaus GJ, Tersmette KW *et al.* Meta-analysis of the risk of gastric stump cancer: detection of high risk patient subsets for stomach cancer after remote partial gastrectomy for benign conditions. *Cancer Res* 1990; **50**: 6486–9.

147. Ikeguchi M, Kondou A, Shibata S *et al.* Clinicopathologic differences between carcinoma in the gastric remnant stump after distal partial gastrectomy for benign gastroduodenal lesions and primary carcinoma in the upper third of the stomach. *Cancer* 1994; **73**: 15–21.

148. Kodera Y, Yamamura Y, Torii A *et al.* Gastric remnant carcinoma after partial gastrectomy for benign and malignant gastric lesions. *J Am Coll Surg* 1996; **182**: 1–6.

149. Greene FL. Management of gastric remnant carcinoma based on the results of a 15-year endoscopic screening program. *Ann Surg* 1996; **223**: 701–6.

150. Stael von Holstein C, Eriksson S, Huldt B & Hammar E. Endoscopic screening during 17 years for gastric stump carcinoma. A prospective clinical trial. *Scand J Gastroenterol* 1991; **26**: 1020–6.

151. Takeda J, Hashimoto K, Koufuji K *et al.* Remnant-stump gastric cancer following partial gastrectomy. *Hepatogastroenterology* 1992; **39**: 27–30.

152. Lacueva FJ, Calpena R, Medrano J *et al.* Follow-up of patients resected for gastric cancer. *J Surg Oncol* 1995; **60**: 174–9.

153. Glimelius B, Hoffman K, Graf W *et al.* Cost-effectiveness of palliative chemotherapy in advanced gastrointestinal cancer (see comments). *Ann Oncol* 1995; **6**: 267–74.

5

SURGICAL MANAGEMENT OF GASTRIC CANCER: THE JAPANESE EXPERIENCE

MITSURU SASAKO

PRINCIPLES OF SURGICAL TREATMENT OF GASTRIC CANCER

Principles of radical surgery and its philosophy

Radical resection for gastric cancer comprises total or at least two-thirds gastrectomy, lymph node dissection, and reconstruction of gastrointestinal continuity. The results of early experience showed a very high incidence of locoregional recurrence, either in the remnant stomach or gastric bed, after simple gastrectomy.[1-3] A certain proportion of these recurrences occur without distant metastases. The philosophical basis of extended gastric resection and lymph node dissection is that gastric cancer often remains a locoregional disease with only local lymphatic spread, which can be cured by gastric resection with sufficient margins and extended lymph node dissection. On this theoretic basis, it is assumed that cancer cells disseminate principally via lymphatic vessels and the removal of metastatic lymph nodes effects a cure by preventing subsequent systemic spread. Lymph nodes are thought to represent a barrier to lymphatic spread – a philosophy introduced by Halsted,[4] but now abandoned in breast cancer. However, the concept still holds true in gastric cancer. As opposed to breast cancer, the incidence of distant metastasis is kept very low until a tumor becomes T3 (**Table 5.1**) and the major pattern of recurrence is either loco-

regional or peritoneal. On the other hand, the frequency of lymph node metastasis is rather high already in T2 tumors, and increases in parallel with the depth of tumor infiltration (**Table 5.2**). There are several possible explanations for the differences between breast and gastric cancers. First, the stomach is a contaminated organ, which has special mucosa associated lymphoid tissue. The number of locoregional lymph nodes of the stomach is much greater than that of breast tissue.[5,6] Secondly, the distance to the lymph–venous confluence at the base of the neck is much greater for stomach than for breast. Thirdly, the venous flow of the stomach is in the portal vein system and blood-borne metastasis other than to the liver is exceptional until the terminal stage of the disease, when metastases occur either via the liver or para-aortic nodes through the thoracic duct.

Lymph node dissection

Lymph node metastasis occurs principally from adjacent nodal stations to more distant nodes. Therefore, the incidence of metastasis to certain nodal stations differs enormously according to the location of the tumor. In the Japanese Classification of Gastric Carcinoma,[7] tumor location is expressed according to its site in the antrum, middle, or proximal stomach (**Figure 5.1**), and locoregional lymph nodes are classified into about 20 stations (**Figure 5.2**). We estimated the incidence of metastasis and

Table 5.1   Incidence of nodal, hepatic and peritoneal metastases (%) according to tumor depth among 4683 patients who underwent laparotomy at NCCH between 1972–91.

DEPTH		LYMPH NODE	LIVER	PERITONEUM	NO. OF PATIENTS
T1	mm	3.3	0	0	1063
	sm	17.5	0.1	0	881
T2	mp	46.8	1.1	0.5	436
	ss	63.7	3.4	2.2	325
T3	se	79.9	6.3	17.8	1232
T4	si	89.8	15.5	41.6	724
Total		47.7	4.5	11.5	4683

mm, mucosa and muscularis mucosa; mp, muscularis propria; sm, submucosal; ss, subserosal; se, serosal; si, surrounding organ invasion.

Table 5.2   Pathologic N-stage distribution according to the tumor depth among 4683 patients who underwent laparotomy at NCCH between 1972–91

DEPTH		N0	N1	N2	N3	N4
T1	mm	96.7	2.2	1.1	0	0
	sm	82.5	12.2	4.9	0.3	0.1
T2	mp	53.0	27.0	16.8	1.8	1.4
	ss	36.3	29.8	25.8	2.5	5.5
T3	se	19.5	24.4	40.1	6.9	9.2
T4	si	7.8	11.6	33.6	21.7	25.2
Total		51.7	15.7	20.3	5.5	6.8

Abbreviations as Table 5.1.

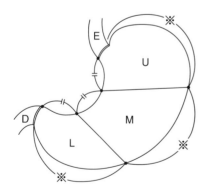

Figure 5.1   The three portions of the stomach. Location of the tumor is described using the three portions as shown. These are delimited by dividing the lesser and greater curvatures at two equidistant points and joining these joints. C, upper third; M, middle third; A, lower third; E, esophagus; D, duodenum. *Reproduced with permission from Reference 7.*

5-year survival rates of the patients with positive nodes station by station, according to the tumor location, using 1281 potentially curable advanced gastric carcinomas. Survival rate was calculated including all the patients with involved nodes in that particular station, irrespective of metastasis to other lymph node stations. Thus, 37 patients with para-aortic nodal metastasis were included. **Figures 5.3–5.6** show the results obtained for antral, middle, and proximal tumors, and those invading all three portions of the stomach. In resecting the left cardial nodes, i.e., station 2, for example, the incidence was 22% for proximal tumor and 7.1% for antral tumors. Similarly, 5-year survival rates were 23.2% and 0%, respectively. This means that station number 2 should be dissected for proximal tumors, but not for antral tumors. In the stations where both the metastatic incidence and 5-year survival rate are high, the effectiveness of dissection is very high. The benefit of dissection of each station is calculated by multiplication of the frequency of metastasis to the station and the 5-year survival rate of patients with metastasis to that station. Thus, survival benefit was calculated without any concept of staging of lymph node metastasis (pN). Generally speaking, the incidence of metastasis to the first-tier nodes is the highest, followed by the second tier. Most of the second-tier stations showed some benefit with dissection. The entire advantage of this so-called D2 dissection is the aggregation of the figures of all second-tier stations.

From the results shown above, the D2 dissection, i.e., dissection of all second-tier stations, is the standard procedure for an advanced gastric carcinoma which can be resected with curative

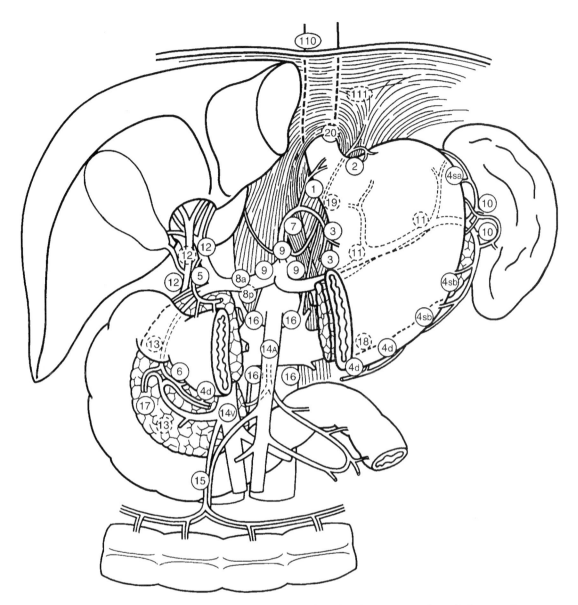

Figure 5.2   Classification of lymph node stations. *Reproduced with permission from Reference 7.*

intent. Extended resection over D2 will be discussed later.

Extent of resection, total or subtotal gastrectomy

The oncologic benefit of total gastrectomy over subtotal gastrectomy is: (i) to gain 2–3 cm longer surgical margins on the lesser curvature and 15 cm on the greater curvature; (ii) to carry out complete dissection of left cardial, splenic hilum, and splenic artery nodes; and (iii) to resect unde-

tected lesions in the proximal stomach which might have remained after subtotal gastrectomy.

In 1994, Meyer *et al.*[8] recommended surgical margins as long as 4 cm for well-circumscribed tumors of the intestinal type, and >8 cm for invasive cancers of the diffuse type. Earlier, Bozzetti *et al.*[9] recommended 6 cm, while in 1993 Arai *et al.*[10] evaluated the differences between macroscopic and microscopic evaluation of the surgical margins of 248 patients with advanced gastric cancer. These latter authors concluded that minimal margins

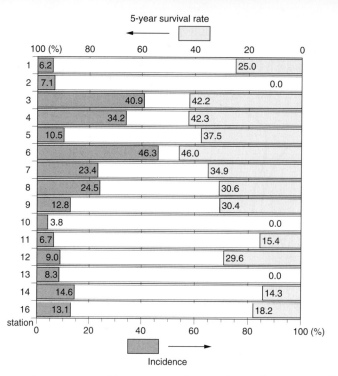

Figure 5.3 Incidence of metastasis and 5-year survival rate in lower-third tumors. The incidence of metastasis to each station is shown by the bar from the left; the 5-year survival rate of those with metastasis is shown by the bar from the right.

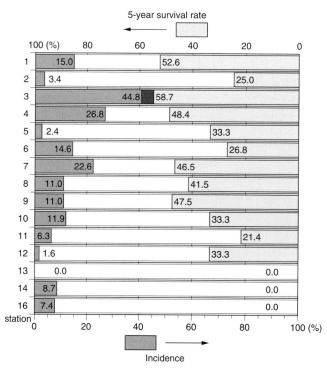

Figure 5.4 Incidence of metastasis and 5-year survival rate in middle-third tumors. The incidence of metastasis to each station is shown by the bar from the left; the 5-year survival rate of those with metastasis is shown by the bar from the right.

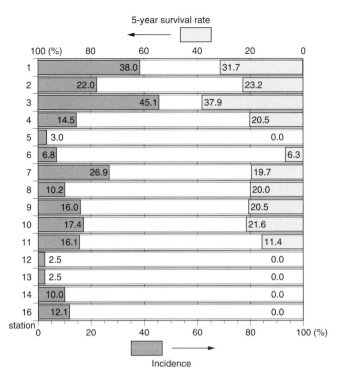

Figure 5.5 Incidence of metastasis and 5-year survival rate in proximal-third tumors. The incidence of metastasis to each station is shown by the bar from the left; the 5-year survival rate of those with metastasis is shown by the bar from the right.

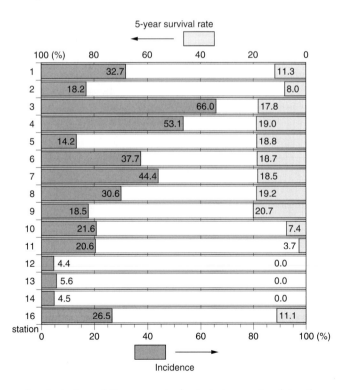

Figure 5.6 Incidence of metastasis and 5-year survival rate in tumors involving three portions of the stomach. The incidence of metastasis to each station is shown by the bar from the left; the 5-year survival rate of those with metastasis is shown by the bar from the right.

should be 3 cm and 6.5 cm in well-circumscribed and diffuse infiltrative tumors, respectively.

As the preoperative diagnosis of proximal extension of the tumor by conventional barium meal study or endoscopy is sometimes difficult – especially in the diffuse infiltrative type – endoscopic ultrasonography (EUS) is very useful for that purpose.[11] Thickening of the wall is easily detected and should be interpreted as tumor invasion. From personal experience, tumors diagnosed as being limited to the distal part of the stomach by gastroenterologists in Western countries often invade up to the gastric body. Without EUS, diffuse submucosal or deeper infiltration beyond the apparent tumor limit can be diagnosed only by experienced endoscopists or radiologists. In our institute, a total gastrectomy is carried out for all linitis plastica type carcinomas, if curable.

As discussed in the previous section, the benefit of dissection of the left cardial or splenic hilum nodes is somewhat limited. These stations are regarded as M (distant nodes) and their dissection is not recommended for antral tumors in the new Japanese Classification. A benefit of dissection of the nodes along the splenic artery is observed for antral tumors; however, dissection should be limited to the proximal half of these (11p), i.e., proximal half of those along the artery.

No study, either prospective or retrospective, has shown any advantage of total gastrectomy over subtotal gastrectomy for antral tumors.[12,13] A study carried out in Hong Kong[14] compared distal gastrectomy with D1 dissection, and total gastrectomy with D3 dissection, including PS (pancreaticosplenectomy). There seems to be no rationale to support this study design, because no study or paper has yet reported benefit for D3 total gastrectomy for antral tumors. There is some misunderstanding of Japanese D2 or D3 dissection. In the Japanese Classification, the D2 associated with total gastrectomy includes complete dissection of splenic hilum, splenic artery, and left cardial nodes, but the D2 associated with subtotal or distal gastrectomy does not include these stations, except the proximal half of the splenic artery nodes. In Japan, a total gastrectomy is indicated only for tumors of the proximal or middle part of the stomach. For tumors of the middle part of the stomach, the decision to perform a total or subtotal resection is determined by the tumor location and observed macroscopic metastasis. If the proximal border of

the lesion is above the line connecting the watershed of right and left gastroepiploic vessels on the greater curvature and the point 3–5 cm below the cardia on the lesser curvature, a total gastrectomy is indicated (**Figure 5.7**).[15]

RESECTION OF NEIGHBORING ORGANS

Resection of organs for T4 tumors

Gastric cancer may invade the left lobe of the liver, the gallbladder, the spleen, the pancreas head, body or tail, the mesocolon, the transverse colon, and the greater or lesser omenta. All of these structures can be resected without causing serious postoperative sequelae. Resection of invaded organs is the only way to achieve a curative resection for T4 tumors, if there is no distant metastasis. Nakajima et al.[16] reported morbidity and mortality of combined resection for various organs. The highest 30-day mortality rate was 7.6%, observed in 532 patients who underwent colectomy, while the morbidity rate in these patients was 33.3%. Thirty-day mortality rates after pancreaticoduodenectomy (117 cases), hepatectomy (101 cases), pancreaticosplenectomy (1670 cases), splenectomy (207 cases), and oophorectomy (23 cases) were 6.7%, 3.0%, 2.9%, 1.3% and 0%, respectively. Morbidity after these procedures was 39.0%, 33.3%, 42.9%, 32.7% and 0%, respectively. The 5-year survival rates of patients who underwent combined resection of organs with gastrectomy were 49.9% after splenectomy, 37.4% after distal pancreatectomy, 44.8% after transverse colectomy and 39.5% after

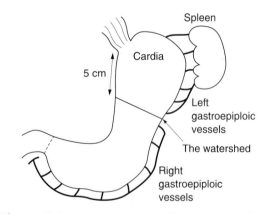

Figure 5.7   Indication of total gastrectomy. If the proximal margin of the tumor is above this line, total gastrectomy is indicated if curable.

hepatectomy.[17] Korenaga et al.[18] reported a 5-year survival rate of 33.1% for distal pancreatectomy with curative intent for T4 tumors, 43% for resection of mesocolon, and 25% for liver resection. If a single neighboring organ is invaded, the 5-year survival rate is rather high, 17.1% in total. On the other hand, if two or more organs are involved, survival after complete resection of these organs is reduced to 4.0% at 5 years. The incidence of subphrenic abscess or pancreatic fistula after pancreatic resection may reach 40%; therefore, a prophylactic drainage tube should be inserted to the left subphrenic space.

Resection of neighboring organs for lymph node dissection

In the standard D2 gastrectomy for advanced cancer, complete resection of greater and lesser omenta and resection of the anterior leaf of the transverse mesocolon are regarded as routine. For early gastric cancer, however, resection of the greater omentum is limited to the area, 3–4 cm from the gastroepiploic vessels, where all lymph nodes are located. The anterior mesocolon is dissected and resected right to the middle colic vessels, the remaining part being left untouched. The lesser omentum is not divided as close to the liver as in advanced cases.

The traditional D2 total gastrectomy includes resection of the pancreatic body and tail, together with the spleen. This extended surgery is the realization of the idea of "en bloc" resection of the gastric bed: lymph nodes along vessels should be dissected together with the vessels themselves "en bloc." The complete form of D2 total gastrectomy is the Appleby operation (**Figure 5.8**),[19] which comprises total gastrectomy, resection of the celiac artery together with the splenic and common hepatic arteries, resection of the pancreas distal to the portal vein, and splenectomy. This operation causes much greater morbidity and mortality, because hepatic arterial blood flow will be supplied by the superior mesenteric artery via the pancreaticoduodenal arcade and gastroduodenal artery. The hospital mortality rate reported by Iizuka[20] was as high as 7.2% (6/83 patients), and thus this procedure is rarely carried out, even in Japan. However, Furukawa et al.[21] reported the

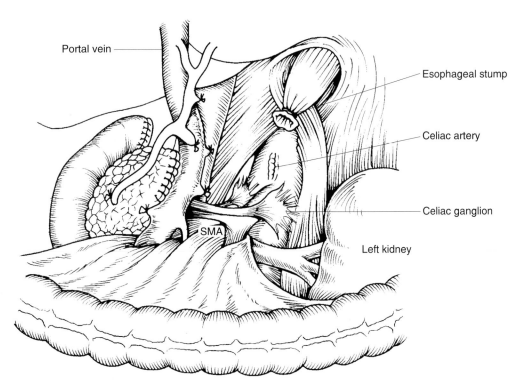

Figure 5.8 View after resection in Appleby's operation. Complete en bloc resection of the gastric bed is realized by this procedure. SMA, superior mesenteric artery.

results of 30 patients treated by this procedure combined with transverse colectomy. Their 30-day postoperative mortality rate was 0%, although they routinely carried out celiac angiography to find patients with the anomaly of branching of this artery and hepatic arteries, in whom the procedure is contraindicated. In conventional extended surgery with pancreaticosplenectomy (PS), hepatic artery nodes are dissected without resection of the common hepatic artery itself, but splenic artery nodes are dissected with ligation and division of the splenic artery at its origin together with the distal half of the organ. Because this incorporates an inconsistency of surgical philosophy, therefore preservation of the splenic artery seems possible, without decreasing the effect of lymph node dissection. In practice, however, it is not easy to carry out sufficient lymph node dissection, preserving this artery up to the splenic hilum, because there are many branches to the spleen, the stomach, and the pancreas parenchyma from the distal portion of this artery. Fortunately, the blood supply to the tail of the pancreas is good enough even after ligation of the splenic artery just distal to the branching of the dorsal pancreatic artery.[22] Based on this approach, "en bloc" dissection of splenic artery and hilar nodes is realized by ligation and division of the splenic artery distal to the dorsal pancreatic artery. In this procedure, so-called pancreas-preserving total gastrectomy (PPTG) described by Maruyama et al.,[22] the spleen is resected together with these vessels and the pancreas is preserved completely. This operation reduced the complication rate of D2 total gastrectomy to half that of the conventional procedure with PS.[22]

Resection of transverse colon may be combined with conventional D2 total gastrectomy, and is termed left upper abdominal evisceration (LUAE). This operation aims to resect the gastric bed "en bloc" to reduce regional recurrence. The middle colic vessels are ligated and divided at their origin to resect the entire mesocolon and omentum together. However, most very advanced cases will recur in other sites, such as the peritoneum, or also the liver. There seems to be little advantage in this operation for T3 tumors, especially because of the higher morbidity of the procedure (Y. Yonemura, personal communication, 1997).

SUPER-EXTENDED SURGERY: PARA-AORTIC LYMPH NODE DISSECTION

The most common pattern of recurrence after D2 gastrectomy for advanced gastric cancer is peritoneal dissemination.[23] However, there are some who develop para-aortic lymph node metastasis, followed by systemic blood-borne metastasis. For several decades, selective sampling or limited resection of para-aortic nodes has been tried by Kajitani.[24] From the same institution, Nishi and Ohta[25] reported that 12 patients with involved nodes at this area survived more than 5 years. Following their report, several surgeons tried systematic wide dissection of para-aortic nodes for advanced gastric cancer. The incidence of metastasis to this area in T3 or T4 tumors is reported to be 21% by Nashimoto et al.,[26] 33% by Kitamura et al.,[27] and 27% by Takahashi et al.[28] The reported 5-year survival rates of node-positive patients treated with curative intent were 15.2% by Takahashi,[29] 23.1% by Nashimoto et al.,[26] and 14% by Aiko et al.[30]

Between 1987 and 1991, 130 patients with advanced gastric cancer underwent wide para-aortic node dissection with curative intent at the NCCH. The results of these patients (group A) were compared with those of 382 patients (group B) who underwent D2 or D3 dissection for advanced cancer with curative intent between 1982 and 1986. Incidence of n2 and n4 was 24.6% and 16.9% for group A, and 39.5% and 2.9% for group B. Thus, by carrying out para-aortic dissection, about 15% of patients shifted from n2 to n4. The long-term survival of these two groups was compared excluding Borrmann type 4 cancer, the incidence of which was significantly different between them. The 5-year survival rate of n2 disease was 51% and 39%, for groups A and B, respectively. Similarly, that of n4 was 38% and 18%, respectively. The 5-year survival rate of pT2 (ss) was 75% and 70% for groups A and B, respectively. Similarly, that of pT3 (se) was 54% and 52%, while that of pT4 was 58% and 27%, respectively. The apparent improvement of survival rate by pN stage (n) after super-extended surgery (group A) was remarkable but it may be largely attributable to a stage migration effect, because improvement was not seen if the results were evaluated by T factor, except in T4. The more than double improvement of 5-year survival observed for T4 tumors should be analyzed further. From this retrospective analysis, the benefit of D4 over D2 dissection is not so large and should be evaluated by a randomized controlled trial. Indeed, we are currently participating in such a trial which is being carried out among 16 leading hospitals in Japan.

LIMITED SURGERY FOR GASTRIC CANCER

Indication for D1 gastrectomy for early gastric cancer

From the results shown in **Table 5.2**, lymph node metastasis to the second tier is observed in 1.1% of cases with mucosal cancer and in 5.4% with submucosal cancer. Therefore, D1 dissection can provide almost the same results as D2 for early gastric cancer. However, those patients with n2 metastasis with early cancer have a good prognosis after D2 dissection; the 5-year survival rate of T1,mm, n2 and T1,sm, n2, was 90% and 78%, respectively. Theoretically, D2 dissection can provide 4% better survival than D1. The reported increase in mortality after D2 dissection in Western populations[31,32] may annul the benefit of the procedure for early gastric cancer. If the surgeons can keep the incidence of postoperative death or severe morbidity as low as in D1 gastrectomy, D2 dissection is still useful even for early gastric cancer because the expectation of a 4–5% increase in survival by adjuvant therapy is not realistic in early gastric cancer. Moreover, the accuracy of preoperative diagnosis regarding the depth of invasion depends on the clinician's experience and seems to be limited in Western countries. "Early gastric cancer" may often invade into the muscularis propria or deeper, and in such cases the incidence of n2 node metastasis is actually 25% for cancer invading the muscularis propria (mp) and 40% for cancer invading the subserosal layer (ss). Therefore, considering that nearly 10% of advanced cancers are underestimated as "early",[33] at least the common hepatic artery nodes, celiac artery nodes, left gastric artery nodes, and proximal splenic artery nodes should be dissected, because this lymphadenectomy can be carried out without splenectomy or pancreatectomy, with minimal increase in morbidity, even in Western populations.[34]

Pylorus-preserving (distal) gastrectomy (PPG) for early gastric cancer

The most important causes of postgastrectomy impairment in quality of life (QOL) are a small volume of the remnant stomach and a loss of reservoir function by resection of the pylorus. Both early and late dumping syndromes are the most frequent and uncomfortable sequelae of gastrectomy. To prevent this, Maki et al.[35] initiated the PPG for benign ulcer disease many years ago. Recently, this operation has been modified and applied to early gastric cancer. In this procedure, 1–3 cm of the prepyloric area of the stomach is preserved, the central part of the organ is resected, and a gastrogastrostomy is made. The hepatic branch and pyloric branch from the anterior vagal trunk are preserved. Some surgeons also preserve the celiac branch from the posterior vagal trunk. There are two methods of preserving antral blood flow: by preserving the posterior pyloric artery (branching either from the gastroduodenal–duodenal or right gastroepiploic artery); or by preserving the right gastric artery. In early gastric cancers located >4 cm proximal to the pylorus and >6 cm distal to the cardia, the incidence of nodal metastasis was 0.5% to the suprapyloric nodes and 1.6% to the infrapyloric ones. From this, it seems wiser to preserve the right gastric artery proximal to the pylorus. All other stations which are dissected in ordinary D2 distal gastrectomy can be dissected without any problem in this procedure. The incidence of postoperative morbidity and mortality is not significantly different from a standard distal gastrectomy. Gastric stasis is observed in 10% of patients in the early postoperative period, but this resolves spontaneously at 3–4 weeks after operation. Dumping is seldom observed, but a detailed evaluation of other factors regarding QOL will be carried out in the near future.

Local excision or endoscopic resection for older patients

In Japan, the average life span for the entire population has been increasing during the past four decades, and is now more than 80 years for females and 76 for males. Naturally, the proportion of older patients is increasing year by year in gastric cancer. On the basis of results reported at NCCH,[36] the 5-year survival rate of patients over 80 years old with early gastric cancer is as low as 53.8%. Most of these died of causes other than gastric cancer. Considering the rather small possibility of metastasis to the second-tier nodes from early gastric cancer (see **Table 5.2**), and less than <10% survival benefit from D2 dissection, it is not useful to carry out D2 dissection for patients aged over 80. Total or proximal gastrectomy for tumors located in the proximal third of the stomach, is associated with a higher mortality than distal gastrectomy, and therefore cannot benefit patients aged over 80 with early gastric cancer. Wedge resection of the stomach (whole layer) or surgical mucosal resection via a gastrotomy is sometimes applied in this situation, depending on the patient's physical condition. If technically possible, endoscopic mucosal resection can be a good option for mucosal cancer.

MORTALITY AND MORBIDITY AFTER RADICAL SURGERY IN JAPANESE PATIENTS

Mortality

Due to the high incidence of gastric cancer in Japan, gastric cancer surgery is common practice. This is in contrast to Western countries, where gastrectomy has become a rare operation after the extensive use of H2 blockers for benign ulcer disease. In many Japanese hospitals, gastrectomy is carried out as part of an educational program. The incidence of mortality depends on surgeons and hospitals. In a historic review, Mine et al.[37] reported a 30-day mortality rate of 8.8% for 438 patients treated between 1955 and 1963. During the next decade, Suehiro et al.[38] reported a 30-day mortality rate of 3.9% for 377 patients, while Imanaga and Nakazato[39] reported a rate of 2.8% for 1628 patients, Yamada et al.[40] 2.4% for 1952 patients, and Nagata et al.[41] 0.7% for 299 patients. Nakajima et al.[42] reported the trend in 30-day mortality rate in 10 485 patients treated between 1946 and 1990 at the Cancer Institute Hospital: 8.6% for 1946–49, 4.8% for 1950–54, 3.3% for 1955–59, 2.8% for 1960–64, 4.1% for 1965–69, 1.4% for 1970–74, 1.0% for 1975–79, 0.2% for 1980–84, and 0.8% for 1985–90. This improvement was due to several factors, including the introduction of total parenteral nutrition, improvement in suture material and the invention of staplers.

Mortality after gastric surgery is different between distal and total gastrectomy. In Japan,

D2 total gastrectomy is usually associated with splenectomy or PS. In 1992, Sowa et al.[43] reported a 7.1% hospital mortality rate for 324 patients undergoing total gastrectomy between 1978 and 1989; the hospital mortality due to surgical complications being 2.5%. In another report, Soga et al.[44] identified a 30-day mortality rate of 6.8% after total or proximal gastrectomy for esophagogastric junction tumors, treated between 1961 and 1987, while the 30-day mortality rate for the same procedure was 3.4% for proximal gastric cancer without esophageal involvement. In 1990, Sasako[45] reported a 4% hospital mortality rate in 348 patients who had undergone total gastrectomy at the National Cancer Center Hospital, with mortality rate due to surgical complications being 3.2%. Nishi and Ohta[25] reported a 2.9% 30-day mortality rate for 1673 patients who underwent total gastrectomy at the Cancer Institute Hospital Tokyo, while Maruyama et al.[22] reported hospital and 30-day mortality rates of pancreas-preserving total gastrectomy and total gastrectomy with PS of 1.6% and 0.3% versus 3.1% and 0.9%, respectively. By comparison, hospital mortality of distal or distal subtotal gastrectomy is much lower. Sasako[44] reported a 0.2% hospital mortality rate for 849 patients who underwent distal (subtotal) gastrectomy, while Nishi and Ohta[25] reported a 30-day mortality rate of 2.1% for 4139 patients with distal gastrectomy.

According to the registration reports from the Japanese Research Society for Gastric Cancer,[46] 30-day mortality rates after gastrectomy according to disease stage were: 0.7% for 1372 stage I patients, 0.5% for 403 stage II, 1.2% for 1148 stage III, and 3.5% for stage IV. In the same report, 30-day mortality rates after gastrectomy according to the level of lymph node dissection were 4.0% for D0, 1.8% for D1, 1.2% for D2, and 2.2% for D3. Among Japanese series, differences in mortality between D1 and D2 are much smaller than are reported from Western countries.

Morbidity

The major morbidity directly related with surgery is anastomotic leakage and intra-abdominal infection. The incidence of each varies according to the type of gastric resection (total or distal) and combined resection of neighboring organs. The results of these complications, as identified at NCCH,[45] are listed in **Tables 5.3** and **5.4**.

Table 5.3 Surgical complications in 1197 patients treated at NCCH between 1982–87

COMPLICATION	TG/PG	DG	OVERALL
Leakage	17.6	2.7	7.0
Pancreatic fistula	19.3	0.6	6.0
Intra-abdominal abscess	5.5	1.3	2.5
Ileus/obstruction	4.3	1.5	2.3
Bleeding	2.9	0.7	1.3
Wound infection	1.1	1.4	1.3
Anastomotic stenosis	0.6	1.3	1.1
Mediastinitis	2.3	0	0.7
Pancreatitis	0.6	0.2	0.4
Empyema	2.0	0	0.6
Wound dehiscence	0.6	0.1	0.3
Acute cholecystitis	0.9	0	0.3

TG, total gastrectomy; PG, proximal gastrectomy; DG, distal gastrectomy.[45]

Table 5.4 Other complications in 1197 patients treated at NCCH between 1982–87

	TG/PG	DG	OVERALL
Liver dysfunction	10.1	3.5	5.4
Pneumonia/atelectasis	2.9	1.8	2.1
Arrhythmia	1.4	0.7	0.9
Ischemic heart disease	0.3	0.3	0.4
Congestive heart failure	0.3	0	0.1
Urinary infection	1.1	0.4	0.6
Drug allergy	0.6	0.1	0.3
Acute enteritis	0.3	0.6	0.5

TG, total gastrectomy; PG, proximal gastrectomy; DG, distal gastrectomy.[45]

Leakage

The incidence of anastomotic leakage at the esophagojejunostomy has decreased remarkably after routine use of stapler guns. Incidence of leakage was analyzed using the patients who underwent esophagojejunostomy or esophagogastrostomy between 1985 and 1991 at NCCH. The overall incidence of leakage, including subclinical minor fistulae, was 15.7% and 19.6%, by one- and two-layer hand suture techniques, respectively. The overall leakage ratio after using staplers was 5.9%, and a clear learning curve was observed: the annual leakage rate decreased from 17% to approximately 6% after 3 years' experience with 80 cases, and with more than 50 such applications annually. Variation between the results of individual surgeons is much less when using staplers than by manual suture (unpublished data). Regarding reconstruction after distal gastrectomy, Billroth type I is the most commonly used technique in Japan. However, this method may be associated with a worse morbidity immediately after operation. The leakage rate is by far the highest and stenosis due to edema is more frequent than when using other methods. The incidence of leakage at gastroduodenostomy (Billroth I) is 3%, and that of gastrojejunostomy (Billroth II or Roux-en-Y) is 0.2–0.3%. As the advantage of Billroth I reconstruction is not clinically evident, this enormous difference cannot be justified, especially in Western countries where the mortality rate after leakage is very high.

In the Dutch Gastric Cancer Trial, comparing D1 versus D2 dissection for curable gastric cancers, leakage after distal gastrectomy was significantly more frequent in D2 than in D1; 7.0% versus 1.9% ($P < 0.05$).[35] It is suggested that the higher incidence of leakage was related to skeletonization of the lesser curvature of the gastric remnant in D2, in which the short gastric vessels, the posterior gastric vessels, and the cardioesophageal branch from the left inferior phrenic vessels are the remaining blood flow of the stomach. As the last two vessels are not constant anatomic structures, the short gastric vessels should be preserved to keep sufficient circulation of the remnant stomach. Blood supply to the lesser curvature and the anastomosis derives mainly from the greater curvature through the intramural vascular network. Subtotal resection of the organ necessitating ligation of short gastric vessels should be avoided for this reason. For high tumors, total gastrectomy should be carried out. Side-to-side gastrojejunal anastomosis on the posterior wall of the gastric stump using linear staplers appears to be dangerous, as it divides the intramural vascular network of the gastric stump, making the small portion of the remnant stomach between the division line of the stomach and the anastomosis ischemic.

Pancreatic fistula and subphrenic abscess

The most frequent complication after D2 total gastrectomy is pancreatic juice leakage (fistula) and associated subphrenic abscess. Occasionally, this leads to digestion of skeletonized arteries which results in a sudden massive intra-abdominal bleed. The incidence of pancreatic complications, which comprises pancreatic fistula, left subphrenic abscess, and acute pancreatitis, was 42.9%, 17.8% and 13.2% after total gastrectomy with PS, PP and simple splenectomy, respectively,[45] while that of distal gastrectomy was 1.1%. In both the Dutch Trial[31] and the MRC Trial,[32] the associated splenectomy was revealed to be a major cause of increased morbidity and mortality after D2 dissection. Indeed, even after PPTG, about one-sixth of patients develop pancreatic complications. The question remains whether this is due to impaired immunity of patients by splenectomy, or to simple injury or ischemia of the pancreas. From the Japanese point of view, dissection of the splenic artery and hilar nodes remains essential for advanced tumors of the upper half of the organ, especially those located near the greater curvature. Rather than avoid PS, various technical devices have been tried: staplers for pancreatic division;[47,48] a filler of the pancreatic duct, Ethibloc®;[49] and latex rubber attached to the pancreas stump for complete drainage.[50] The development of PPTG decreased morbidity and mortality with full dissection of splenic artery and hilar nodes. With any technique, the prophylactic insertion of a drainage tube to the subphrenic space or pancreatic stump is essential to prevent reoperation. By checking the amylase concentration of the drainage fluid on the first, third, and fifth postoperative days, the prediction of development of pancreatic complication is feasible. If there is no enzyme-rich drainage on the fifth postoperative day, the tube can be removed.[51] In obese patients, the border of pancreas is unclear and surgical complications after these procedures should be higher than in others. In principle, surgeons who treat gastric cancer should have sufficient knowledge and experience of treating pancreatic diseases and of handling complications of pancreatic surgery.

Pneumonia

A gastrectomy with extended surgery is usually associated with massive fluid loss to the extravascular space, either in the abdominal free cavity or retroperitoneal connective tissue. This is partly due to lymphorrhea from divided lymphatics, and partly to the wide dissection of the retroperitoneum and membrane structures including the pancreatic capsule and anterior sheet of the mesocolon. Thus, patients require a much larger quantity of fluid repletion after extensive surgery than following simple gastrectomy in order to maintain their circulatory volume and renal function. We inject 2–3 ml/kg/h of fluid on the day of operation and on the first postoperative day. This often results in overhydration when the body fluid returns to the vascular bed, and in extreme cases causes acute cardiac insufficiency or lung edema. If this does not occur, pneumonia may ensue. Prophylactic use of low-dose catecholamines is useful to maintain good urinary function and prevent overhydration when body fluid returns to the circulation after 3–4 days following surgery. The routine use of epidural anesthesia with morphine chloride for pain control is effective to prevent pulmonary complications. Patients can walk from the first or second postoperative days with minimum pain.

PRINCIPLES OF POSTOPERATIVE CARE

Prophylactic drainage tube

In view of the high incidence of infectious complications after total gastrectomy with splenectomy or PS, routine drainage of the left subphrenic space is recommended. In the case of distal pancreatectomy, another drainage tube should also be placed close to the stump of the pancreas. These tubes should be retained until 5–7 days postoperatively, when the possibility of pancreatic fistula or subphrenic abscess can be denied from the clinical course and amylase level of the exudate. When the amylase level is high, the tube should be retained for 12–14 days, at which time a fistulography is performed. Subsequent handling of the drainage tube is as per the normal drainage tube in the abscess cavity. However, aggressive irrigation may often be performed after 14 postoperative days if a large amount of purulent discharge is apparent and/or the amylase level of the discharge is very high.

Pain control and physiotherapy

Epidural anesthesia using morphine chloride is carried out routinely in many Japanese hospitals. This helps patients both psychologically and physically in that patients can walk from the early postoperative period and ventilate and cough easily. For normal-risk Japanese patients, the blowing of a simple wind instrument, an increased dead space and use of an expiratory pressure breather (e.g., Souffle©), to give higher end-expiratory pressure, and inhalation of some expectorants are sufficient to prevent pulmonary complications.

Oral intake of food

After distal gastrectomy, fluid intake is started on the fourth postoperative day, after which semi-solid and then solid foods are given gradually. Most patients can ingest near-normal solid food by the 11th postoperative day. In order to prevent rupture of the anastomosis due to overeating, patients are told not to take more than one-third of their normal amount of diet. This situation should be maintained until 14–16 days post-operatively.

After total or proximal gastrectomy, a radiographic study using a water-soluble material is carried out to confirm continuity and passage of the esophagojejunostomy. If continuity is normal, fluid intake will be commenced on the same day. Patients begin to eat solid food on 13–15 days post-operatively. They are requested to eat slowly, but the quantity of food ingested is not restricted, unlike those undergoing a distal gastrectomy.

SURGICAL TREATMENT OF GASTRIC CANCER INVADING THE OESOPHAGUS

As opposed to Western populations, reflux esophagitis is seldom seen in the Japanese population. Therefore, adenocarcinoma of the lower esophagus associated with Barrett's epithelium is also rare. Most tumors involving the gastroesophageal junction are either cardia cancer or gastric cancer of the body invading up to the esophagus, corresponding to Types II and III tumors, respectively.[52]

There are two commonly applied operations for these tumors: a left thoracoabdominal oblique approach, or an abdominal approach with wide incision of the diaphragm, enabling easy access of the lower mediastinum.[53,54] The former provides the best operative field, enabling a wide resection of esophageal hiatus, including crura, complete dissection of lower mediastinal lymph nodes and safe esophagojejunostomy under direct vision.[55] The reported incidence of lower mediastinal nodal involvement from these tumors is between 14 to 40%.[56–59] However only a few patients with positive mediastinal nodes survived for more than 5 years after surgery. The best 5-year survival rate reported is 16%,[60] with three out of 31 patients

with mediastinal lymph node metastasis surviving more than 5 years. The recent advancement of staple guns made intrathoracic or mediastinal anastomosis without thoracotomy as safe as when using a thoracoabdominal approach. For this reason, effectiveness of both techniques is now being investigated in a randomized controlled trial in Japan, evaluating morbidity, mortality, post-operative quality of life, and survival.

PRINCIPLES AND INDICATIONS OF NON-CURATIVE RESECTION

Non-curative resection is indicated when remarkable symptoms require resection, or when survival benefit is expected. In many antral tumors, a stenosis at the gastric outlet requires a resection or gastrojejunal bypass.[61] The choice of these two treatment options is made according to the patient's risk factors (age, sex, associated diseases, obesity index, nutritional state) and the surgeon's skill and experience. The safety of operation depends largely on the degree of duodenal invasion. If more than 2 cm of the first portion of the duodenum is invaded macroscopically, resection is of high risk and should be avoided. Tumors causing severe anemia or acute hemorrhage necessitate resection. Bleeding requiring frequent blood transfusions disturbs any kind of medical treatment. If a distal gastrectomy can include the main tumor site and a safe anastomosis is achievable, then resection is the first step of the entire treatment schedule. For bleeding tumors requiring a total gastrectomy, the decision to resect is made according to patient's risk factors, tumor site, the amount of residual unresected metastasis, and to the surgeon's skill and experience.

Many linitis plastica tumors do not cause either stenosis or hemorrhage. The role of surgery in non-curative linitis plastica is controversial. We compared the results of 104 patients with linitis plastica who underwent non-curative resection and 43 patients who underwent exploratory laparotomy alone, most of whom subsequently underwent chemotherapy.[62] There were eight hospital deaths, two due to surgical complications, and six from cancer. If all cases were included, the survival curves showed a statistically significant difference ($P < 0.05$ by Log-rank test) between the two groups. To minimize the background differences between two groups, linitis plastica with diffuse

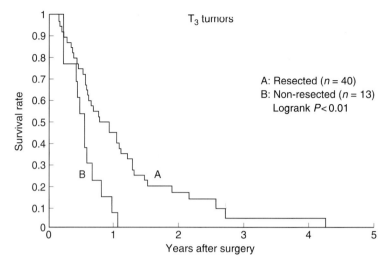

Figure 5.9 Survival curves of patients with linitis plastica. Survival after non-curative resection is evaluated between resected and non-resected tumors.

peritoneal dissemination (P3) were exclusively compared. There was no statistical difference between two survival curves; however, if survival time spent at home was compared, patients who underwent resection had a significantly longer time at home (*P* < 0.05 by Log-rank test). Median survival time at home was one and four months for the non-resected and resected groups, respectively, while mean survival time was 2.7 and 6.0 months, respectively. Of the 104 patients, eight (7.7%) could not be discharged from the hospital and did not benefit from the resection. Selection of patients is, therefore, of paramount importance, and the benefit of resection in T3 tumors is evident (**Figure 5.9**). In the future, when no doubt more effective adjuvant treatment will appear, resection will be attempted after neoadjuvant treatment.

REFERENCES

1. Wangensteen OH, Lewis FJ, Arhelger SW *et al.* An interim report upon the "second look" procedure for cancer of stomach, colon and rectum and for "limited intraperitoneal carciniomatosis". *Surg Gynecol Obstet* 1954; **99**: 257–67.
2. Papachristou DN & Fortner JG. Local recurrence of gastric adenocarcinoma after gastrectomy. *J Surg Oncol* 1981; **18**: 47–53.
3. Gunderson LL & Sosin H. Adenocarcinoma of the stomach: areas of failure in a re-operation series (second or symptomatic look) clinico-pathologic correlation and implications for adjuvant therapy. *Int J Radiat Oncol* 1981; **8**: 1–11.
4. Halsted WS. The results of operations for the cure of cancer of the breast performed at the Johns Hopkins Hospital from June, 1889 to January, 1894. *Johns Hopkins Hosp Bull 1894–1895* 1895; **4**: 297.
5. Bunt AMG, Hermans J, van de Velde CJH *et al.* Lymph node retrieval in a randomized trial on western-type versus Japanese-type surgery in gastric cancer. *J Clin Oncol* 1996; **14**: 2289–94.
6. Fisher CJ, Boyle S, Burke M *et al.* Intraoperative assessment of nodal status in the selection of patients with breast cancer for axillary clearance. *Br J Surg* 1993; **80**: 457–8.
7. Japanese Gastric Cancer Association. Japanese Classification of Gastric Carcinoma, 2nd edn. *Gastric Cancer* 1998; **1**: 10–24.
8. Meyer HJ, Jähne J & Pichlmayr R. Strategies in the surgical treatment of gastric carcinoma. *Ann Oncol* 1994; **5**: s33–6.
9. Bozzetti F, Bonfanti G, Bufalino R *et al.* Adequacy of margins of resection in gastrectomy for cancer. *Ann Surg* 1982; **196**: 685–90.
10. Arai K, Kitamura M & Miyashita K. Studies on proximal margin in gastric cancer from the standpoint of discrepancy between macroscopic and histological measurement of invasion. *Jpn J Gastroenterol Surg* 1993; **26**: 784–9 (in Japanese with English abstract).
11. Maruta S, Tsykamoto Y, Niwa Y *et al.* Endoscopic ultrasonography for assessing the

horizontal extent of invasive gastric cancer. *Am J Gastroenterol* 1993; **9**: 555–9.

12. Gennari L, Bozzetti F, Bonfanti G *et al.* Subtotal versus total gastrectomy for cancer of the lower two-thirds of the stomach: a new approach to an old problem. *Br J Surg* 1986; **73**: 534–8.

13. Gouzzi JL, Huguier M, Fagnier PL *et al.* Total versus subtotal gastrectomy for adenocarcinoma of the gastric antrum. *Ann Surg* 1989; **209**: 162–6.

14. Robertson CS, Chung SCS, Woods SDS *et al.* A prospective randomized trial comparing R1 subtotal gastrectomy with R3 total gastrectomy for antral cancer. *Ann Surg* 1994; **220**: 176–82.

15. Sasako M, Kinishita T, Maruyama K *et al.* Quality control of surgical technique in a multicenter, prospective, randomised, controlled study on the surgical treatment of gastric cancer trial. *Jpn J Clin Oncol* 1992; **22**: 41–8.

16. Nakajima T, Nishi M & Kajitani T. Improvement in treatment results of gastric cancer with surgery and chemotherapy: experience of 9700 cases in the Cancer Institute Hospital, Tokyo. *Semin Surg Oncol* 1991; **7**: 365–72.

17. Maruyama K, Sasako M, Kinoshita T *et al.* Surgical treatment for gastric cancer: the Japanese experience. *Semin Oncol* 1996; **23**: 360–8.

18. Korenaga D, Okamura T, Baba H *et al.* Results of resection of gastric cancer extending to adjacent organs. *Br J Surg* 1988; **75**: 12–15.

19. Appleby LH. The coeliac axis in the expansion of the operation for gastric carcinoma. *Cancer* 1953; **6**: 704–7.

20. Iizuka I. Collateral circulation after division of the common hepatic artery – clinical study concerning Appleby's operation. *J Jpn Surg Soc* 1990; **91**: 631–8 (in Japanese with English abstract).

21. Furukawa H, Hiratsuka M & Iwanaga T. A rational technique for surgical operation on Borrmann type 4 gastric carcinoma: left upper abdominal evisceration plus Appleby's method. *Br J Surg* 1988; **75**: 116–19.

22. Maruyama K, Sasako M, Kinoshita T *et al.* Pancreas-preserving total gastrectomy for proximal gastric cancer. *World J Surg* 1995; **19**: 532–6.

23. Katai H, Maruyama K, Sasako M *et al.* Mode of recurrence after gastric cancer surgery. *Dig Surg* 1994; **11**: 99–103.

24. Ohashi I, Konishi T, Izumoi S *et al.* Gastric cancer patients with paraaortic node metastasis who survived more than five years. *Jpn J Gastroenterol Surg* 1976; **9**: 112–16 (in Japanese with English abstract).

25. Nishi M & Ohta K. Rationalization and limit of gastric cancer surgery. In: Idezuki Y, Kawashima Y, Sugimachi K *et al.* (eds) *Surgery of the Stomach and the Duodenum IV*. Tokyo: Nakayama-Shoten 1987: 162–70 (in Japanese).

26. Nashimoto A, Sasaki T & Akai S. A study of lymphatic routes to the abdominal paraaortic lymph nodes and the significance of these lymph node dissection for advanced gastric cancer. *Jpn J Gastroenterol Surg* 1991; **16**: 1169–78 (in Japanese with English abstract).

27. Kitamura M, Arai K & Iwasaki Y. Clinico-pathological studies on paraaortic lymph node metastasis and post-operative quality of life in gastric cancer patients. *Jpn J Gastroenterol Surg* 1994; **27**: 2071–8 (in Japanese with English abstract).

28. Takahashi S, Tokuda H, Matsushige H *et al.* Evaluation of super extensive lymph node dissection (R4) for advanced gastric cancer. In: Takahashi T (ed.) *Recent Advances in Management of Digestive Cancers*. Tokyo: Springer-Verlag 1993: 297–9.

29. Takahashi S. Study of paraaortic lymph node metastasis of gastric cancer subjected to superextensive lymph node dissection. *Jpn J Gastroenterol Surg* 1990; **91**: 29–35 (in Japanese with English abstract).

30. Aiko T, Hokita S, Saihara T *et al.* Indication and long-term results in treatment of gastric cancer with paraaortic lymph node metastasis. *Rinshougeka* 1991; **46**: 1075–82 (in Japanese).

31. Bonenkamp JJ, Songun I, Hermans J *et al.* Randomised comparison of morbidity after D1 and D2 dissection for gastric cancer in 996 Dutch patients. *Lancet* 1995; **345**: 745–8.

32. Cuschieri A, Fayers P, Fielding J *et al.* Postoperative morbidity and mortality after D1 and D2 resections for gastric cancer: preliminary results of MRC randomised controlled surgical trial. *Lancet* 1996; **347**: 995–9.

33. Sano T, Okuyama Y, Kobori O *et al.* Early gastric cancer – Endoscopic diagnosis of depth of invasion. *Digest Dis Sci* 1990; **35**: 1340–4.

34. Maki T, Shiratori K, Ono H *et al.* Pylorus preserving gastrectomy as an improved operation for gastric ulcer. *Surgery* 1967; **61**: 838–45.

35. Sasako M for the Dutch Gastric Cancer Study Group. Risk factors of surgical treatment for gastric cancer in Dutch patients – Analysis of morbidity and hospital mortality in the Dutch gastric cancer trial. *Br J Surg* 1997; **84**: 1567–71.

36. Sasako M, Kinoshita T & Maruyama K. Prognosis of early gastric cancer. *Stomach and Intestine*

1993; **28**: 139–46 (in Japanese with English abstract).

37. Mine M, Majima S, Haraden M *et al.* End results of gastrectomy for gastric cancer: effect of extensive lymph node dissection. *Surgery* 1970; **68**: 753–8.

38. Suehiro S, Nagasue N, Abe S *et al.* Carcinoma of the stomach in atomic bomb survivors. A comparison of clinico-pathologic features to the general population. *Cancer* 1986; **57**: 1894–8.

39. Imanaga H & Nakazato H. Results of surgery for gastric cancer and effect of adjuvant mitomycin C on cancer recurrence. *World J Surg* 1977; **1**: 213–21.

40. Yamada E, Miyaishi S, Nakazato H *et al.* The surgical treatment of cancer of the stomach. *Int Surg* 1980; **65**: 387–99.

41. Nagata, T, Ikeda M & Nakayama F. Changing state of gastric cancer in Japan: histologic perspective of the past 76 years. *Am J Surg* 1983; **145**: 226–33.

42. Nakajima T, Ota K, Ishihara S *et al.* Progress of treatment of gastric cancer in Cancer Institute Hospital. *Jpn J Cancer Chemother* 1994; **21**: 1734–44.

43. Sowa M, Kato Y, Nakanishi I *et al.* Total gastrectomy - with special reference to anastomotic failure following total gastrectomy for gastric cancer. *Gekachiryou* 1992; **66**: 125–30 (in Japanese).

44. Soga J, Ohyama S, Suzuki T *et al.* Carcinomas involving the esophagogastric junction. *Int Surg* 1990; **75**: 205–7.

45. Sasako M. Gastric cancer. In: Hojo K (ed.) *Complications and its Management after Cancer Surgery of the Digestive Tract.* Tokyo: Kanehara 1990: 39–53 (in Japanese).

46. Registration Committee of the Japanese Research Society for Gastric Cancer & Miwa Gastric Cancer Registration Center. Vol 20, Report of end results of gastric cancer patients from National Registration. Tokyo: National Cancer Center Press, 1986.

47. Pachter HL, Pennington R, Chassin J *et al.* Simplified distal pancreatectomy with the Auto Suture stapler: preliminary clinical observations. *Surgery* 1979; **85**: 166–70.

48. Sasako M, Kinoshita T & Maruyama K. Distal pancreatectomy using staplers. *Shujutu* 1991; **45**: 1133–7 (in Japanese).

49. Takagi M. Pancreatic duct occlusion by Ethibloc® after distal pancreatectomy. *Shujutu* 1989; **43**: 267–71 (in Japanese).

50. Arai K. Studies on leakage of pancreatic juice following distal pancreatectomy from the standpoint of transition of amylase and trypsin values in exudate. *Jpn J Gastroenterol Surg* 1994; **95**: 56–65 (in Japanese with English abstract).

51. Sano T, Sasako M, Katai H *et al.* Amylase concentration of drainage fluid after total gastrectomy. *Br J Surg* 1997; **84**: 1310–12.

52. Hölscher AH, Bollschweiler E & Siewert JR. Carcinoma of the cardia. *Ann Chirurg Gynecol* 1995; **84**: 185–92.

53. Okamura T, Korenaga D, Baba H *et al.* Thoracoabdominal approach for cure of patients with an adenocarcinoma in the upper third of the stomach. *Am Surg* 1989; **55**: 248–51.

54. Tanigawa N, Shimomatsuya T, Horiuchi T *et al.* En bloc resection for cancer of the gastric cardia without thoracotomy. *J Surg Oncol* 1993; **54**: 23–8.

55. Kawaura Y, Mori Y, Nakajima H *et al.* Total gastrectomy with left oblique abdominothoracic approach for gastric cancer involving the esophagus. *Arch Surg* 1988; **123**: 514–18.

56. Husemann B. Cardia carcinoma considered as a distinct clinical entity. *Br J Surg* 1989; **76**: 136–9.

57. Takeshita K, Ashikawa T, Tani M *et al.* Clinicopathological features of gastric cancer infiltrating the lower oesophagus. *World J Surg* 1994; **18**: 428–32.

58. Arai K, Kitamura M & Iwasaki Y. Rational lymph node dissection for upper third gastric cancer with oesophageal invasion. *Jpn J Gastroenterol Surg* 1994; **27**: 1899–1903 (in Japanese with English abstract).

59. Hashimoto K & Kakegawa T. Left thoracoabdominal approach for gastric cancer with oesophageal invasion. *Gastroenterol Surg* 1992; **15**: 1611–19 (in Japanese).

60. Kajiyama Y, Tusrumaru M, Udagawa H *et al.* Prognostic factors in adenocarcinoma of the gastric cardia: pathologic stage analysis and multivariate regression analysis. *J Clin Oncol* 1997; **15**: 2015–21.

61. Shone DN, Nikoomanesh P, Smith-Meek MM *et al.* Malignancy is the most common cause of gastric outlet obstruction in the era of H2 blockers. *Am J Gastroenterol* 1995; **90**: 1769–70.

62. Sasako M, Maruyama K, Katai H *et al.* Is palliative gastrectomy for linitis plastica effective? *Gastroenterol Surg* 1996; **19**: 1445–52 (in Japanese).

6

COMBINED MODALITY THERAPY

DAVID KELSEN

INTRODUCTION

Only 50–60% of all newly diagnosed patients with gastric cancer can undergo potentially curative resections. While the resection rate among asymptomatic, screened Japanese patients is higher (approximately 85–95%), even in Japan, many patients are not part of screening programs, and may be found to have more advanced cancers. For any patient, following resection, the risk of recurrence is directly related to stage. Patients with tumor penetration through the gastric wall (T3 or T4), or lymph node metastasis are at particularly high risk for subsequent failure. Whether or not the cure rate is affected by the type of operation performed (especially the extent of lymph node dissection, D1 versus D2) is controversial. Even patients undergoing more extensive node dissections are at substantial risk for failure. This chapter will review currently available data for the use of postoperative chemotherapy, used either alone or with immunotherapy, and more recent investigational studies involving either preoperative (neoadjuvant) chemotherapy or postoperative intraperitoneal chemotherapy. Some of these trials have also employed pre- or postoperative radiation therapy, more recently with concurrent chemotherapy.

FAILURE PATTERN

Complete resection of all gross disease with negative margins on histologic review is the mainstay for potentially curative therapy for gastric carcinomas. The reason for proposing adjuvant therapy (either pre- or postoperatively) in this disease is the high distant failure rate, as well as a significant risk for local recurrence with any single modality.

Knowing the most likely sites of recurrence helps in planning the best strategy for a patient with resected (or resectable) gastric cancer. Using systemic therapy is a rational approach for tumors with a high likelihood for systemic failure with or without local recurrence. Neoadjuvant chemotherapy (also known as preoperative or primary chemotherapy) is an attractive concept in gastric cancer, since curative resection of the primary tumor is often difficult or impossible, and systemic metastases are common. The failure pattern for gastric cancer has been studied both by second-look laparotomies and, perhaps less usefully, by autopsies. The most important data came from patients who had undergone potentially curative resection.

Gunderson and Sosin reviewed a series of second-look laparotomies which had been performed at the University of Minnesota during the period 1949–1971.[51] Most patients who underwent a second procedure had had lymph node metastases at initial operation. While 39 patients had symptoms strongly suggestive of recurrent disease (thus not truly fitting the criteria for "second-look" laparotomy), most were asymptomatic. It should be recognized that the incidence of extra-abdominal disease reported in this series probably substantially underestimates the real incidence, since second-look laparotomies were not performed in a patient who has obvious extra-abdominal cancer. In this respect, autopsy series may offer a better reflection of the incidence of extra-abdominal failure. In autopsy and the University of Minnesota series, regional relapse for gastric cancer was usually defined as tumor in perigastric tissues (e.g., in the retroperitoneal "gastric bed," perigastric lymph nodes, gastric remnant). The most common metastatic sites in both types of reviews were lymph nodes within the abdomen, the liver, or the peritoneal surface. Overall, peritoneal or hepatic recurrence was an extremely common finding. Extra-abdominal disease was seen in approximately 20–40% of patients, with no single organ system being distinctly at higher risk. In two autopsy series, the rate of local regional failure following potentially curative resection was 40–80%.[2,3]

Theoretical rationale for neoadjuvant therapy

The rationale for neoadjuvant chemotherapy has been reviewed.[4] Primary chemotherapy can cause early tumor regression, thus improving local control rates after subsequent surgery and/or radiation. For some tumors, organ conservation may be possible following chemotherapy (usually given with radiation). Finally, responding patients may benefit from subsequent (postoperative) chemotherapy. Negative factors include the potential that early use of systemic treatment allows resistant tumor cell clones to develop. There may be a delay in local control measures and, if the response is substantial, there may be uncertainty as to how extensive a resection is appropriate. Occasionally, responding patients may refuse curative surgery or radiation. Importantly, neoadjuvant chemotherapy can mount a simultaneous assault on both distant metastases and the primary tumor, and can be employed when the patient is best able to tolerate potential toxicities.

However, since the chemotherapy currently used in gastric cancer has substantial toxicities, the ability to identify before an operation patients with a good chance of cure with surgery alone, as opposed to those in whom a multimodality approach would be reasonable, would be valuable.

SELECTING PATIENTS FOR ADJUVANT THERAPY

The TNM staging system for gastric tumors is based on depth of penetration through the bowel wall, the presence or absence of regional nodal metastasis, and the presence of distant metastasis. Patients at especially high risk for recurrence have TNM stage T 3–4,N any M 0 tumors (stage II, IIIa, or IIIb). For example, even patients without nodal metastases (T3N0 gastric cancers) have at least a 50% chance of dying within 5 years, and those with lymph node metastases have an even more ominous prognosis. Most (70–80%) American patients are at high risk; even so, the preoperative identification of low-risk patients is difficult. In selected areas of Japan, up to 30–40% of all newly diagnosed gastric cancer patients have stage Ia or Ib cancers (T1–2N0–1M0).[4,5] Cure rates with surgery alone for these patients are high (>80% for 5-year survival).[6] Unfortunately, only a small proportion (10–20%) of newly diagnosed American gastric cancer patients have such early-stage disease. If a neoadjuvant approach is employed, sparing patients who have an excellent outcome with surgery alone from the potential toxicities of chemotherapy or chemotherapy plus radiation is important. Most preoperative screening tests, including computed tomography (CT) or magnetic resonance imaging (MRI) scans of the abdomen and chest, do not accurately stage the depth of tumor invasion (T stage), nor do they accurately identify regional nodal involvement (N stage). Two other techniques may be more useful. Endoscopic ultrasonography (EUS) has been shown to be more accurate in assessing T stage, and shows promise for improving staging of nodal disease. More recently, laparoscopy and laparoscopic ultrasound have been shown to be additional techniques to select high-risk patients who still are potentially curable. Positron emission tomography (PET) scans, while promising, are more experimental.

Postoperative adjuvant chemotherapy

The conventional approach to adjuvant therapy (especially for patients with gastric cancer) is to use postoperative treatment.

Adjuvant therapy should be considered to be additional treatment for patients who have already undergone potentially curative therapy. For gastric cancer, this means a surgical procedure in which all gross disease has been removed, no distant (M1) tumor was present, and the margins of resection are negative. As noted above, curative resections are possible in only a relatively small number of patients with gastric cancer: several recent large surgical series indicated that only 30–50% of patients with gastric cancer undergoing exploration have a potentially curative resection.[7,8] The other 50–70% either have unresectable disease or have a palliative resection of the primary, leaving behind either gross tumor or microscopically positive margins. If gross residual gastric cancer or positive margins are left behind, postoperative therapy should not be considered as adjuvant treatment.

Timing of postoperative adjuvant therapy

The time from surgery to the start of postoperative therapy varies widely. In some centers, especially in Japan, postoperative treatment (if employed) for gastric cancer patients begins immediately after surgery. In the United States, treatment usually starts 4–6 weeks after resection. Sound theoretical reasons exist for initiating adjuvant therapy very soon after resection. Studies such as those by Fisher et al.[9] showing an increased labeling index of metastasis following resection of the primary (suggesting a potential for increased cell kill) have led some investigators to emphasize that adjuvant treatment should begin immediately per- or postoperatively.[9,10] A biologic explanation for this phenomenon may be the observations of Folkman and colleagues,[11] who identified antiangiogenesis substances secreted by primary tumors. It is possible that resection of the primary causes a sharp drop in circulating antiangiogenesis proteins, allowing metastatic sites to develop an adequate blood supply and to enlarge and spread. With any mechanism of tumor progression, delays of 4–8 weeks following surgery may allow metastases to grow to the point where eradication is much more difficult, or impossible.

Data developed from several animal models suggest that the risks of peritoneal implantation and of intra-abdominal tumor dissemination following laparotomy are high.[12,13] Therefore, particularly with intraperitoneal chemotherapy, a strong theoretical rationale exists for immediate postoperative treatment.

DOES CHEMOTHERAPY CHANGE OUTCOME IN PATIENTS WITH ADVANCED DISEASE?

Before discussing the data currently available for adjuvant chemotherapy in gastric cancer, it may be useful to review recent studies which examined the effectiveness of chemotherapy in the palliative setting. While many Phase II trials have demonstrated that systemic chemotherapy can cause tumor regression, and Phase III studies have compared one type of chemotherapy with another, there has been considerable controversy as to whether any chemotherapy treatment for gastric cancer offered either a survival or quality of life advantage over best supportive care. If systemic therapy, compared with the natural history of gastric cancer in untreated patients, was ineffective, its role in increasing the cure rate when used in the adjuvant setting would be weakened.

Data from four random assignment trials in which patients with advanced incurable gastric cancer began therapy with supportive care only, or received systemic chemotherapy at time of study entrance are shown in **Table 6.1**. In one of these studies (no. 3), a crossover from best supportive care to chemotherapy soon after study entrance occurred in a number of patients. While several of these trials have relatively small numbers of patients (which is understandable considering the type of randomization to a treatment or no treatment arm) the results are strikingly similar. Patients randomly assigned to best supportive care had a median duration of survival of 3–4 months in studies in which no rapid crossover was allowed. One-year survival was seen in only 5–10% of patients and, when reported, no 2-year survivors were seen for those randomized to best supportive care. Patients beginning treatment with systemic chemotherapy had a clinically and statistically significantly longer median duration of survival. Perhaps more importantly, the 1-year survival rate was 35–40%, and some patients (5–10%) were alive at 2 years. This type of data indicates that systemic chemotherapy, even when using regimens with modest effectiveness, can have a substantial effect on the natural history of gastric cancer. These findings, plus those from other solid tumors such as breast cancer or colorectal cancer, support the concept of systemic chemotherapy as an integral part of combined modality therapy for high-risk patients with gastric cancer.

Table 6.1 Gastric cancer. Chemotherapy for advanced disease: treatment versus best supportive care (BSC)

STUDY NO.	REGIMEN	NO. OF PATIENTS	MEDIAN SURVIVAL (MONTHS)	SURVIVAL RATE (%)	
				1-YEAR	2-YEAR
1.	FAMTX	30	10	40	6
	BSC	10	3	10	0
2.	FAMTX	17	12	NS	NS
	BSC	19	3	NS	NS
3.	E(top)LF	10	10	NS	NS
	BSC	8	4	NS	NS
4.	E(pirub)LF	52	10.2	34.6	9.6
	BSC	51	5	7.8	0

Modified from Ref. 14.
FAMTX, fluorouracil, doxorubicin, methotrexate; FEMTX, fluorouracil, epirubicin, methotrexate; E (top) LF – eptoside, leucovorin; fluorouracil; E (pirub) LF – epirubicin, leucovorin, fluorouracil; BSC – best supportive care
NS, not specified.

POSTOPERATIVE ADJUVANT THERAPY REGIMENS

The results of selected prospective random assignment trials in gastric cancer, some of which date back to the 1960s, are summarized in **Table 6.2**.

Two early Veteran's Administration Study Group (VASOG) trials investigated the use of single agent thiotepa or of 5-fluorodeoxyuridine (FUdR) after surgical resection,[15,16] though neither demonstrated a treatment benefit.

Nitrosurea-containing adjuvant regimens

Four studies have used chemotherapy combinations which included 5-fluorouracil (5-FU) and the nitrosourea methyl-CCNU following gastric resection. Interestingly, 5-FU and methyl-CCNU had only minimal effectiveness in patients with advanced cancer, and the combination was an inferior arm in a random assignment trial. The Gastrointestinal Tumor Study Group (GITSG) assigned patients following surgery to receive either no additional treatment or to 18 months (originally 2 years) of methyl-CCNU and 5-FU.[17] In the initial GITSG report, a trend for improved overall survival for the chemotherapy arm was noted ($P = 0.07$). While the difference in survival distribution eventually reached statistical significance, still in favor of the chemotherapy arm, a second

study with an identical design using 5-FU and methyl-CCNU was used by the Eastern Cooperative Oncology Group (ECOG). In a slightly larger group of 180 patients (89 control, 91 treated), no significant differences in disease-free or overall survival were seen (median survival 32.7 and 36.6 months and 2-year survival rate 57% for both groups).[18] A third study by the Veteran's Administration Surgical Oncology Group (VASOG), used the same agents on a different schedule; this was also a negative trial.[19]

More recently, Estrada *et al.*[20] added doxorubicin to methyl-CCNU and 5-FU in a small group of 66 evaluable patients. Of these patients, 31 received 12–18 months of adjuvant chemotherapy, while 35 patients were followed expectantly. At 5 years there was no difference in disease-free (29% treated versus 34% observed) or overall survival rate (29% versus 37%). There were two treatment-related deaths. A fifth study used a different nitrosurea, BCNU, plus 5-FU. Again, no improvement in survival was noted in comparison with those patients undergoing resection alone. Since methyl-CCNU has a small but definite increased risk of inducing acute non-lymphocytic leukemia, and since there is a lack of confirmed adjuvant efficacy for the combination, use of 5-FU and methyl-CCNU as adjuvant treatment for gastric cancer is not appropriate.

Table 6.2 Gastric cancer. Adjuvant therapy: selected Phase III trials

REFERENCE	REGIMEN	NO. OF PATIENTS	MEDIAN SURVIVAL	5-YEAR SURVIVAL RATE (%)
Allum et al.[23]	Mito-FU	141	16 months	28
	Mito-FU CMFV	140	16 months	10
	Control	130	15 months	18
Nakajima et al.[24]	Mito-FU-AraC	81	>5 years	68
	Mito-UFT-AraC	83	>5 years	63
	Control	79	>5 years	51
Panettiere et al.[53]	FAM	83	32 months	NS
	Control	93	28 months	NS
Coombes et al.[25]	FAM	133	NS	46
	Control	148	NS	35
GITSG[17]	MeCCNU-FU	71	56 months	50
	Control	71	33 months	31
ECOG[18]	MeCCNU-FU	91	33 months	57
	Control	89	37 months	57
VASOG[19]	MeCCNU-FU	66	2.1 years	39
	Control	68	2.2 years	38
Estape et al.[21]	Mitomycin	33	Not reached	76
	Control	37	12 months	30
Carrato et al.[22]	Mito-UFT	69	2.3 years	NS
	Control	75	2.6 years	NS

A, doxorubicin LE; araC, cytosine arabinoside; FU, 5-fluorouracil; Mito, mitomycin C; MeCCNU, methyl CCNU; NS, not specified; UFT, uracil, ftorafur.

Mitomycin-containing regimens

Many trials, including Japanese studies, have used mitomycin, an anti-tumor antibiotic. One Spanish study included high-dose mitomycin C alone following surgical resection.[21] Mitomycin C $(20 \, mg/m^2)$ was given once every 6 weeks for four doses. In this small trial (only 33 patients received chemotherapy and 37 comprised a control group), a striking difference in survival was noted (seven relapses in the treated arm, 23 in the control arm; $P < 0.001$). A 1991 update continues to show a significant survival advantage for the mitomycin-treated group.[21] However, a larger study also involving mitomycin reached an opposite conclusion. In a preliminary report, 144 evaluable patients were randomized after gastrectomy to receive (within seven days of surgery) mitomycin C $(10 \, mg/m^2)$ monthly for six doses plus oral UFT or to expectant observation.[22] Sixty-nine patients received chemotherapy and 75 were in the control arm. With a median follow-up of 3 years, there was no difference in disease-free or overall survival (median survival for chemotherapy patients was 2.3 years, and

for observation 2.6 years). In comparing these two studies, it should be noted that although the total dose in the second trial was similar $(80 \, mg/m^2$ versus $60 \, mg/m^2)$, the dose intensity was different.

Allum et al.[23] performed a three-arm random assignment trial including a mitomycin arm. Postoperative 5-FU and mitomycin C with or without cyclophosphamide, 5-FU, vincristine, and methotrexate induction were compared with surgery alone. The study allowed treatment to begin as late as 12 weeks after surgery, while the design called for 2 years of chemotherapy. This mature study (median follow-up of 100 months), found an overall median survival of 15.5 months, with no significant differences between the treated or control groups.

Japanese studies involving mitomycin have also been reported. Nakajima et al.[24] treated a group of 243 patients with either mitomycin C, 5-FU, and cytosine arabinoside, or a similar regimen in which 5-FU was replaced by Ftorafur, an oral compound. Control patients had surgery alone. While there was a trend for better outcome for chemotherapy patients ($P = 0.09$), there was no significant differences in overall 5-year survival. A subgroup analysis found a significant improvement in survival for treated patients with earlier-stage disease (stages I and II), but these were retrospective (unplanned) analyses.

Doxorubicin-containing regimens

Doxorubicin-containing combination chemotherapy regimens have also undergone extensive study, with some trials also including mitomycin. Coombes et al.[25] reported the results of a study in which patients who had undergone potentially curative resection were randomized to receive 5-FU, doxorubicin, and mitomycin (FAM) or no postoperative therapy. Some 281 patients were evaluable, with adjuvant chemotherapy being started up to 6 weeks after surgery. In total, 133 patients were randomized to FAM and 148 to the control arm. With a median follow-up of over 5 years, there was no significant difference in overall survival rates: (FAM 45.7%, control 35.4%). Several subgroup analyses were performed. Patients with T3 or T4 tumors and positive lymph nodes who received adjuvant therapy had a better survival ($P = 0.07$ in favor of the FAM group). Three chemotherapy patients died from suspected treatment-related complications. In a second FAM study, the Southwest Oncology Group also found no advantage to adjuvant treatment with this regimen.[26] Both groups of investigators concluded that FAM adjuvant chemotherapy should be considered investigational.

Krook et al.[27] used a different doxorubicin-containing combination. After curative resection, 125 evaluable patients were randomized to either observation alone ($n = 64$) or to three cycles of 5-FU ($350 \, mg/m^2/day$) for five days plus doxorubicin ($40 \, mg/m^2$). Three cycles of therapy were given, with treatment able to be started up to 6 weeks following resection. There were no differences in overall survival between the two groups [median 31 months (observation) versus 36 months (treated)], while 5-year survival rates were almost identical (33% versus 32%). Two treatment-related deaths were reported, both due to neutropenic sepsis. Recently, Neri et al.[28] reported a significant benefit to an epirubicin-containing chemotherapy regimen in treatment of patients with stage III disease. In this trial, patients having undergone potentially curative surgery (with either a D1 or D2

resection) who were found to have lymph node metastases were randomly assigned to expectant observation or to receive epirubicin–5-FU–leucovorin adjuvant chemotherapy. Patients could enter the study between the fourth and sixth week after surgery, and chemotherapy was given for 7 months. Some 103 patients were randomized, 55 to observation and 48 to receive chemotherapy. The two arms were well balanced for site of the primary, T stage and N stage tumors, and most patients had undergone a D1 resection. The median survival ($P < 0.01$) for patients randomly assigned to observation was 13.6 months, while for those undergoing adjuvant therapy it was 20.4 months ($P = 0.01$). Hepatic metastases were the most common site of recurrence. After 36 months of follow-up, 25% of patients receiving adjuvant therapy were alive compared with 13% of those undergoing expectant observation. Especially in view of the lack of benefit seen in the trial by Krook et al.,[28] these encouraging results require a larger confirmatory trial.

Several large-scale phase III randomized studies are now under way investigating new regimens in the post- or perioperative setting for patients with gastric cancer. The European Organization for Research and Treatment of Cancer (EORTC-40905) has completed a trial comparing postoperative FAMTX (high-dose 5-FU and methotrexate plus doxorubicin) versus no additional therapy after potentially curative resection. This large study has a projected accrual in excess of 700 patients. A second study performed by the MRC in the United Kingdom uses perioperative therapy with epirubicin, cisplatin and 5-FU versus operation alone for patients with resectable disease. The study design involves both pre- and postoperative chemotherapy. A total of 500 patients are planned for study entrance. The EORTC study will clarify the role of postoperative therapy using a "second-generation" regimen with a higher response rate than seen in some earlier chemotherapy treament plans. The MRC study, like the U.S. trials discussed below, will involve neoadjuvant and postoperative chemotherapy.

CHEMOTHERAPY PLUS CONCURRENT RADIATION

The strategy of increasing local control with chemotherapy plus concurrent radiation, has also undergone Phase III trial, as has a single study of postoperative radiation without chemotherapy. Dent et al.[29] treated 142 patients, randomly assigned to either no additional therapy or to 2000 cGy given in eight treatment fractions over 10 days plus 5-FU daily for four days immediately prior to radiation. A second cycle of 5-FU was given on day 28. In this study, some patients had incomplete resections, presumably with positive margins, though the others in this subgroup ("Division One") had curative resections. In this small trial, 31 patients were in the control group and 35 in the chemotherapy/radiation group, and there was no difference in overall survival between the two groups. Indeed, the control arm had a slight survival advantage.

In a second small chemotherapy-radiotherapy trial, Moertel and co-workers[30] treated a group of 62 curatively resected patients who received either no additional treatment or 5-FU plus radiation therapy. No patients had residual cancer. Therapy was initiated from 4–10.5 weeks postoperatively. This trial used a pre-randomization design, with 39 patients randomized to treatment and 23 to control. Some 23% of those randomized to chemoradiotherapy were long-term survivors, compared with only 4% of control patients ($P = 0.052$). However, some patients randomized to chemoradiation refused treatment, and 30% of these were alive at 5 years. On the basis of these two small studies, the usefulness of radiation therapy plus 5-FU remains open to question, and is the subject of a current USA national intergroup trial, Intergroup 116. This study has completed accrual.

Postoperative radiation

Hallissey et al.[31] reported the outcome of a study in which patients with locally advanced but resectable gastric cancer underwent no treatment after operation, received postoperative chemotherapy, or were assigned to undergo postoperative radiation therapy. Some patients with stage IV resected disease were allowed entrance into this trial and comprised approximately one-third of all patients. The chemotherapy involved a modified FAM regimen. A total radiation therapy dose of 4500 cGy in 25 fractions was delivered. Although a 500 cGy boost was allowed, it was rarely employed. After a 5-year follow-up, there were no significant differences between any of the three arms.

Intraperitoneal chemotherapy

Since peritoneal failure is so common, the use of postoperative intraperitoneal (IP) chemotherapy has been extensively studied. The pharmacokinetic advantages of IP chemotherapy have been well described.[32] In addition, Sugarbaker et al.[33] and others have reviewed the theoretical advantages of immediate postoperative IP therapy. Preclinical models also support IP therapy.[12,13] Clinically, Sugarbaker and colleagues treated a small group of patients with colon cancer with either intravenous or IP treatment, and demonstrated a change in the failure pattern with a marked decrease in peritoneal metastasis with intraperitoneal chemotherapy when compared with intravenous treatment. However, there was no survival advantage to IP therapy.[34] Recently, the Gynecological Oncology Group (GOG) published the results of a large-scale trial in women with ovarian cancer who had undergone resection with minimal residual disease.[35] In this trial, all patients received intravenous chemotherapy using cyclophosphamide. Patients were then randomized to receive either intravenous or IP cisplatin chemotherapy. In this trial, a significant survival advantage was seen for women who received part of their therapy intraperitoneally versus all their treatment intravenously, thus supporting the concept of regional IP treatment in diseases in which peritoneal recurrence is a common event.

These observations in gastrointestinal and other malignancies have led to similar studies in gastric cancer. Both Western and Japanese investigators have explored the role of intraperitoneal treatment using a variety of regimens.

Atiq et al.,[36] at the Memorial Sloan-Kettering Cancer Center, treated 35 patients who had undergone resection of all visible disease, using intraperitoneal cisplatin and 5-FU plus systemic 5-FU. The majority of patients had stage IIIA or IIIB tumors, and received IP cisplatin ($25 mg/m^2$) and 5-FU ($750 mg/m^2$) during days 1–4, plus concurrent systemic 5-FU as a 96-h infusion for a planned five cycles. Each cycle was given once monthly. With a median follow-up of 42 months, 40% of patients were alive and free of disease. While in general toxicity was acceptable, an unusual side effect of sclerosing encapsulating peritonitis was noted in 15% of patients. Additional studies performed by the same investigators revealed that solutions containing 5-FU had a pH >8.5. In the initial trial, cisplatin and 5-FU were mixed in the same container prior to IP instillation. The authors speculated that this resulted in hydrolysis of cisplatin to a reactive alkylating species. In order to avoid sclerosing peritonitis, subsequent patients received IP cisplatin and 5-FU in separate solutions, and no further episodes of SEP were seen.

Several small Phase III trials of IP therapy for gastric cancer have been reported. Kaibara et al.[37] used hyperthermic peritoneal perfusion for high-risk gastric cancer patients with mitomycin C as the cytotoxic agent, therapy being given immediately after resection. Some 42 patients received IP treatment, while 40 underwent resection alone. Overall, a trend to improved survival was seen, though this did not reach statistical significance (64.3% for IP therapy versus 52.5% for the control group). Peritoneal recurrence was seen more frequently in the control group. Hagiwara et al.[38] also used IP mitomycin C following curative resection in high-risk patients. In their study, mitomycin C adsorbed to a carbon-containing solution was infused at the end of the operative procedure. Twenty-four patients received mitomycin, and 25 were followed expectantly following surgery. In this trial, all patients had tumors which infiltrated the serosa. A highly significant difference in favor of the intraperitoneal treated group was reported (2-year survival rate 68.6% versus 26.9%; this difference was maintained at 3 years).

Schiessel et al.[39] used IP cisplatin alone in a group of 31 patients, though this was not a truly adjuvant study as some patients had only palliative resections, with gross residual tumor. Thirty-three other patients were randomized to receive no additional therapy after surgery. IP therapy was begun within 4 weeks of therapy. While toxicity was acceptable, there was no survival advantage for the IP group.

Sautner et al.[40] performed a similar random assignment Phase III trial, using IP cisplatin, in which 67 patients with gastric cancer were treated. Cisplatin ($90 \, mg/m^2$) was given intraperitoneally once monthly. Some patients in this trial had documented peritoneal metastases. There was no difference in survival between the two groups. While the authors concluded that IP cisplatin had no significant impact on recurrence, the inclusion of patients with advanced disease and small sample size limited the power of this study.

In summary, the strategy of using IP chemotherapy in the adjuvant setting has been demonstrated to be tolerable using several different regimens. Phase III trials reported to date have generally involved such small numbers of patients that the power to detect significant differences is quite weak. Furthermore, the chemotherapy regimens have varied substantially. Additional studies to better define the most effective IP regimen (including studies using new agents such as Paclitaxel), and most importantly, large-scale studies should be performed prior to making a definitive decision as to the role of this approach.

Immunochemotherapy

Adjuvant immunochemotherapy following curative resection of gastric cancer has been studied by both Japanese and Korean investigators. Several trials used a protein-bound polysaccharide extracted from *Coriolus versicolor* (PSK), either alone or combined with chemotherapy. PSK's mechanism of action is not fully understood. In most of these trials, patients in the control arm also received chemotherapy, though only a few trials had an observation-alone control arm. Nakazato et al.[41] treated 262 patients who received mitomycin C plus 5-FU (given by mouth) or the same chemotherapy plus PSK. Immunotherapy was given for 36 months. To enter the study, patients had to have a positive PPD. Both groups received up to ten cycles of chemotherapy. With a minimum follow-up of 5 years, a significant survival advantage was seen for patients given PSK: 70.7% of the PSK plus chemotherapy group versus 59.4% of those receiving chemotherapy alone were alive and disease-free at 5 years ($P = 0.047$). Ochiai and colleagues[42] compared chemotherapy with chemoimmunotherapy, using a *Nocardia rubra* cell wall skeleton extract. Both groups received chemotherapy, including mitomycin C, 5-FU, and cytosine arabinoside. Therapy was started immediately following surgery, with patients receiving mitomycin C on postoperative day 1. This was followed by weekly mitomycin C, 5-FU and cytosine arabinoside. Ninety patients were given chemotherapy alone, and 97 received chemoimmunotherapy. There was no difference in overall survival for those patients having had curative resections. A subgroup analysis of 71 patients who had had palliative resections was performed separately. A survival advantage was noted for patients receiving chemoimmunotherapy.

Korean investigators performed several studies of OK432 plus chemotherapy following potentially curative resection. In one trial,[43] chemotherapy (mitomycin C, 5-FU, and cytosine arabinoside) plus OK432 (a *Streptococcus pyogenes* preparation) was given to 74 patients; a control group of 64 patients underwent surgery alone. At 5 years, 44.6% of those receiving chemoimmunotherapy were alive, as opposed to 23.4% of those randomized to surgery only. In a follow-up study, resected patients were randomized to receive either immunotherapy with OK432 plus chemotherapy (mitomycin C and 5-FU),[43] chemotherapy alone, or expectant observation. At 5 years, 45.3% of the immunochemotherapy group were alive as opposed to 29.8% of the chemotherapy group, and 24.4% of the surgery only group.

In summary, these studies suggest that postoperative immunochemotherapy may decrease recurrence in patients with locally advanced but resected gastric cancer. The mechanism for action for this approach is not fully understood.

Hormonal therapy with tamoxifen

Harrison *et al.*[44] studied the use of hormonal therapy in 100 patients in a random assignment trial using tamoxifen as a single agent. Since this study allowed entrance of patients who had residual gross disease, it was also not truly adjuvant therapy. Some 55.8% of tumors were estrogen receptor-positive. There was no effect of tamoxifen on survival outcome; indeed, the control group did slightly better than those receiving hormonal therapy.

Neoadjuvant chemotherapy

The rationale for using chemotherapy preoperatively (neoadjuvant therapy) prior to attempted resection in high-risk gastric cancer patients has been discussed above. Several Phase II pilot studies have now been reported, and Phase III trials are planned. The following is a summary of selected Phase II and small-scale Phase III studies (**Table 6.3**).

Ajani *et al.*[45] studied 48 patients with potentially resectable gastric cancer. Three cycles of EAP (etoposide, adriamycin, cisplatin) chemotherapy were given prior to operation; two additional courses were planned postoperatively. Following chemotherapy, 85% of patients underwent operation; 77% had potentially curative resections. Toxicity (usually neutropenia) was substantial but generally manageable, although there was one chemotherapy-related death. The median duration of survival for all patients was 15.5 months. In a second study by the same group of investigators, Ajani *et al.*[46] used a similar regimen of cisplatin, 5-FU and etoposide (EFP). Five cycles (two preoperative and three postoperative courses) were planned. In total, 25 patients were treated, with one postoperative death. Some 72% of patients had potentially curative resections. The median duration of survival was similar to the first trial (15 months), though the authors noted that the most common site for recurrent disease was peritoneal carcinomatosis either found at surgery or developing subsequently.

Leichman *et al.*[47] treated 38 patients with resectable gastric tumors with two cycles of preoperative chemotherapy followed by surgery and IP postoperative treatment. 5-FU ($200\,mg/m^2$) per day

Table 6.3 Neoadjuvant therapy of gastric cancer: Phase II–III trials

REFERENCE	REGIMEN	NO. OF PATIENTS	OPERATION (%)	RESECTION (%)	MEDIAN SURVIVAL (MONTHS)	2-YEAR SURVIVAL RATE (%)
Ajani *et al.*[45]	EAP	48	85	77	16	42
Ajani *et al.*[46]	EFP	25	100	72	15	44
Leichman *et al.*[47]	FP-IP Rx	38	92	76	17+	NS
Kelsen *et al.*[48]	FAMTX-IP Rx	56	89	61	15	40
Ajani *et al.*[45,46]	FP-INF	30	90	80	16+	NS
Kang *et al.*[49]	EFP	53	89	71	33	55
	Control	54	100	61	32	55

EAP, etoposide, adriamycin, cisplatin; EFP, etoposide, fluorouracil, cisplatin, 5-FU, cisplatin; FAMTX, high-dose 5-fluorouracil and methotrexate plus doxorubicin; FP-INF, fluorouracil, cisplatin; IP, intraperitoneal; NS, not specified.

was given over 3 weeks with weekly intravenous leucovorin ($20\,mg/m^2$) and cisplatin ($100\,mg/m^2$) on postoperative day 1. After a 1-week break, a second course of treatment, also lasting 21 days, was given. After resection, IP therapy with FUdR ($3000\,mg$ total daily dose) for three days plus cisplatin ($200\,mg/m^2$) with intravenous sodium thiosulfate was given. Some 92% of patients underwent laparotomy, while 87% had resection. Among the study patients, 68% received postoperative IP therapy. There was one treatment-related death. The median survival had not been reached at 17+ months. However, this trial was not limited to high-risk patients, and pretreatment clinical staging was not provided. Postoperative staging showed 14 patients with either stage 0 (one patient) or stage I disease, while seven patients had stage II tumors.

Kelsen et al.[48] used preoperative FAMTX in 56 high-risk patients, with three cycles of FAMTX being given prior to operation, followed by IP chemotherapy using 5-FU and cisplatin with concurrent intravenous 5-FU. High-risk patients were defined as those with T3NanyM0 tumors, using endoscopic ultrasonography (EUS): most had stage IIIA or IIIB tumors. While toxicity in general was tolerable, myelosuppression was seen frequently. Neutropenic fever led to admission on at least one occasion in 60% of patients. In this study, efficacy was determined as change in EUS stage compared with pathologic stage; downstaging was shown in 51% of patients. The surgical outcome was defined as operability and resectability; operability rate was 89%, and resectability rate 81% (61% curative, 20% palliative). With a median follow-up of 28 months, the median duration of survival for all patients was 15.3 months; for those having curative resections, the median duration of survival was 31 months.

More recently, Kang et al.[49] reported the results of a small-scale Phase III random assignment trial comparing neoadjuvant therapy with cisplatin, etoposide and 5-FU versus surgery alone. As shown in **Table 6.3**, in this study the potentially curative resection rate was slightly higher for patients receiving neoadjuvant chemotherapy, but no differences in median or 2-year survival were seen at the time of the preliminary report.[49]

In summary, preoperative chemotherapy, given with or without postoperative treatment, is now undergoing study at a number of institutions in the United States. To date, none of these trials has shown an increase in operative morbidity or mortality. Antineoplastic activity resulting in downstaging has been suggested by EUS data, and by the higher than expected number of patients found at surgery to have stage I and II tumors. While promising, the strategy of using neoadjuvant chemotherapy requires definitive testing using adequately sized random assignment Phase III trials before firm conclusions regarding its value can be made. Multicenter Phase II pilot neoadjuvant therapy trials are now under way in the United States, and a Phase III study including GE junction patients is under way in the UK.

SUMMARY

Postoperative adjuvant chemotherapy has been studied in many random assignment trials, though, to date, there are no confirmed Western trials in which systemic (intravenous) adjuvant therapy has clearly increased the cure rate in resectable gastric cancers compared with expectant observation. While the trend toward improved survival seen in several of these trials is encouraging, a recent meta-analysis failed to demonstrate convincingly any benefit.[50] However, it should be noted that there are serious methodologic criticisms of many of these earlier trials, particularly in the delay in starting therapy and the use of less than optimal chemotherapy regimens. In addition, almost all Phase III gastric adjuvant trials have involved relatively small numbers of patients (<100–200 per arm), so that the power to detect clinically important differences in outcome is quite weak.

Several important trials, currently under way both in the United States and in Europe, use newer potentially more effective chemotherapy combinations with larger numbers of patients. Among these trials is an EORTC random assignment study of the FAMTX regimen versus observation only in the immediate postoperative period. The USA Intergroup trial compares chemotherapy and concurrent radiation with observation to decrease local and distant failure. Both studies plan to accrue substantially more patients than earlier trials.

Several other strategies are being tested. There are sound theoretical grounds for using immediate postoperative IP chemotherapy in patients with gastric cancer. Asian investigators have performed several Phase II and small Phase III studies using IP chemotherapy, with or without hyperthermia. These small trials suggest improvement in disease-free survival in patients with established peritoneal metastasis or in patients at high risk (T3 or T4) to have distant micrometastases. American investigators have also shown that postoperative IP chemotherapy is tolerable, and does not increase operative morbidity or mortality. Postoperative intraperitoneal therapy after neoadjuvant chemotherapy is undergoing study at several centers.

Neoadjuvant chemotherapy without any postoperative IP treatment is also being explored by several groups. Recent studies have shown that, with careful dose adjustment, toxicity is acceptable and that there is no increase in operative morbidity or mortality. An important goal for neoadjuvant therapy is to increase the number of potentially curative resections, since as noted above only half of those currently explored can be resected with negative margins and no visceral disease. The preliminary data from several of these trials is quite encouraging; however, until definitive Phase III studies accruing enough patients have been performed, it is too early to recommend neoadjuvant

therapy as a standard of care. Such a large-scale study is under way in the UK.

Finally, data from Asian investigators suggest that there is a role for chemoimmunotherapy in the treatment of patients with advanced gastric cancer. While the mechanism of action has not yet been defined, immunochemotherapy merits additional study.

These new approaches are encouraging, and entrance of patients with newly diagnosed gastric cancer into such investigational trials is strongly encouraged. For now, the standard of care in the United States has not yet changed. For patients with operable gastric cancer who have undergone careful staging as described above, operation alone remains the treatment of choice. Patients with positive microscopic margins or documented distant metastasis have a particularly dismal prognosis, and postoperative chemotherapy with or without radiation should be considered. An algorithm for care of operable patients and the role of adjuvant therapy is shown in **Figure 6.1**.

ACKNOWLEDGEMENTS

The author gratefully acknowledges the expert assistance of Adrienne Scodary in the preparation of the manuscript.

REFERENCES

1. Fein R, Kelsen DP, Geller N, Bains M, McCormack P & Brennan MF. Adenocarcinoma of the esophagus and gastroesophageal junction. Prognostic factors and results of therapy. *Cancer* 1995; **56**: 2512–18.

2. McNeer G, Vanderberg H, Donn F *et al*. A critical evaluation of subtotal gastrectomy for the cure of cancer of the stomach. *Ann Surg* 1951; **134**: 1–7.

3. Wisbeck WM, Becher EM & Russell AH. Adenocarcinoma of the stomach: autopsy observations with therapeutic implications for the radiation oncologist. *Radiother Oncol* 1986; **7**: 13–18.

4. Yamazaki H, Oshima A, Murakami R, Endoh S & Ubukata T. A long-term follow-up study of patients with gastric cancer detected by mass screening. *Cancer* 1989; **63**: 613–17.

5. Kaneki E, Nakamura T, Umeda N *et al*. Outcome of gastric carcinoma detected by gastric mass survey in Japan. *Gut* 1977; **18**: 626–30.

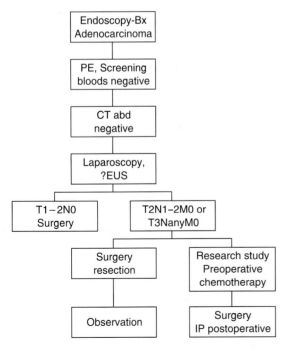

Figure 6.1 Gastric cancer treatment algorithm for locoregional disease. EUS, endoluminal ultrasonography.

6. Noguchi Y, Imada T, Matsumoto A, Coit DG & Brennan MF. Radical surgery for gastric cancer. A review of the Japanese experience. *Cancer* 1989; **64**: 2053–62.

7. Rohde H, Gebbensleben B, Bauer P, Stutzer H & Zieschang J. Has there been any improvement in the staging of gastric cancer? Findings from the German Gastric Cancer TNM Study Group. *Cancer* 1989; **64**: 2465–81.

8. Wanebo H, Kennedy BJ, Chmiel J, Steele G, Winchester D & Osteen R. Cancer of the stomach. A patient care study by the American College of Surgeons. *Ann Surg* 1993; **218**: 583–92.

9. Fisher B, Gunduz N & Saffer EA. Influence of the interval between primary tumor removal and chemotherapy on kinetics and growth of metastases. *Cancer Res* 1983; **43**: 1488–92.

10. Gunduz N, Fisher B & Saffer E. Effect of surgical removal on the growth and kinetics of residual tumor. *Cancer Res* 1979; **39**: 1361–5.

11. Ingber D, Fujita T, Kishimoto S *et al*. Synthetic analogues of fumagillin that inhibit angiogenesis and suppress tumor growth. *Nature* 1990; **348**: 555–7.

12. Eggermont AMM, Steller EP & Sugarbaker PH. Laparotomy enhances intraperitoneal tumor growth and abrogates the antitumor effects of interleukin-2 and lymphokine-activated killer cells. *Surgery* 1987; **102**: 71–8.

13. Murthy SM, Goldschmidt RA, Rao LN, Ammirati M, Buthmann T, Scanlon EF. The influence of surgical trauma on experimental metastasis. *Cancer* 1989; **64**: 2035–44.

14. Wils J. The treatment of advanced gastric cancer. *Seminars in Oncology* 1996; **23**: 397–406.

15. VA Cooperative Surgical Study Group. Use of thiotepa as an adjuvant to the surgical management of carcinoma of the stomach. *Cancer* 1965; **18**: 291–7.

16. Serlin O, Wolkoff J, Amandeo J *et al*. Use of the 5-fluorodeoxyuridine as an adjuvant to the surgical management of carcinoma of the stomach. *Cancer* 1969; **25**: 223–8.

17. Gastrointestinal Tumor Study Group. Controlled trial of adjuvant chemotherapy following curative resection for gastric cancer. *Cancer* 1982; **49**: 1116–22.

18. Engstrom PF, Lavin PT, Douglass HO, Jr & Brunner KW. Postoperative adjuvant 5-fluorouracil plus methyl-CCNU therapy for gastric cancer patients. Eastern Cooperative Oncology Group study (EST 3275). *Cancer* 1985; **55**: 1868–73.

19. Higgins GA, Amadeo JH, Smith DE, Humphrey EW & Keehn RJ. Efficacy of prolonged intermittent therapy with combined 5-FU and methyl-CCNU following resection for gastric carcinoma. A Veterans Administration Surgical Oncology Group report. *Cancer* 1983; **52**: 1105–12.

20. Estrada E, Lacave L, Valle M *et al*. Methyl-CCNU, 5-fluorouracil, and adriamycin (MeFA) as adjuvant chemotherapy in gastric cancer. *Proc Am Soc Clin Oncol* 1988; **7**: 94 (abstract).

21. Estape J, Grau JJ, Alcobendas F *et al*. Mitomycin C as an adjuvant treatment to resected gastric cancer. A 10-year follow-up. *Ann Surg* 1991; **213**: 219–21.

22. Carrato A, Diaz-Rubio E, Medrano J *et al*. Phase III trial of surgery versus adjuvant chemotherapy with mitomycin C and tegafur plus uracil, starting within the first week after surgery, for gastric adenocarcinoma. *Proc Am Soc Clin Oncol* 1995; **14**: 198 (abstract).

23. Allum WH, Hallissey MT & Kelly KA. Adjuvant chemotherapy in operable gastric cancer. 5 year follow-up of first British Stomach Cancer Group trial. *Lancet* 1989; **1**: 571–4.

24. Nakajima T, Takahashi T, Takagi K, Kuno K & Kajitani T. Comparison of 5-fluorouracil with ftorafur in adjuvant chemotherapies and combined inductive and maintenance therapies for gastric cancer. *J Clin Oncol* 1984; **2**: 1366–71.

25. Coombes RC, Schein PS, Chilvers CE *et al*. A randomized trial comparing adjuvant flourouracil, doxorubicin, and mitomycin with no treatment in operable gastric cancer. International Collaborative Cancer Group. *J Clin Oncol* 1990; **8**: 1362–9.

26. Gagliano R, McCracken J & Chen T. Adjuvant chemotherapy with FAM in gastric cancer: A SWOG study. *Proc Am Soc Clin Oncol* 1983; **2**: 1141 (abstract).

27. Krook JE, O'Connell MJ, Wieand HS *et al*. A prospective, randomized evaluation of intensive course 5-fluorouracil plus doxorubicin as a surgical adjuvant chemotherapy for resected gastric cancer. *Cancer* 1991; **67**: 2454–8.

28. Neri B, De Leonardis V, Romano S *et al*. Adjuvant chemotherapy after gastric resection in node-positive cancer patients: a multicentre randomised study. *Br J Cancer* 1996; **73**: 549–52.

29. Dent D, Werner I, Novis B *et al*. Prospective randomized trial of combined oncological therapy for gastric carcinoma. *Cancer* 1979; **44**: 385–91.

30. Moertel CG, Childs DS, O'Fallon JR, Holbrook MA, Schutt AJ & Reitemeier RJ. Combined 5-fluorouracil and radiation therapy as a surgical adjuvant for poor prognosis gastric carcinoma. *J Clin Oncol* 1984; **2**: 1249–54.

31. Hallissey MT, Dunn JA, Ward LC & Allum WH. The second British Stomach Cancer Group trial of adjuvant radiotherapy or chemotherapy in resectable gastric cancer: five-year follow-up. *Lancet* 1994; **343**: 1309–12.

32. Markman M. Intraperitoneal chemotherapy for malignant diseases of the gastrointestinal tract. *Surg Gynecol Obstet* 1987; **164**: 89–93.

33. Sugarbaker PH, Cunliffe WJ, Belliveau J *et al.* Rationale for integrating early postoperative intraperitoneal chemotherapy into the surgical treatment of gastrointestinal cancer. *Semin Oncol* 1989; **16**: 83–97.

34. Sugarbaker PH, Gianola FJ, Speyer JL, Wesley R, Barofsky I & Myers CE. Prospective randomized trial of intravenous versus intraperitoneal 5-FU in patients with advanced primary colon or rectal cancer. *Semin Oncol* 1985; **12**: 101–11.

35. Alberts DS, Liu PY, Hannigan EV *et al.* Intraperitoneal cisplatin plus intravenous cyclophosphamide versus intravenous cisplatin plus intravenous cyclophosphamide in stage III ovarian cancer. *N Engl J Med* 1996; **335**: 1950–3.

36. Atiq OT, Kelsen DP, Shiu MH *et al.* Phase II trial of postoperative adjuvant intraperitoneal cisplatin and fluorouracil and systemic fluorouracil chemotherapy in patients with resected gastric cancer. *J Clin Oncol* 1993; **11**: 425–33.

37. Kaibara N, Hamazoe R, Iitsuka Y, Maeta M & Koga S. Hyperthermic peritoneal perfusion combined with anticancer chemotherapy as prophylactic treatment of peritoneal recurrence of gastric cancer. *Hepatogastroenterology* 1989; **36**: 75–8.

38. Hagiwara A, Takahashi T, Kojima O *et al.* Prophylaxis with carbon-adsorbed mitomycin against peritoneal recurrence of gastric cancer. *Lancet* 1992; **339**: 629–31.

39. Schiessel R, Funovics J, Schick B *et al.* Adjuvant intraperitoneal cisplatin therapy in patients with operated gastric carcinoma: results of a randomized trial. *Acta Medica Austriaca* 1989; **16**: 68–9.

40. Sautner T, Hofbauer F, Depisch D, Schiessel R & Jakesz R. Adjuvant intraperitoneal cisplatin chemotherapy does not improve long-term survival after surgery for advanced gastric cancer. *J Clin Oncol* 1994; **12**: 970–4.

41. Nakazato H, Koike A, Saji S, Ogawa N & Sakamoto J. Efficacy of immunochemotherapy as adjuvant treatment after curative resection of gastric cancer. *Lancet* 1994; **343**: 1122–6.

42. Ochiai T, Sato H, Hayashi R *et al.* Randomly controlled study of chemotherapy versus chemoimmunotherapy in postoperative gastric cancer patients. *Cancer Res* 1983; **43**: 3001–7.

43. Kim JP, Kwon OJ, Oh ST & Yang HK. Results of surgery on 6589 gastric cancer patients and immunochemosurgery as the best treatment of advanced gastric cancer. *Ann Surg* 1992; **216**: 269–79.

44. Harrison JD, Morris DL, Ellis IO, Jones JA & Jackson I. The effect of tamoxifen and estrogen receptor status on survival in gastric carcinoma. *Cancer* 1989; **64**: 1007–10.

45. Ajani JA, Mayer RJ, Ota DM *et al.* Preoperative and postoperative combination chemotherapy for potentiall resectable gastric carcinoma. *J Natl Cancer Inst* 1993; **85**: 1839–44.

46. Ajani JA, Ota DM, Jessup JM *et al.* Resectable gastric carcinoma. An evaluation of preoperative and postoperative chemotherapy. *Cancer* 1991; **68**: 1501–6.

47. Leichman L, Silberman H, Leichman CG *et al.* Preoperative systemic chemotherapy followed by adjuvant postoperative intraperitoneal therapy for gastic cancer: a University of Southern California pilot program. *J Clin Oncol* 1992; **10**: 1933–42.

48. Kelsen D, Karpeh M, Schwartz G *et al.* Neoadjuvant and postoperative chemotherapy for high-risk gastric cancer. *Proc American Society of Clinical Oncology* 1994; **13**: A566 (Abstract).

49. Kang YK, Choi DW, Im YH *et al.* A phase III randomized comparison of neoadjuvant chemotherapy followed by surgery versus surgery for locally advanced stomach cancer. *Proc American of Clinical Oncology* 1996; 215 (Abstract).

50. Kelsen D, Ilson D, Minsky B, Lipton R. Phase I trial of combined modality therapy for localised esophageal cancer: radiation therapy plus concurrent cisplatin and escalating doses of 96 hour infusional paclitaxel. Proceedings of ASCO 1998; **17**: 260a (Abstract).

51. Gunderson LL, Sosin H. Adenocarcinoma of the stomach: areas of failure in a re-operation series (second or symptomatic look) clinicopathologic correlation and implications for adjuvant therapy. *Int J Radiat Oncol Biol Phys* 1992; **8**: 1–11.

52. Panettiere FJ, Haas C, McDonald B *et al.* Drug combinations in the treatment of gastric adenocarcinoma: a randomized Southwest Oncology Group Study. *J Clin Oncol* 1984; **2**: 420–4.

7
EARLY GASTRIC CANCER

J. RÜDIGER SIEWERT
ANDREAS SENDLER
KNUT BÖTTCHER

INTRODUCTION

Patients with gastric cancer have a collective crude 5-year survival rate of about 25–30%.[1,2] However, there is a subset of patients with an excellent prognosis; namely those patients with early gastric cancer who have, following appropriate treatment, a survival rate equivalent to that of healthy age-matched controls.[3,4] Despite the excellent outlook for this group of patients, questions remain regarding the diagnostic modalities, the optimal extent of gastric resection and lymphadenectomy, or the need for adjuvant treatment.[5]

Definition

The current definition of early gastric cancer (EGC) dates from the 1962 publication of the Japanese Society of Gastroenterological Endoscopy,[6] which specified adenocarcinoma of the stomach confined to the mucosa or submucosa irrespective of lymph node involvement. A tumor superficial to the muscularis propria with metastatically involved lymph nodes is still considered "early gastric cancer."

Classification

The pathologic identification of early gastric neoplasms dates back more than a century. In 1883, Hauser[7] described epithelial invasion limited to the muscularis mucosae on serial sections of a gastric carcinoma specimen. Versé presented a detailed description of the development of gastric adenomas and polyps and the association with carcinoma in a series of 10 000 autopsies. There were 12 patients who had gastric cancer confined to the mucosa.[8] In 1938, the Japanese surgeon Saeki[9] demonstrated the correlation between long-term survival and the histologic depth of tumor invasion. Among 202 patients who had a gastrectomy for tumor confined to the mucosa or submucosa, irrespective of regional lymph node involvement, there was a 91.5% survival rate. Before "early gastric cancer" was established as a distinct form of gastric carcinoma, it became apparent from retrospective studies in Japan that these patients had an excellent prognosis. The terms "superficial carcinoma," "le cancer de l'estomac au debut," or "Frühkarzinom" correspond to early gastric carcinoma of the Japanese classification.[4]

In 1963, to establish uniform criteria for the treatment of gastric carcinoma, the Japanese Society for Gastric Cancer issued "The general rules for gastric cancer study in surgery and pathology".[6] Differing from Borrmann's classification, which focuses on the different forms of invasiveness and is used in advanced gastric cancer, the classification rules of the Japanese Society are based on the growth appearance on the mucosal surface. Early gastric carcinomas are defined as those whose invasion is limited to either the mucosa or the submucosa irrespective of lymph node metastases. Basically, early gastric cancer is classified into three main types (**Figure 7.1**):

- **Type I:** protruded lesion, the tumor is a tall, nodular or polypoid lesion that often shows an irregular surface with crevices between papillary projections.

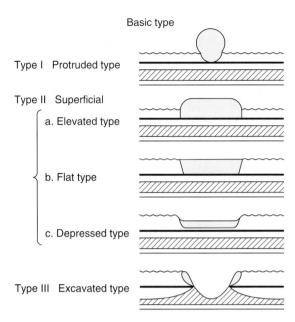

Basic type

Type I   Protruded type

Type II   Superficial

a. Elevated type

b. Flat type

c. Depressed type

Type III   Excavated type

Figure 7.1 Macroscopic classification of basic types of early gastric cancer.

- **Type II**: (superficial) carcinomas are further divided into three subtypes:
  - **i.** Type IIa: superficial and slightly elevated lesions consist of a slight elevation of the lesions approximately twice or greater the thickness of the mucosa up to 5 mm. Generally, the elevation of type IIA is less than twice the thickness of the adjacent mucosa.
  - **ii.** Type IIb: superficial and flat lesions are approximately at the level with the surrounding mucosa.
  - **iii.** Type IIc: superficial and slightly depressed lesions have a shallow depression. The depression is only erosion or ulcer-like, leaving a flattened mucosa layer on its base.
- **Type III:** excavated lesion, the malignant change surrounds an ulceration of variable depth.

A distinction is drawn between types I and IIa according to the following criteria: a lesion with a protrusion that is more than twice as high as the normal mucosal width is classified as type I, and a lesion with a lesser degree of protrusion is classi-

fied as type IIa. In addition, early gastric cancer often has complex morphologic features. For example, a combination of shallow and deep depression (types IIc and III) or a shallow depression and a slight protrusion (types IIc and IIa). The first Roman numeral indicates the predominant type. Combinations of the three types are fairly common.[10]

In reviewing 1600 cases of early gastric cancer, Chia *et al.*[11] found that flat, elevated, and depressed tumors occurred in a ratio of $1:2:4$. Nishi and colleagues[12] reported that approximately 80% of early gastric cancers belong to the depressed type. The relative frequency of the different macroscopic types of early gastric cancer varies with different authors and different countries. The protuberant (type I) carcinoma accounts for about 10–15%, but the incidence reported by European authors[4,13] is rather higher than the Japanese experience.[12] Superficial type II carcinoma is more common than type I, but these are mostly type IIC (superficial depressed). However, European authors report a much higher incidence of all superficial type early gastric cancers than their Japanese colleagues. It has already been pointed out that the type III early gastric cancer in its pure form is rare, but all combinations with the other types are common. Thus, the combination forms account for about 75% of all early gastric cancers in Japan and for 40–50% in the main European publications (**Figure 7.2**).[10]

Following the rules of the International Union Against Cancer (UICC) and the American Joint Commission on Cancer (AJC), staging of early gastric cancer is performed according to the TNM system.[14] Early gastric cancers are T1 carcinomas, which includes stage IA (T1 N0), stage IB (T1 N1), and stage II (T1 N2) tumors. The term "stage T1 gastric cancer" has also been used to describe early gastric cancer, given this heterogeneity using the AJC and UICC staging systems. The Japanese staging system[6] is heavily based on lymph node involvement. The extent of resection (D) denotes the level of lymph nodes (N) excised. The nodal stations differ according to the site of primary tumor. Higher-numbered nodal routes are more distant from the cancer, and therefore less likely to be involved in early gastric cancer.

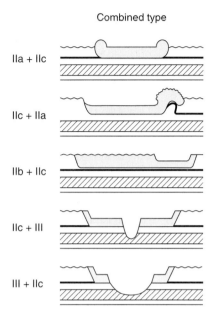

Combined type

IIa + IIc

IIc + IIa

IIb + IIc

IIc + III

III + IIc

Figure 7.2 Macroscopic classification of combined types of early gastric cancer.

EPIDEMIOLOGY

In most published reports on early gastric cancer, men outnumber women by a ratio of 1:5 to 1:2. This ratio is almost constant in world mortality statistics, regardless of the prevalence of gastric cancer in each country. In North American studies, the patients are typically middle-aged, with the mean age at diagnosis at 63 years (ranging from 44 to 70 years).[3] The average Japanese patient is 5 to 10 years younger at diagnosis (mean age approximately 55 years).[15] A slight increase in patients over 60 years of age has been noted since the early 1970s. According to mass surveillance health data in Japan, there is a female predominance until the fourth decade. Men predominate in their forties and fifties, and the peak is reached in the sixties for both men and women.[16] This difference may also reflect the aggressive screening practice in Japan. **Figure 7.3** displays the age distribution at time of presentation at the NCC Tokyo, the German Gastric Cancer Study (GGCS), and our own centre (Tu-Munich).

The comparison of crude, rather than disease-specific survival rates between Japan and the other countries, is hampered by this difference in patients' age. In comparison with Japan, the incidence of gastric carcinoma in the Western world is approximately eight-fold lower.[17] It remains unknown whether such epidemiologic differences are explained by differences in tumor biology, or whether they solely represent a selection phenomenon. Several pieces of evidence suggest that survival rates and frequency of early gastric cancer may be underestimated in Western countries.[18]

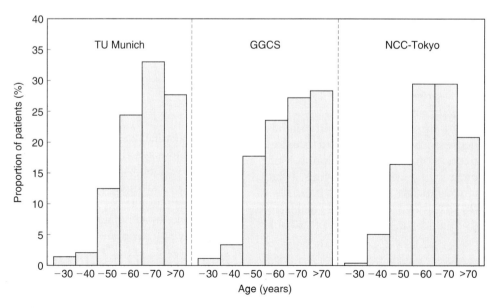

Figure 7.3 Distribution of age at time of presentation with early gastric cancer. Data from the Technische Universität München, the German Gastric Cancer Study, and the National Cancer Center Tokyo.

Data from Europe and the United States are derived mainly from patient populations investigated at cancer referral centers, whereas most gastric cancers in Japan are diagnosed during mass survey of asymptomatic patients. Secondly, the more aggressive diagnostic approaches in Japanese patients with upper intestinal symptoms may lead to more frequent detection of small gastric cancers. However, Eckardt et al.[19] reported from a German medical practice, that in their patient population of 16 000 upper gastrointestinal endoscopies, they found 241 patients with gastric cancer, 51 of whom (21.2%) had early gastric cancer.

Helicobacter pylori has been suggested to be a risk factor for gastric carcinogenesis.[20] Endo et al.[21] found *H. pylori* infection in 40 out of 68 cases with EGC, though a significantly higher incidence of infection was found in intestinal-type cancer. *H. pylori* infection may have a crucial relationship to the early stages of carcinogenesis of intestinal-type cancer.[20]

PATHOLOGY AND GROWTH PATTERNS

Endoscopic biopsies are limited and, therefore, can only suggest EGC. A gastric malignancy can be correctly staged and diagnosed only after a meticulous pathologic examination of the surgical specimen. EGC is defined as a carcinoma, which is confined to the mucosa or mucosa and submucosa, regardless of the presence of lymph node metastases. It has to be emphasized that this is a classification of the growth or macroscopic appearance. EGC can also be subdivided by microscopic criteria into two groups: intramucosal carcinoma and submucosal carcinoma, both with potential for lymph node metastases. Surface carcinoma and superficial carcinoma are terms which have been used synonymously with intramucosal carcinoma. The expression "superficial spreading carcinoma" was introduced by Inokuchi[22] to describe that type of carcinoma which spreads superficially into the mucosa and submucosa without penetrating the deep muscle layers, until it has covered a considerable surface area. It could be regarded as an early manifestation of linitis plastica.

According to "The general rules for gastric cancer study in surgery and pathology" of the Japanese Research Society for Gastric Cancer,[6] the stomach is divided into the upper (cardia region), middle, and lower (antrum) thirds. Data from the Tokyo National Cancer Center showed the highest rate of occurrence in the middle region (46.4%), followed by the antrum. In the whole series of patients subjected to surgery for gastric cancer in the Japan Registry, including advanced cases, tumors in the antrum were most common (45%), followed by the middle and the cardia regions. EGC occurs more frequently in the lesser curvature (50%), followed by the posterior wall (25%), anterior wall, and greater curvature.[10] **Table 7.1** shows a comparison of the localization of EGC at time of diagnosis between The National Cancer Center Tokyo (1981–1992), the German Gastric Cancer Study (1986–1989), and the data of our own institution (1982–1993).

Table 7.1 Localization of early gastric cancer at time of presentation in three different institutions (Technische Universität München, National Cancer Center Tokyo, and data from the German Gastric Cancer Study)

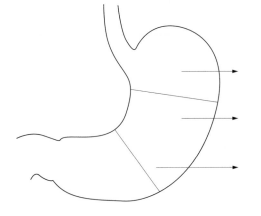

TU MUNICH (%)	GGCS (%)	NCC TOKYO (%)
20.9	15.4	14.3
32.7	35.5	46.4
46.4	48.7	38.7 0.6*

*Whole stomach.

The classification of EGC can be used for lesions of any size, although most of them are about 2.0 cm diameter, or less. Larger areas up to 5 cm diameter are not uncommon. In the early 1960s, 86% of EGC were larger than 2 cm, but smaller lesions have been increasingly diagnosed in recent years, reflecting the progress in diagnostic methods. The diagnosis of small cancers (<10 mm in size) and particularly the so called "minute" cancer (<5 mm) is important, not only in its potential for a complete cure but also in its contribution to the understanding of premalignant lesions.[23] Type IIB cancer consists of 60% of tumors <5 mm in diameter, and none larger than 5 mm, which indicates that as the tumor grows, the originally flat lesion becomes either protruding or depressed.[24]

About 5–15% of gastrectomy specimens for EGC will show multifocal lesions.[25] Multiple carcinoma was found in 8.3% of 500 EGC cases at the National Cancer Center in Tokyo,[26] and in 77% of these, two lesions coexisted in the stomach, while coexistence of three lesions was found in 20%, and more than four lesions in 3%. The 5-year survival rate of these patients was 85.8%. Interestingly, in patients aged over 65 years the range of multiple tumors was 13%, twice that of the group under 65 years. The background gastric mucosa giving rise to multiple gastric carcinoma frequently revealed extensive distribution of intestinal metaplasia in the stomach.

Histologic features and classification

The classification proposed by Laurén[27] and the World Health Organization (WHO)[6] are often used. Following the Laurén classification of gastric cancer, tumors are divided into two main histologic patterns: (i) neoplasm with gland formation (intestinal type); and (ii) tumors devoid of glandular characteristics (so-called non-intestinal type).[27] The intestinal type occurred predominantly among elderly men in areas with a high incidence of gastric cancer ("epidemic": Japan, Costa Rica). The diffuse type of gastric cancer, described as "endemic," occurs more often in women and younger patients and frequently exhibits transmural invasion (**Figure 7.4**). These different subtypes of the Laurén classification have different routes of metastases. While the intestinal-type metastasizes predominantly into the liver and lymph nodes, the diffuse type spreads into the peritoneum.[28] However, the histologic pattern has no value as an independent predictor of the patient's outcome in early gastric cancer.[24]

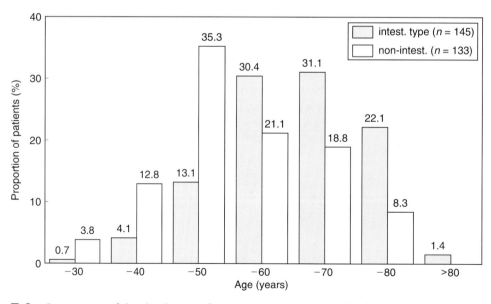

Figure 7.4 Comparison of the distribution of age and the Laurén classification in early gastric cancer. Data from the German Gastric Cancer Study.

Using the WHO International Histological Classification, the following main types of EGC can be identified:

- Papillary adenocarcinoma: the carcinoma consists of papillary and villous proliferation of cuboidal to high-cylindrical-shaped carcinoma cells.
- Tubular adenocarcinoma: in this type, glandular formation is distinct.
- Poorly differentiated adenocarcinoma: few, if any, glandular formations are seen. Acinar or microglandular structures may be seen only in a small number of areas.
- Signet-ring cell carcinoma: within the cytoplasm of the tumor cells, a large amount of mucus is present. The name of the carcinoma refers to the shape, which resembles a signet ring. This type can be further divided into goblet-cell, classical, and eosinophilic cytoplasm types.
- Mucinous adenocarcinoma: the carcinoma cells float in this type within mucus pools, exhibiting nodular patterns of various sizes.

Special types of early gastric carcinoma are adenosquamous carcinoma, squamous cell carcinoma, carcinoid tumor, and undifferentiated carcinoma.

An overview of the histologic types of EGC is given in **Table 7.2**, which comprises data from around 2000 cases with 2675 lesions from the National Cancer Center Hospital Tokyo (1962–1969).

Type I protuberant and type IIa (superficial elevated) early gastric carcinomas are almost differentiated adenocarcinomas. Among the type IIC

(superficial flat) carcinomas, highly differentiated, poorly differentiated, signet ring cell, and undifferentiated lesions are all seen. The degree of differentiation in any one lesion is often variable. The relative frequency of poorly differentiated and undifferentiated carcinomas is much higher among the type III (excavated) EGCs than any of the other types. In general, elevated carcinomas are usually very differentiated, flat ones contain all histologic types, and depressed and excavated cancers have the highest incidence of poorly differentiated and undifferentiated carcinomas. Mucinous adenocarcinomas are rare and are located mainly in submucosal or deeper layers, so that these account for only 0.7% of EGC in a Japanese study.[10]

Lymph node involvement

It is reported that even EGC showed lymph node metastases with a frequency ranging from 0% to 17% in intramucosal carcinomas and from 13% to 30% in submucosal carcinomas in Japan.[29–31] The corresponding ranges in Europe were 1.5–7% and 4–12.3%, respectively. In a literature review, the average incidence of lymph node metastases was 13.8%,[29] while at the National Cancer Center Tokyo, lymph node metastases were seen in 2.1% of cases, with tumors limited to the mucosa and in 13.9% of cases with submucosal invasion. The respective percentages in other reports based on the data from multiple Japanese institutions were 4% and 19%.[32]

The rate of lymph node metastases is related to the gross type and size of the primary tumor: 4% in tumors <1 cm in diameter, and 18% in tumors >4 cm. Metastases from mucosal cancer were limited to primary regional nodes, but the submucosal cancers may spread to the N2 or even M1 (lym) nodes.[33] The frequency of metastases to lymph nodes also varied depending on the presence or absence of ulceration in the carcinoma. Among cases with tumors limited to the mucosa, metastases were found in no cases without ulceration but in 2–3% of cases with ulceration. Conversely, in cases with submucosal invasion, lymph node metastases were found in 23.3% of those with ulceration.[10] Maehara *et al.*[34] showed in a multivariate analysis of 396 cases, that the independent risk factors for lymph node involvement in EGC were tumor size, lymphatic vessel involvement, and submucosal involvement.

Table 7.2 Occurrence of different histologic types in early gastric cancer. Data from the National Cancer Center Tokyo[10]

HISTOLOGIC TYPE	NO. OF LESIONS	(%)
Papillary adenocarcinoma	172	(6.4)
Tubular adenocarcinoma	1453	(54.3)
Poorly differentiated adenocarcinoma	355	(13.3)
Signet-ring cell carcinoma	676	(25.3)
Mucinous adenocarcinoma	19	(0.7)
Total	2675	(100)

Early gastric cancer <10 mm in maximum diameter rarely metastasizes to regional lymph nodes. However, cancers measuring ≥30 mm in maximum diameter have a high risk of lymph node metastasis. Importantly, lymph node metastases were observed in 30% of cases with lesions >50 mm in maximum diameter, and remote nodes were involved in some of these cases. Therefore, particular caution has to be exercised in the surgical treatment of EGC of the superficial spreading type (see below).[33]

It is generally accepted that the risk of skip metastases is higher in early stages compared with advanced stages.[35] Hiki[36] reported an incidence of skip metastases of 4.1% in EGC (8/195), while Sowa et al.[29] reported an incidence of 6.6% but only in cases with undifferentiated submucosal cancer. The differences in patient presentation according to gender, tumor type, lymph node metastases, and distant metastases of a Japanese center, the GGCS, and our own center is shown in **Table 7.3**.

Secondary ulceration in early gastric cancer

Secondary ulcer formation seems to occur frequently with the early gastric carcinoma. In a Japanese study,[10] ulceration was seen in about 65% of the whole group of EGC and in 80% of patients below the age of 65 years; ulceration was less frequently observed in elderly patients (70%). In a Japanese study,[37] the frequency of ulceration and/or ulcer scar has decreased from 94% in 1962 to 72% in 1983. At the National Cancer Center in Tokyo, a large number of early gastric carcinomas with submucosal invasion were found in the group with ulceration (360/529 cases, 68.1%).[10] The presence of an ulcer appears to contribute to the development of submucosal invasion in type IIc carcinomas measuring <3 cm, while in carcinomas

Table 7.3 Patient presentation at time of diagnosis at the NCC Tokyo (1981–1992, n = 1259), the GGCS (1986–1989, n = 279) and our own institution (1982–1993, n = 153)

	NCC TOKYO (%)	GGCS (%)	TU MUNICH (%)	P-VALUE
Depth of invasion				
Mucosa	56.1	50.9	50.3	
Submucosa	43.9	49.1	49.7	NS
Tumor diameter (mm)				
≤ 40	77.8	76.8	84.3	
41–60	13.8	14.5	11.1	
61–80	5.2	6.9	4.6	
>80	3.2	1.8	0	NS
Grading				
G1/2	65.4	61.9	46.4	
G3/4	34.6	38.1	53.6	<0.001
Laurén classification				
Intestinal	65.4	52.3	53.6	
Non-intestinal	34.6	47.7	46.4	<0.001
Lymph nodes				
pN0	89.1	83.5	92.8	NS
pN1	7.5	7.5	3.3	<0.001
pN2	3.4	9.0	3.9	NS
Distant metastases				
M0	99.8	96.4	96.7	
M1	0.2	3.6	3.3	<0.001
Gender				
Male	68.7	60.9	58.8	
Female	31.3	39.1	41.2	0.0048
Concurrent disease				
Pulmonary	9.1	15.4	6.5	NS
Cardiovascular	17.5	26.2	24.8	<0.001
Renal	3.7	6.8	2.0	NS
Diabetes	15.4	9.0	7.2	NS

>3 cm, pronounced submucosal invasion was found in the absence of ulceration.

Growth types of early gastric cancer

Early gastric cancer usually grows in two directions, horizontally within the mucous membrane, and vertically into the deeper layers. However, some lesions spread superficially within the mucosa, and feature virtually no deep invasion (superficial spreading or "SUPER" type), whereas others have a strong tendency to invade deeply (penetrating or "PEN" type).[38]

SUPER type

As stated, the SUPER type of EGC spread superficially, eventually covering a wide portion of the mucous membrane, but they do not penetrate into the deeper layers. It was designated the superficial type of carcinoma by Stout.[39] In Japan, SUPER-type gastric carcinoma is defined as an m or sm carcinoma that covers an area of 25 cm or more, as estimated by multiplying the longest diameter by that perpendicular to it. SUPER-type EGC is predominant in women, especially young women.[22] Among lesions of this type, those classified macroscopically as depressed (poorly differentiated) carcinomas and protruded (well-differentiated) carcinomas are located in the middle stomach and in the antrum, respectively. The proportion of the SUPER-type cases in the population with EGC varies widely in reports (from 8% to 21%).[22,33] When classified by depth of invasion, sm cancer is more frequent in this type (68%) than in the entire group of patients with EGC (48%).[38] Two groups reported that sm carcinomas accounted for as many as 58% of protruded lesions of SUPER-type and 67% of depressed lesions,[33] while the depth of invasion of sm cancer usually was slight. Metastatic nodal involvement with the SUPER-type is 2.6-fold as frequent as metastasis in the entire group of patients with EGC.[38]

PEN type

The PEN-type early gastric carcinomas are defined as those measuring ≤4 cm in maximum diameter, and invading the submucosa extensively and deeply.[22] PEN-type early gastric carcinomas were recognized as relatively small lesions of type IIa and IIc microscopically, and as well-differentiated adenocarcinomas histologically. In a report by Hirayama and colleagues,[40] many such lesions metastasized

through the vascular system, often resulting in liver involvement. The 5-year survival rate of their patients with PEN-type lesions was 65%, which was lower than that of patients with SUPER-type lesions. Macroscopically, many PEN-type lesions are of the depressed type and they display an infiltrative growth pattern; moreover, hematogenous metastasis occurs frequently. Poorly differentiated lesions of this type are predominantly seen in female patients in their fifth or sixth decades, the lesions being highly infiltrative.[22,40]

These observations raise the possibility that poorly differentiated PEN-type EGC is a precursor of linitis plastica, and appears to be consistent with the fact that poorly differentiated type IIc EGC occasionally advances to linitis plastica.[33] Studies of the proliferative activity of cancer cells have demonstrated that epidermal growth factor and transforming growth factor-β are less activated in the SUPER-type than in PEN-type carcinoma.[31] Late recurrence in the stomach remnant was common in the SUPER-type cases, while early recurrence in the liver was often seen in cases of the penetrating type.

Natural history of early gastric cancer

Whether or not EGC will develop to advanced cancer is a critical problem for clinicians, since most patients with this condition are treated on the presumption of its being a prestage of advanced gastric cancer.[23,41] The follow-up of patients with EGC is one of the most important ways of clarifying the process from early to advanced gastric cancer. However, when patients have been diagnosed as having EGC, they cannot – for ethical reasons – be followed-up without treatment. Most reports on the natural history of gastric cancer have been based on retrospective follow-up studies,[23] though Tsukuma *et al.*[42] were able to follow 43 of 56 patients in whom EGC was diagnosed endoscopically and cancer confirmed by histology, and in whom surgical resection was delayed or had not been carried out. They reported that, among 56 eligible cases, 50% of such patients progressed to advanced cancer within 37 months, and in 80–90% within 4–5 years. After 77 months, 50% of all patients had died from gastric cancer, the estimated 5-year survival rate being 64.5%. Bodner and colleagues[43] reported on seven patients with EGC who were untreated. Three of these patients died (at 36, 30 and 11 months after diagnosis) from reasons other than cancer. The autopsies revealed no tumor progression, the tumor being unchanged in size and depth of invasion. Three patients were still alive (at 18, 14, and 12 months after diagnosis) without endoscopic evidence of tumor growth, an observation which suggested that progression from early to advanced gastric cancer sometimes may take years. In conclusion, EGC will develop into advanced cancer in most cases if it is left untreated or is inadequately treated. Thus, the most reasonable management of EGC is adequate surgical resection.[23,24]

DIAGNOSIS

Most EGC patients have symptoms that mimic those of peptic ulcer disease.[3,4] Epigastric pain or dyspepsia was noted by approximately two-thirds of patients, about 40% of whom experience nausea and vomiting. One-fourth of patients develop anorexia, but have a negligible weight loss. Clinical signs of upper gastrointestinal hemorrhage (either hematemesis or melaena) occur in one-fourth of patients. In contrast, patients with advanced gastric cancer often present with significant weight loss, anorexia, and hematemesis, in addition to abdominal pain.

The mean duration of symptoms is usually longer than in advanced gastric cancer. In two reports, the mean duration of symptoms in patients with EGC was 21 and 36 months compared with 6 and 8 months in patients with advanced gastric cancer.[3,44] Chronic symptoms, although suggestive of EGC, will not distinguish this favorable form of cancer from advanced gastric cancer. However, radiologic or endoscopic evaluation of the stomach is required to diagnose early gastric cancer. Physical examination of patients with EGC is usually unremarkable, as there will not be signs of distant metastasis. Blood tests, including complete blood counts and serum chemistries, are routinely normal.

For decades, the "gold standard" for evaluating patients with symptoms of peptic ulcer disease was barium upper gastrointestinal radiography.[45] However, because of improved flexible endoscopy equipment and more accurate tissue diagnosis with multiple biopsy samples, physicians have increasingly chosen esophagogastroduodenoscopy as the initial diagnostic test for dyspepsia.[46] Several clinical reports have documented both a lower sensitivity of upper tract radiography for superficial gastric mucosal abnormalities, and the inability to differentiate benign from malignant gastric ulcers on upper gastric intestinal radiology.[13,47–49] With inspection alone, endoscopy correctly diagnoses EGC in only 50% of cases,[50] but with multiple directed biopsies, gastroscopy is highly sensitive and specific for early carcinoma. To improve diagnostic sensitivity, multiple (up to 10) biopsies in each case and dye-spraying endoscopy with Congo red and methylene blue are sometimes recommended.[51,52]

Screening

A high incidence of gastric carcinoma, coupled with strong public and physician cooperation in the screening practices, enable the Japanese to institute a national effort to diagnose gastric cancer. Up to 65% of cases are consequently diagnosed as early gastric cancer,[53] and an average of 16 cases of gastric cancer per 1000 persons has been detected in the asymptomatic Japanese population. The overall long-term survival has therefore improved by 20%.[53] However, the prevalence of EGC as a proportion of total cases remains low in Europe (6.5% of 40 000 gastric cancers) and North America.[54] Mass screening for gastric cancer is therefore economically impractical in the Western hemisphere, given its low rate of incidence. The availability of esophagogastroduodenoscopy with biopsies is a highly sensitive and accurate diagnostic procedure, and mandates that high-risk patients (patients with persistent epigastric discomfort despite medical therapy, and those with gastric polyps, pernicious anemia or a family history of gastric cancer) should be screened by endoscopy without unnecessary delay. In the Western world, with its low incidence of EGC, the so-called "open access endoscopy" is promoted. Using this approach, patients with unspecified gastric symptoms can be investigated by specialized gastrointestinal centers without prior consultation with a general practitioner. Using this approach, O'Hanlon et al.[55] reported that among 1902 patients, 85 were identified with gastric cancer, and 10 (12%) of these had EGC. Furthermore, 187 patients with potentially premalignant lesions were entered into surveillance programs. Thus, the detection of gastric cancer at the earliest stage is paramount in the improvement in patient survival.

Staging

Staging of gastric cancer is the exact evaluation of the tumor stage, which means the depth of tumor infiltration into the organ wall (T category), the lymph node status (N category), and the presence of distant metastases (M category) according to the criteria of the UICC.[14]

T category: primary tumor

In the patient care study of the American College of Surgeons, diagnosis of gastric cancer was established in 94% of patients by endoscopy and biopsy.[56] Using these two procedures, the location of the tumor and its macroscopic appearance should also be clarified. The first biopsy will determine the histopathologic type of the tumor. Gastric cancer is predominantly adenocarcinoma, though gastric lymphoma (MALT) must be excluded before beginning treatment because this entity is treated completely differently. The histopathologic subclassification according to the Laurén classification of tumor growth (intestinal versus non-intestinal type) must also be determined, as this provides additional important information about the luminal extent of the surgical resection which is necessary. The grade of differentiation (G 1–3, i.e., well to poor), should also be reported in this first biopsy.

As the depth of infiltration is most important to ensure the diagnosis of EGC, endosonography (EUS) is the first step for further diagnostic planning. The crucial point in the decision for or against limited surgery is the preoperative differentiation between carcinomas of mucosal or submucosal type. In Japan, with a high incidence of gastric cancer and with extensive experience in endoscopy, this differentiation is already made solely on the basis of the macroscopic appearance during the investigation.[57,58] In our opinion a more objective decision using EUS would be preferable.

The overall sensitivity of T staging using EUS is about 85%. Problems still arise in the differentiation of T2 (subserosal invasion) from the T3 stage. This distinction is crucial, since it separates local from the locally advanced tumor growth. Sano *et al.*[58] reported accurate prediction of tumor depth by endoscopic inspection alone in 71.9% of patients; however, the accuracy in staging sm cancer was only 60.2%. The cumulative results of six studies (451 tumors) which used conventional endosonoscopes indicate that accuracy for diagnosis of mucosal disease is in the range of 90%, whereas that for submucosal disease is about 70% (**Table 7.4**).[59] Yasuda[60] reported the experience in more than 600 cases of gastric cancer in which the overall staging accuracy was divided into mucosal, submucosal, muscularis propria, and invasion deeper than the subserosal layer, with accuracy rates of 79.5%, 72.7%, 58.3% and 91.6%, respectively. The use of EUS is hampered by the problem of over- or understaging. It is often difficult, especially in ulcerated gastric cancer, to differentiate between carcinoma, inflamed surrounding soft tissue, or even fibrosis. Furthermore, EUS cannot detect microinvasive cancer.[61,62]

It should be mentioned that the use of EUS is strongly dependent on the training and experience of the investigator. The excellent results published in various studies are obtained by very well-trained, specialized "endosonografters." Until now, the use of EUS has been restricted to centers which have already accumulated sufficient experience with this sophisticated technique, and further evaluation of the method must be carried out with respect to clinical consequences. EUS is still far superior to upper gastrointestinal radiography with double-contrast barium meals and computed tomography (CT) for the determination of the overall T stage. Lightdale[63] found a 92% concordance between EUS and surgical pathology, but only 42% concordance between CT scanning and surgical pathology.

N category: nodal involvement

As stated previously, the incidence of metastases in EGC is, besides the depth of infiltration, dependent on growth type, macroscopic appearance, and

Table 7.4 Accuracy of endoluminal ultrasound in locoregional staging in early gastric cancer (TNM system)

REFERENCE	STAGE	NO. OF PATIENTS	EUS ACCURACY (%)
Pollack *et al.*[59]		451	
	T1a		90
	T1b		70
Yasuda[60]	T1a	234	79.5
	T1b	132	72.7

tumor diameter. Protruded-type carcinomas (type I, type IIA) with a diameter <25 mm and excavated types (type IIC) with a diameter <20 mm rarely produce lymph node metastases.[36]

Using EUS, the diagnostic accuracy for N category in gastric cancer is reported to be between 65% and 87%.[61] However, in our own study,[64] we found an accuracy of only 65% in N1-stage and 52% in N2-stage tumors. The diagnosis of lymph node metastases is problematic due to a low rate of detected lymph nodes and a high rate of false-positive findings. EUS can only visualize lymph nodes in close proximity to the gastric wall. The N2 stage is obviously difficult to diagnose. As with other imaging methods, EUS can detect only enlarged lymph nodes, and not those which are invaded but not enlarged.

Overall, EUS appears to be more accurate than percutaneous ultrasound or CT for the evaluation of N stage. Chin et al.[65] reported an accuracy of 70% in assessing regional lymph node metastases using dynamic CT. The detection rate of lymph nodes was low when perigastric lymph nodes were close to the primary tumor, but was relatively high in the case of extraperigastric nodes because enlarged lymph nodes were clearly distinguished from adjacent, highly enhanced vessels in the early phase of dynamic CT. It seems possible that dynamic CT could close the gap in the evaluation of the N2 stage.

M category: distant metastases

Early gastric cancer is rarely reported to metastasize to the lymph nodes around the celiac axis and the retroperitoneal space along the large abdominal vessels. For that, only rare liver metastases should be excluded by ultrasonography.

Percutaneous abdominal ultrasound has problems similar to those known for CT scanning. Although it is fairly sensitive for detecting metastases of >15 mm in diameter (sensitivity 80.5%), the sensitivity of detecting liver metastases of <10 mm diameter is only 37%.[66] Percutaneous ultrasound ought to be used as a screening method.

Surgical treatment

The aim of any surgical approach for early and advanced gastric carcinoma should be a complete resection with no residual tumor left behind at the end of the operation. This situation corresponds to the R0 category of the UICC, and complete tumor resection in this respect refers to:

- the primary tumor, i.e., no residual tumor at the oral and aboral resection margins and the tumor bed (the so-called third dimension); and
- the lymphatic drainage, i.e., as a minimal requirement no residual tumor in the peripheral or border lymph nodes

Despite the varied surgical management for early gastric cancer, the worldwide survival statistic has been excellent (**Tables 7.5** and **7.6**). Although the crude 5-year survival rates range from 60% to 100%,[4,13,15,69] the age-adjusted survival rates match that of controls. Nevertheless, controversy over surgical management persists.[70,71]

In order to improve the prognosis of a patient, the tumor must be removed with an adequate safety margin, the extent of which depends on the growth pattern of the tumor, i.e., the Laurén classification, the grading, and the T category. Gastric carcinoma with a diffuse-type growth pattern requires a larger oral and aboral safety margin as compared with tumors with an intestinal-type growth pattern. This is also true for the tumor bed, i.e., the so-called third dimension of the resection.

The clearance needed for surgical margins when performing a subtotal gastrectomy for EGC is still debatable. A gross margin of 2 cm has been deemed sufficient by some clinicians, but most surgeons strive for proximal and distal margins of 5 cm.[72] On the other hand, excellent survival results have been reported for patients with margins as narrow as 5 mm.[73] However, while a gross margin of 2 cm will nearly always provide microscopic clearance in intestinal-type tumors, a margin of 3–5 cm is recommended in non-intestinal-type lesions.[74]

In some studies, multicentricity has been used as a rationale for routine total gastrectomy.[73,75] However, collective studies from Japan, Europe, and the U.S. (see **Tables 7.5** and **7.6**) involving subtotal gastrectomy show a low recurrence rate and excellent patient survival. These data show that dissection of gross disease and inspection of the gastric remnant is sufficient for tumor control, despite the high incidence of multifocal disease. In conclusion, subtotal gastrectomy is sufficient for EGC only at the middle and distal part of the

Table 7.5 Results of treatment of early gastric cancer in Europe

REFERENCE	NO. OF PATIENTS	INVASION		POSITIVE LN (%)	RECURRENCE (%)	OPERATIVE MORTALITY RATE (%)	CRUDE 5-YEAR SURVIVAL RATE (%)
		MUCOSA (%)	SUBMUCOSA (%)				
Moreaux and Bougaran[4]	101	32	68	18.8	5.9	1	88
Pinto et al.[67]	142	53	47	9.8	7.7	2.1	84 (93, N0) (57, N+)
Gebhardt et al.[47]	130	50	50	8	NR	8	76
Oleagiotta et al.[99]	142	63	37	14	5	1	93
Marczell et al.[72]	103	59	41	10	4	2	84
GGCS[2]	279	51	49	16.5	NR	1.6	83 (88 m) (78 sm)
TU Munich[2]	153	50	50	11	NR	1	88

LN, lymph nodes; NR, not reported.

Table 7.6 Treatment results of early gastric cancer in Japan

REFERENCE	NO. OF PATIENTS	INVASION		POSITIVE LN (%)	RECURRENCE (%)	OPERATIVE MORTALITY RATE (%)	CRUDE 5-YEAR SURVIVAL RATE (%)
		MUCOSA (%)	SUBMUCOSA (%)				
Itoh et al.[84]	109	49	51	10	5	0	96
Mori et al.[68]	21	62	38	10	5	0	NR
Ohta et al.[31]	1412	49	51	13	2	1	94
Endo & Habu[17]	374	50	50	8	NR	1	89
Nishi et al.[12]	2152	53	47	11.4 / 2.5 (m) / 21.4 (sm)	1.5	NR	94.5 (m) / 91.3 (sm)

NR, not reported.

stomach, especially in type I and type IIa lesions. However, if the lesion has located in the proximal part of the stomach, total gastrectomy has to be carried out (**Table 7.7**).[29]

Subtotal gastrectomy

The luminal extent of the subtotal gastrectomy resection specimen comprises about four-fifths of the stomach. Along the lesser curvature, the resection should reach up to about 2 cm below the anatomic cardia, while along the greater curvature the resection must extend beyond the right and left gastroepiploic veins extending to the hilus of the spleen. The small remaining fundus is fed through the short gastric vessels from the splenic hilus. In all cases, the dissection of the duodenum should be extended beyond the border of the gastroduodenal artery into the extraperitoneal space, after which the duodenal stump can be closed with a stapler. Closure of the remaining proximal stomach can also be performed with a stapler (TA 90), thus preventing contamination of the surgical field. The extraluminal extent of resection and lymphadenectomy must be performed as radically as with a total gastrectomy. Limitations exist only with respect to lymph node station 2 (left of the cardia). Lymph node station 1 along the lesser curvature must be included in the lymphadenectomy. In order to perform the lymphadenectomy in the correct layer, i.e., the adventitia of the arteries, the lymph node dissection should be started along the gastroduodenal artery which has already been

dissected when closing the duodenal stump. From there it is easy to find the correct dissection layer of the common hepatic artery, which is the starting point for the lymphadenectomy to the center and the periphery. Towards the periphery, the lymphadenectomy should always be continued beyond the bifurcation of the hepatic artery. The right gastric artery should be ligated at its origin. In addition to compartments 1 and 2, a lymphadenectomy of lymph node station 13 and of the right para-aortic and paracaval nodes (lymph node station 16) should always be performed, together with a subtotal gastrectomy. This requires sufficient mobilization of the duodenum according to Kocher. Lymph node station 13 represents the border lymph node towards the periphery. This lymph node is marked and pulled through the foramen of Winslow behind the hepatoduodenal ligament. The surgeon's left index finger is then inserted into the foramen of Winslow to push the portal vein cephalad and anterior towards the surgeon. Further dissection of the lymph nodes can be continued on the adventitia of the portal vein.

Medially, the left gastric artery is ligated and severed at its origin, while the left gastric vein is similarly ligated and cut. The posterior dissection is continued to the diaphragmatic crura, and the left and right phrenic arteries are then ligated. After severing the vagus nerve, the entire lymphatic and fatty tissue block can be pulled aborally. Further dissection along the lesser curvature is performed using the technique of a vagotomy, i.e., the

Table 7.7   Choice of surgical procedure, lymph node dissection and R status in NCC Tokyo (1981–1992, $n = 1259$), the GGCS (1986–1989, $n = 279$) and our own institution (1982–1993, $n = 153$)

	NCC (%)	GGCS (%)	TU MUNICH (%)	P-VALUE
Extent of resection				
Subtotal gastrectomy	80.5	40.9	43.1	<0.001
Total gastrectomy	4.8	52.0	41.8	<0.001
Enlarged gastrectomy	8.7	4.0	11.1	NS
Various	6.0	3.2	3.9	
Lymph node (LN) dissection				
D1 ($\leq$ 25 LN)	45.0	41.6	23.7	
D2 (>25 LN)	55.0	58.4	76.3	<0.001
R-status				
R0	99.9	96.8	98.0	
R1/2	0.1	3.2	2.0	<0.001

NS, not significant.

anterior and posterior sheath of the hepatogastric ligament are divided step by step. This allows complete removal of the lymph nodes along the lesser curvature.

Resection of lymph node station 11 is performed at the upper border of the pancreas towards the splenic hilus. This lymph node station should be dissected with great care, since a splenectomy would compromise the blood supply of the gastric stump. Resection of the greater omentum is obligatory.

Extent of lymphadenectomy

The degree of lymphadenectomy needed for EGCs is also controversial.[76,77] In Japan,[16] the principal surgical procedure for early as well as advanced gastric cancer is a total resection with complete excision of group I and II lymph nodes. **Figure 7.5** shows the lymph nodes that should be removed during lymphadenectomy.

The rate of lymph node metastasis in EGC is low for mucosal cancer, but much higher for submucosal cancer. The rate of metastasis to group I lymph nodes was reported to be 0.7–4.7% for mucosal and 10.6–18.9% for submucosal cancer.[78] The rate of metastasis to group II lymph nodes were lower than those to group I lymph nodes, being 0–2.4% for mucosal cancers, and 2.3–8.9% for submucosal cancers. Metastasis to group III or IV lymph nodes may also occur, but only in a very small number of patients.[79] As indicated above, accurate intraoperative or preoperative determination of the presence

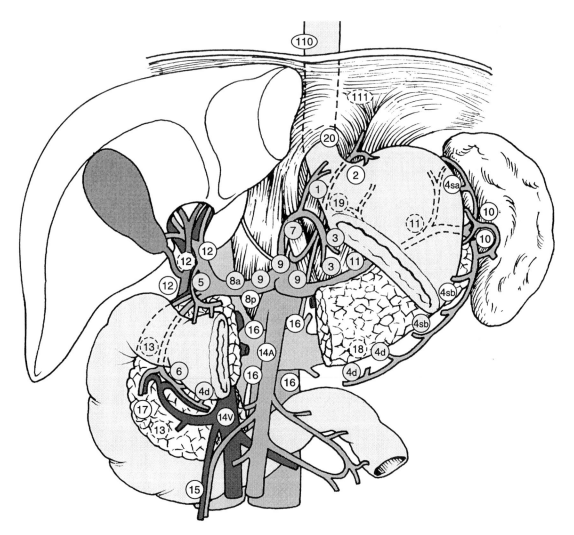

Figure 7.5 Schema of lymph nodes that should be dissected during lymphadenectomy in early gastric cancer.

or absence of lymph node metastasis is difficult. Since lymphatic metastases are predicted to occur in 3% of mucosal cancer and about 20% of submucosal cancer, the conventional view is that D2 lymphadenectomy should be the standard surgical procedure. However, it is also argued that a selective policy should be adopted depending on the depth of the primary.

Suzuki et al.[80] compared the extent of lymph node dissection with survival rates. In the group without lymph node metastasis there was no significant difference in survival rates according to the extent of lymphadenectomy. However, in the group with lymph node metastasis, the results of D2 resection were significantly higher at 5–10 years than the D1 operation. Nonetheless, the main dilemma lies in the staging of the depth of the primary tumor, as radical surgery would be indicated in many submucosal early gastric cancers. On the other hand, Baba and colleagues[81] reported a study of 373 surgically treated patients with EGC and without microscopic nodal involvement. The 5-year survival rates for patients treated with D2 gastrectomy were 97.3% and 95.4%, respectively, these values being significantly higher than the 90.1% and 81.1% noted for D1 gastrectomy. Although no difference was found in morbidity and mortality, the incidence of death from a recurrence of the gastric cancer was significantly higher in patients treated with D1 gastrectomy than those with D2. Multivariate analysis revealed patient's age and D2 gastrectomy to be independent prognostic factors in patients with node-negative EGC. Another argument promoting D2 lymphadenectomy is the prognostic impact of the so-called microinvolvement of lymph nodes which were negative by routine histology but positive using immunohistologic methods.[82] In our own study, the presence of three or more tumor cells in more than 10% of the lymph nodes in pN0 cases was revealed by multivariate analysis to be an independent prognostic factor,[83] and this was confirmed for EGC in a study by Maehara et al.[82] The prognosis for node-negative patients with microinvolvement identified by cytokeratin-staining was significantly poorer when compared with patients without involvement.

In taking all these data together, limited (D1) lymphadenectomy can only be recommended for cancer with a low risk for lymph node metastases, namely tumors confined to the mucosa, the elevated type I and IIa lesions, small cancers and well-differentiated adenocarcinomas.[78]

Lymph node metastases are common in patients with submucosal or elevated EGC, particularly if they are ≥4 cm in diameter and poorly differentiated with vascular invasion.[44,79,84] Women aged under 50 years tend to have unfavorable EGC,[80] and in such patients D2 lymphadenectomy, as for advanced cancers, should be advised. Early gastric cancers which are most likely to recur are the IIa and IIc or elevated submucosa cancers, well-differentiated tumors, those positive for lymph node metastasis, or those in which there is vascular invasion.[15,69,85,86] Surprisingly, differentiated EGCs have more extensive lymph node metastasis. Malignant cells quickly replace most of these nodes and invade the perinodal fatty tissue.[30] These high-risk groups should be treated in the same way as those with advanced cancer by means of complete lymph node dissection.

Reconstruction

Analyses of the quality of life after total gastrectomy support reconstruction using a pouch.[87] Since the advantages observed after pouch reconstruction are only important for long-term outcome, in EGC this should be the procedure of choice. For the construction of a pouch, a side-to-side anastomosis over a distance of 10–15 cm between the ascending and descending portion of the first jejunal loop is usually sufficient (the Hunt–Rodino pouch). A jejunoplication can be added to the pouch, though whether a Roux-en-Y biliary diversion should be added to the pouch to avoid alkaline reflux into the pouch and the distal esophagus is controversial.

The esophageal–intestinal anastomosis can easily be performed with a CEA stapler, a type of reconstruction which has been shown in controlled studies to be superior to a manual anastomosis.[87]

The reconstruction of alimentary tract continuity following subtotal gastrectomy can be performed with a retrocolic or antecolic jejunal loop, with an isoperistaltic orientation of the gastroenterostomy. A side-to-side jejunojejunostomy (according to Braun) is recommended. Analyses of quality of life and patient satisfaction after total and subtotal gastrectomy[88] have shown that symptoms and objective signs of alkaline reflux into the esophagus are a common sequela of this reconstruction.

Consequently, we have modified the reconstruction to a Roux-en-Y configuration.

ENDOSCOPIC TREATMENT AND LIMITED SURGERY

There are three possibilities for limited treatment in EGC:

- laser therapy;
- endoscopic mucosal resection; and
- combined endoscopic–laparoscopic wall resection of the stomach (so-called "wedge" resection).

Endoscopic surgical techniques have been evaluated in Japan for elderly or other poor-risk patients and in those refusing operative resection.[89–91] Using strict selection criteria and careful follow-up, disease-free survival rates approaching 100% have been reported.[78] Recently, it was considered that for selected patients with EGC this procedure may be justified to achieve a radical cure. The problem in performing endoscopic surgery is that staging must be very accurate, because metastatic lymph node involvement cannot be treated by this technique. Evaluation of the efficacy of treatment requires long-term follow-up with repeated biopsies. For both endoscopic and conventional surgical treatment, an accurate description of the histologic diagnosis is essential to predict the likely pattern of lymph node involvement and local infiltration which will determine optimum therapy. However, following laser therapy and mucosectomy no "full wall" specimen is available. A distinct histologic examination is therefore not possible, and whether the specimen represents a true mucosa-type carcinoma may remain doubtful.

When considering endoscopic mucosal resection or laser therapy, selection should ideally be for tumors that rarely metastasize to lymph nodes. The following tumors may fulfil these criteria:[36,92,93]

- Confined to the mucosa (type I).
- Less than 1.5 cm in diameter.
- Macroscopically elevated (type IIa).
- Macroscopically depressed, without intramural ulcers or ulcer scars (type IIc).
- Well-differentiated adenocarcinoma (G1).

Laser therapy

Laser surgery is most widely used as it is easier than the other methods, but requires expensive equipment. Hiki and colleagues[94] accumulated data in a Japanese nationwide study on the endoscopic laser treatment of EGC from 71 hospitals, in which 1436 cases were studied. The proportion with no evidence of local recurrence for more than one year after treatment was 85% for laser therapy. In 1993, Yasuda and co-workers[95] presented a study with 111 early carcinomas of types I, IIA, and IIC, 99 of which were treated with endoscopic laser therapy. There was no difference in the success rate in relation to endoscopic classification, tumor location, and histologic type of cancer. After 2.7 years, 81% of the patients had no recurrence. In comparison, 12 patients were treated with laser therapy followed by operation and, of these, 75% were tumor-free after 2.7 years. However, laser therapy cannot always be performed completely, depending on the location and size of the lesion. Furthermore, the main disadvantage of laser therapy is the lack of a resected specimen for histologic evaluation. For this reason, this type of therapy should only be used for palliative treatment or for treatment of high-risk patients.

Mucosal resection (strip biopsy)

In contrast, histologic examination of the resected mucosa is possible with endoscopic mucosal resection. Histologic examination of the resected mucosa allows confirmation of the integrity of the resection in determination of vascular invasion, as well as histologic type of malignancy. However, this technique is also not appropriate for all anatomic regions of the stomach. Mucosectomy was introduced by Tada and co-workers[96] and developed to obtain biopsies as large as 2–3 cm in diameter. The technique involves injections of physiologic saline into the submucosa under the lesion to create a small swelling, which is resected using a high-frequency snare. This procedure permits resection en bloc of tissue 1–2 cm in diameter. Tada et al.[93] reported a collective of 82 patients with 87 lesions, which were resected endoscopically, and compared these with a group of 27 patients with 29 lesions undergoing surgery. Results indicated that there was no difference in 5-year survival.

Laparoscopic wedge resection

Endoscopic resection is a minimally invasive option for the treatment of mucosal gastric cancer. However, even if the selected cancer region has little possibility of lymph node metastasis, the indication for performing resection is limited and depends on the size and location of the lesion. Ohgami *et al.*[97] have developed an innovative, minimally invasive method: the laparoscopic wedge resection for early gastric cancer (**Figure 7.6**). In this operation, a specimen of the whole gastric wall is resected, which can be examined according to the pathohistologic work-up mentioned below. The diagnosis of mucosal carcinoma must be confirmed, otherwise an open resection of the stomach must follow.

The entire surgical procedure is performed laparoscopically and under general anesthesia. The location of the cancerous lesion is confirmed from inside of the stomach with the guidance of a gastroscope. If the lesion is in the greater curvature or in the posterior wall of the stomach, the gastric wall of the lesion should be exposed laparoscopically. The gastric wall in the vicinity of the lesion is pierced with a catheter which has a built-in straight needle, and is introduced through the working channel of the gastroscope. The needle and catheter are pulled to outside of the gastric wall and a small metal rod is connected by string to the end of the catheter, and introduced into the stomach. Finally, the lesion is lifted upward by the string, with support from the metal rod. Wedge resection

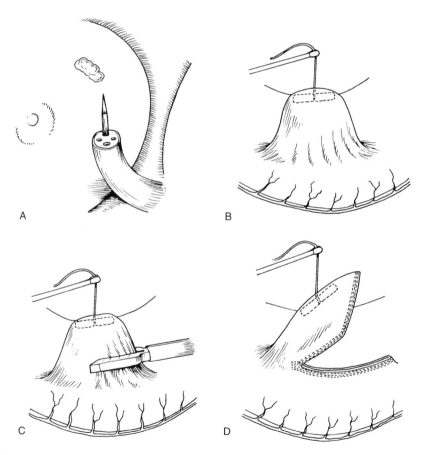

Figure 7.6 Laparoscopic wedge resection in early gastric cancer. A. The gastric wall in the vicinity of the lesion is pierced with a catheter which has a built-in straight needle and is introduced through the working channel of the gastroscope. B. The cancerous lesion is lifted up with the support of a small metal rod (lesion lifting method). C. Wedge resection of the stomach is carried out using a stapling device, such as an ENDIO-GIA. D. Water-tightness of the stapling line is secured. During resection, the absence of any severe deformity or severe stenosis of the stomach is confirmed by gastroscopy.[36]

of the stomach is carried out using a stapling device such as an ENDO-GIA (see **Figure 7.6**).

If necessary, perigastric lymph nodes can also be dissected laparoscopically in an en-bloc fashion. However, because complete lymph node dissection by this method is still limited, the absolute indication of this method should be for the lesion which has little possibility of lymph node metastasis. The indications for this procedure are:

- mucosal cancer;
- an elevated lesion (type IIa) <25 mm or depressed lesion (type IIc) <15 mm without ulcer; and
- a lesion which is not at the lesser curvature or near to the cardia or pylorus.

The advantages of this method are: (i) that it is minimally invasive; (ii) that the cancerous lesion is resected at a sufficient distance from any surgical margin; and (iii) that a detailed histologic examination is feasible. The disadvantages are that it requires general anesthesia and there is a limitation of its application, depending on the location of the lesion.

In conclusion, laser therapy and mucosal strip biopsy should only be recommended in the very high-risk patients. In most cases, combined laparoscopic wedge resection should be the procedure of choice if limited surgery can be applied.

PROGNOSIS AND RECURRENCE

Numerous variables have been evaluated as prognostic factors for early gastric cancer, but only a few reliable predictors of patients' outcome exist. Part of the difficulty in detecting statistical significance for patient survival lies in the small sample size in most reports and the outstanding overall survival rate. At present, no meta-analyses to overcome these problems exist.

Microscopic examination to identify histologic features that predict patients' outcome remain inconsistent. Although some investigators have noted improved survival in early gastric cancer of the intestinal type,[98] most studies show no difference in long-term survival rate according to the Laurén classification.[13,99] In one study, well-differentiated tumors had a better outlook,[100] but in other reports patients with high-grade tumors fared as well as those having low-grade tumor.[46,69] Although several American studies[31,69]

have shown no survival benefit according to depth of invasion, several large Japanese studies[15,71,78] demonstrated better patient outcome if the tumor was limited to the mucosa. Ichiyoshi et al.[101] documented higher risk of recurrence with submucosal early gastric cancer. The absence of mucosal lymphatic tissue would explain the low incidence of lymph node metastases and of local recurrences seen with intramucosal early gastric cancer. Folli et al.[102] evaluated the prognostic factors in 223 patients with EGC. Multivariate analysis showed the significant difference in survival rates between patients with and without involved nodes. Ranaldi et al.[103] investigated 414 cases of early gastric cancers. In multivariate analysis, the size of the tumor, lymph node metastasis, and the level of penetration were unfavorable prognostic factors. However, a small number of patients died despite the presence of several prognostic factors. These authors presumed that other biologic factors may therefore be important in determining the aggressive behavior of certain early gastric cancers.

Few investigators have evaluated the effect of gastric tumor size on patient prognosis. Friesen et al.[104] showed that patients with gastric carcinoma of any diameter involving only the mucosa fared well. In contrast, Shiu and colleagues[105] reported a statistically significant survival advantage for patients with gastric carcinoma <1.5 cm in diameter. These findings were consistent with Japanese data which showed that large tumors (>4 cm) typically have deeper gastric wall penetration and are more likely to have lymph node metastasis.[78] Large studies have identified a survival advantage for node-negative patients.[13,105] Among the 232 patients reported by Endo and Habu[17] there were 5- and 10-year survival rates of 90% and 84%, respectively, for patients without nodal metastasis. In contrast, for patients with positive lymph nodes, a 5-year survival rate of 79% and a 10-year survival rate of 65% was documented. With most patients doing well after surgical resection currently available data offer little information to predict treatment failure.

The value of measuring tumor cell DNA content remains controversial. Several retrospective studies have shown no difference in patient survival according to ploidy status,[106,107] while others have demonstrated that patients with aneuploid tumors are more susceptible to recurrence.[108,109] De Aretxabala et al.[110] noted a poor prognosis if

>10% of the tumor cells were polyploid, but these patients more commonly had also submucosal tumor involvement.

To date, the value of molecular biology in identifying prognostic factors remains doubtful. Fonseca et al.[111] reported a significantly worse prognosis for patients with p53-positive staining in the tumor. In this investigation, the patients' ($n = 129$) survival rate was 92.1% for those with p53-negative tumors, and 71.2% with positive malignancies. In a multivariate analysis, p53 detection and lymph node involvement emerged as independent prognostic factors, including other clinical and pathologic criteria. Proliferating Cell Nuclear Antigen (PCNA) is an auxiliary protein of DNA polymerase δ, and is considered to correlate with cell proliferation state. In a study by Maeda et al.,[112] the PCNA labeling index in patients with lymph node metastases was significantly higher than in those without metastases. Multivariate analysis indicated that PCNA labeling is an independent indicator for lymph node metastasis. Previously, Kamata et al.[113] had demonstrated in vivo determination of proliferation using bromodeoxyuridine labeling, and reported lymph node-negative patients with a labeling index <12% in the primary tumor. It was concluded that this method could provide a useful indicator for lymph node status, though the data were not confirmed. Prognostic factors are summarized in **Table 7.8**. For the evaluation of prognostic factors, only prospective research following complete tumor resection is acceptable. Multivariate analysis must be performed to evaluate the impact of a single factor on overall survival. Unpredictable therapeutic effects should be excluded, and only those patients who are treated according to standardized and strict treatment protocols should be taken into account. Indeed, only when following such standards can the value of any factor be proven. The sometimes conflicting results obtained from studies in the evaluation of prognostic factors can often be traced to the inclusion of incompletely resected patients, or to the retrospective evaluation of paraffin-embedded material.[114]

Sano and colleagues[15] reported on the follow-up of 1475 patients and performed a review of the Japanese literature to elucidate recurrence in EGC. In their investigation, excluding operative death and cases of non-curative resections, 1.4% of the patients died from recurrent disease. The death

Table 7.8 Prognostic factors in early gastric cancer

FACTORS	CERTAIN	UNCERTAIN
Tumor-related	Depth of invasion Nodal involvement	Laurén classification Grading Tumor size Growth type Ploidy Tumor biology (p53, PCNA, BrdU)
Patient-related		Gender Age Morbidity
Therapy-related	Lymph node dissection (D1 versus D2)	Subtotal versus total resection

BrdU, bromodeoxyuridine; PCNA, proliferating cell nuclear antigen.

rate associated with other causes (6.6% of patients), including other malignant diseases, surpassed that associated with disease recurrence. Late recurrence after 5 years was seen in only seven patients. By combining data from patients in 20 published reports, the authors estimated a recurrence rate for EGC of at least 1.9%, exclusive of cancers arising in the gastric stump. The incidence of recurrence was significantly higher in submucosal (3.6%), node-positive (10.7%) and histologically differentiated carcinomas (2.3%), than in mucosa, node-negative and undifferentiated groups, respectively. Hematogenous metastasis was the most common mode of recurrence. The mean survival period of patients with recurrent disease was 40 months and 23% of patients died more than 5 years after surgery. **Table 7.9** shows the analysis of 20 reports dealing with recurrence of EGC.

ADJUVANT THERAPY

Minimal data have been published on the use of adjuvant therapy for early gastric cancer. With an impressive surgical success rate and with standard cancer chemo- and radiotherapy regimens being physically demanding, no randomized prospective trials exist to assess the efficiency of adjuvant therapy. Although some Japanese investigators[78,115] recommend adjuvant chemotherapy even for EGC,

Table 7.9 Analysis of 20 reports dealing with recurrent disease in EGC[15]

	TOTAL NO. OF PATIENTS	NO. OF RECURRENCES (%)	*P*-VALUE
Depth of invasion			
Mucosa	5851	38 (0.6)	
Submucosa	5438	195 (3.6)	<0.0001
Node involvement			
Negative	7340	77 (1.1)	
Positive	816	87 (10.7)	<0.0001
Histologic type			
Differentiated	4127	95 (2.3)	
Undifferentiated	2742	37 (1.3)	<0.0001

no objective data support this treatment. It must be mentioned however, that even in case of advanced gastric cancer, adjuvant treatment is controversial following R0 resection.

CONCLUSIONS

Early gastric cancer is a unique form of gastric carcinoma with an excellent prognosis, though whether it is a definite precursor of advanced gastric cancer is, in some cases, still doubtful. The tumor is most commonly diagnosed in Japan secondary to aggressive screening practices. Early detection is dependent upon a low threshold for endoscopic investigation with multiple biopsies. Specific symptoms, physical findings, or diagnostic laboratory testing are rarely present with EGC. Following diagnosis, subtotal gastrectomy in distal EGC achieves survival rates equivalent to those of age-matched controls; however, total gastrectomy is necessary with lesions in the proximal stomach or multicentric carcinoma. Radical (D2) lymphadenectomy should be undertaken in all patients, although an exclusion might be made in patients with a small lesion confined to the mucosa (so-called type I lesion) or those with a small, type IIa lesion. In recent studies, D2 lymphadenectomy has shown better survival among node-negative patients, and following operation, the patient outcome is usually excellent. In elderly, high-risk patients, limited surgery such as endoscopic strip biopsies and laser treatment should be the method of choice while laparoscopic wedge resection may be an alternative in favorably located mucosal lesions.

REFERENCES

1. Boring CC, Squires TS & Tong T. Cancer statistics 1991. *Bol Asoc Med P R* 1991; **83**: 225–42.
2. Roder JD, Böttcher K, Siewert JR, Busch R, Hermanek P, Meyer H and the German Gastric carcinoma study 1992. Prognostic factors in gastric carcinoma. *Cancer* 1993; **72**: 2089–97.
3. Farley DR & Donohue JH. Early gastric cancer. *Surg Clin North Am* 1992; **72**: 401–21.
4. Moreaux J & Bougaran J. Early gastric cancer. A 25-year surgical experience. *Ann Surg* 1993; **217**: 347–55.
5. Kennedy BJ. Cure for early gastric cancer (editorial). *Cancer* 1993; **72**: 3139–40.
6. Japanese Research Society for Gastric Cancer. The general rules for the gastric cancer study in surgery and pathology I: Clinical classification. *Jpn J Surg* 1981; **11**: 127–39.
7. Hauser G. Das chronische Magengeschwür, sein Vernarbungsprocess und dessen Beziehungen zur Entwicklung des Magenkarzinoms. Leipzig: FCW Vogel, 1883.
8. Versé M. Über die Entstehung, den Bau und das Wachstum der Polypen, Adenome und Karzinome des Magen-Darmkanals. *Arb Pathol Inst Leipzig* 1908; **1**: 40–52.
9. Saeki J. Über die histologische Prognostik des Magenkarzinoms. *Mitteil Med Gesellschaft zu Tokyo* 1938; **52**: 191.
10. Hirota T, Ming S-C & Itabashi M. Pathology of early gastric cancer. In: Nishi M, Ichikawa H, Nakajima T, Maruyama K & Tahara E (eds) *Gastric Cancer*. Tokyo, Berlin, Heidelberg: Springer-Verlag 1993: 66–87.
11. Chia MM, Langman JM, Hecker R, Lew WY, Rowland R & Fock KM. Early gastric cancer: 52 cases of combined experience of two south

Australian teaching hospitals. *Pathology* 1988; **20**: 216–26.

12. Nishi M, Ishihara S, Nakajima T, Ohta K, Ohyama S & Ohta H. Chronological changes of characteristics of early gastric cancer and therapy: experience in the Cancer Institute Hospital of Tokyo, 1950–1994. *J Cancer Res Clin Oncol* 1995; **121**: 535–41.

13. Lawrence M & Shiu MH. Early gastric cancer Twenty-eight-year experience. *Ann Surg* 1991; **213**: 327–34.

14. Hermanek P & Sobin LH. *UICC TNM Classification of Malignant Tumors*. 4th edn. Berlin, New York: Springer, 1992.

15. Sano T, Sasako M, Kinoshita T & Maruyama K. Recurrence of early gastric cancer. Follow-up of 1475 patients and review of the Japanese literature. *Cancer* 1993; **72**: 3174–8.

16. Maruyama K, Sasako M, Kinoshita T, Sano T & Katai H. Surgical treatment for gastric cancer: the Japanese approach. *Semin Oncol* 1996; **23**: 360–8.

17. Endo M & Habu H. Clinical studies of early gastric cancer. *Hepatogastroenterology* 1990; **37**: 408–10.

18. Craanen ME, Dekker W, Blok P, Ferwerda J & Tytgat GN. Time trends in gastric carcinoma: changing patterns of type and location. *Am J Gastroenterol* 1992; **87**: 572–9.

19. Eckardt VF, Giessler W, Kanzler G, Remmele W & Bernhard G. Clinical and morphological characteristics of early gastric cancer. A case-control study. *Gastroenterology* 1990; **98**: 708–14.

20. Craanen ME, Blok P, Dekker W & Tytgat GN. *Helicobacter pylori* and early gastric cancer. *Gut* 1994; **35**: 1372–4.

21. Endo S, Ohkusa T, Saito Y, Fujiki K, Okayasu I & Sato C. Detection of *Helicobacter pylori* infection in early stage gastric cancer. A comparison between intestinal- and diffuse-type gastric adenocarcinomas. *Cancer* 1995; **75**: 2203–8.

22. Inokuchi K. Early gastric cancer viewed from its growth patterns. *Surg Annu* 1986; **18**: 111–28.

23. Yoshimori M. The natural history of early gastric cancer. *Jpn J Clin Oncol* 1989; **19**: 89–93.

24. Leocata P, Gallo P, Chiominto A *et al.* Is early gastric cancer diffuse type a forerunner of advanced gastric cancer. *Tumori* 1993; **79**: 108–11.

25. Isozaki H, Okajima K, Hu X, Fujii K & Sako S. Multiple early gastric carcinoma. *Cancer* 1996; **78**: 2078–86.

26. Noguchi Y, Ohta H, Takagi K *et al.* Synchronous multiple early gastric carcinoma: a study of 178 cases. *World J Surg* 1985; **9**: 786–93.

27. Laurén P. The two histological main types of gastric carcinoma: diffuse and so-called intestinal type carcinoma: an attempt at a histoclinical classification. *Acta Pathol Microbiol Scand* 1965; **64**: 31–43.

28. Weiss M, Eder M & Bassermann R. Charakterisierung verschiedener Magenkarzinomtypen mit unterschiedlicher Metastasierung in Leber, Peritoneum und Knochen. *Pathologe* 1993; **14**: 260–4.

29. Sowa M, Kato Y, Nishimura M, Kubo T, Maekawa H & Umeyama K. Surgical approach to early gastric cancer with lymph node metastasis. *World J Surg* 1989; **13**: 630–5.

30. Boku T, Nakane Y, Okusa T *et al.* Strategy for lymphadenectomy of gastric cancer. *Surgery* 1989; **105**: 585–92.

31. Ohta H, Noguchi Y, Takagi K, Nishi M, Kajitani T & Kato Y. Early gastric carcinoma with special reference to macroscopic classification. *Cancer* 1987; **60**: 1099–106.

32. Sakita T. Early gastric cancer registry in Japan. *Gastroenterol Endosc* 1983; **25**: 317–22.

33. Sowa M. Early gastric cancer. In: Wanebo HJ (ed.) *Surgery for Gastrointestinal Cancer.* Philadelphia, New York: Lippincott-Raven 1996: 335–46.

34. Maehara Y, Orita H, Okuyama T *et al.* Predictors of lymph node metastasis in early gastric cancer. *Br J Surg* 1992; **79**: 245–7.

35. Maruyama K, Gunven P, Okabayashi K, Sasako M & Kinoshita T. Lymph node metastases of gastric cancer. General pattern in 1931 patients. *Ann Surg* 1989; **210**: 596–602.

36. Hiki Y. Endoscopic treatment of early gastric cancer. In: Nishi M, Ichikawa H, Nakajima T, Maruyama K & Tahara E (eds) *Gastric Cancer.* Tokyo, Berlin, Heidelberg: Spinger-Verlag 1993: 392–403.

37. Hirota T, Itabashi M, Daibo M *et al.* Chronological changes in the morphological features of early gastric cancer, especially recent changes in macroscopic findings. *Jpn J Clin Oncol* 1984; **14**: 181–99.

38. Inokuchi K & Sugimachi K. Growth pattern of early gastric cancer. In: Nishi M, Ichikawa H, Nakajima T, Maruyama K & Tahara E (eds) *Gastric Cancer.* Tokyo, Berlin, Heidelberg: Springer-Verlag 1993: 88–101.

39. Stout AP. Superficial spreading type of carcinoma of the stomach. *Arch Surg* 1942; **44**: 651–62.

40. Hirayama D, Fujimori T, Arao M & Maeda S. Clinicopathological and immunohistochemical study on penetrating and superficial spreading

type of early gastric cancers (in Japanese). *Nippon Shokakibyo Gakkai Zasshi* 1990; **87**: 2434–43.

41. Shimizu S, Tada M & Kawai K. Early gastric cancer: its surveillance and natural course. *Endoscopy* 1995; **27**: 27–31.

42. Tsukuma H, Mishima T & Oshima A. Prospective study of "early" gastric cancer. *Int J Cancer* 1983; **31**: 421–6.

43. Bodner E, Pointner R & Glaser K. Natural history of early gastric cancer (letter). *Lancet* 1988; **2**: 631.

44. Green PH, O'Toole KM, Weinberg LM & Goldfarb JP. Early gastric cancer. *Gastroenterology* 1981; **81**: 247–56.

45. Ichikawa H. X-ray diagnosis of early gastric cancer. In: Nishi M, Ichikawa H, Nakajima T, Maruyama K and Tahara E (eds) *Gastric Cancer*. Tokyo, Berlin, Heidelberg: Springer-Verlag 1993: 232–45.

46. Longo WE, Zucker KA, Zdon MJ & Modlin IM. Detection of early gastric cancer in an aggressive endoscopy unit. *Am Surg* 1989; **55**: 100–4.

47. Gebhardt C, Husemann B, Hermanek P & Gentsch HH. Clinical aspects and therapy of early gastric cancer. *World J Surg* 1981; **5**: 721–4.

48. Traynor OJ, Lennon J, Dervan P & Corrigan T. Diagnostic and prognostic problems in early gastric cancer. *Am J Surg* 1987; **154**: 516–19.

49. Ikeda Y, Mori M, Kamakura T, Haraguchi Y, Saku M & Sugimachi K. Improvements in diagnosis have changed the incidence of histological types in advanced gastric cancer. *Br J Cancer* 1995; **72**: 424–6.

50. Ballantyne KC, Morris DL, Jones JA, Gregson RH & Hardcastle JD. Accuracy of identification of early gastric cancer. *Br J Surg* 1987; **74**: 618–19.

51. Iishi H, Tatsuta M & Okuda S. Diagnosis of simultaneous multiple gastric cancers by the endoscopic Congo red–methylene blue test. *Endoscopy* 1988; **20**: 78–82.

52. Yoshida S, Yamaguchi H, Saito D & Kido M. Endoscopic diagnosis: latest trends. In: Nishi M, Ichikawa H, Nakajima T, Maruyama K & Tahara E (eds) *Gastric Cancer*. Berlin, New York, Tokyo: Springer-Verlag 1993: 246–62.

53. Hisamichi S, Fukao A & Tsubono Y. Evaluation of mass screening for stomach cancer. In: Nishi M, Ichikawa H, Nakajima T, Maruyama K & Tahara E (eds) *Gastric Cancer*. Berlin, New York, Tokyo: Springer-Verlag 1993: 16–25.

54. Winslet M, Mohsen Y, Fielding JWL & Hallissey MT. Early gastric cancer: diagnosis, treatment and outcome. *GI Cancer* 1995; **1**: 123–7.

55. O'Hanlon D, Karat D, Scott D, Raimes S & Griffin SM. Open access endoscopy (OAE) is effective in detecting early gastric cancer (abstract). *GI Cancer* 1997; **2**: 81.

56. Wanebo HJ, Kennedy BJ, Chmiel J, Steele G, Jr, Winchester D & Osteen R. Cancer of the stomach. A patient care study by the American College of Surgeons. *Ann Surg* 1993; **218**: 583–92.

57. Kawaura Y, Kanehira E, Ohta Y & Nakano I. Predicting histologic findings from endoscopic appearance of early gastric cancer. *J Clin Gastroenterol* 1991; **13**: 517–20.

58. Sano T, Okuyama Y, Kobori O, Shimizu T & Morioka Y. Early gastric cancer. Endoscopic diagnosis of depth of invasion. *Dig Dis Sci* 1990; **35**: 1340–4.

59. Pollack BJ, Chak A & Sivak MV, Jr. Endoscopic ultrasonography. *Semin Oncol* 1996; **23**: 336–46.

60. Yasuda K. EUS probes and mucosectomy for early gastric carcinoma. In: Sivak MV (ed.) 10th International Symposium on Endoscopic Ultrasonography. *Gastrointest Endosc* 1995; **43**: 29–31.

61. Rösch T. Endosonographic staging of gastric cancer: a review of literature results. *Gastrointest Clin North Am* 1995; **3**: 549–57.

62. Abe S, Lightdale, CJ & Brennan MF. The Japanese experience with endoscopic ultrasonography in the staging of gastric cancer. *Gastrointest Endosc* 1993; **39**: 586–91.

63. Lightdale CJ. Endoscopic ultrasonography in the diagnosis, staging and follow-up of esophageal and gastric cancer. *Endoscopy* 1992; **24**(Suppl 1): 297–303.

64. Maruyama M & Baba Y. Gastric carcinoma. *Radiol Clin North Am* 1994; **32**: 1233–52.

65. Chin SY, Lee BH, Kim KH, Park ST, Do YS & Cho KJ. Radiological prediction of the depth of invasion and histologic type in early gastric cancer. *Abdom Imaging* 1994; **19**: 521–6.

66. Zocholl G, Kuhn FP, Augustin N & Thelen M. Diagnostic value of sonography and computed tomography in liver metastases (in German). *ROFO Fortschr Geb Rontgenstr Nuklearmed* 1988; **148**: 8–14.

67. Pinto E, Roviello F de SA & Vindigni C. Early gastric cancer: report on 142 patients observed over 13 years. *Jpn J Clin Oncol* 1994; **24**: 12–19.

68. Mori M, Kitagawa S, Iida M et al. Early carcinoma of the gastric cardia. A clinicopathologic study of 21 cases. *Cancer* 1987; **59**: 1758–66.

69. Bringaze WL, III, Chappuis CW, Correa P & Cohn I, Jr. Early gastric cancer 21-year experience. *Ann Surg* 1986; **204**: 103–107.

70. Heesakkers JP, Gouma DJ, Thunnissen FB, Bemelmans MH & Von Meyenfeldt MF. Non-radical therapy for early gastric cancer. *Br J Surg* 1994; **81**: 551–3.

71. Abe S, Yoshimura H, Nagaoka S *et al.* Long-term results of operation for carcinoma of the stomach in T1/T2 stages: critical evaluation of the concept of early carcinoma of the stomach. *J Am Coll Surg* 1995; **181**: 389–96.

72. Marczell AP, Rosen HR & Hentschel E. Diagnosis and tactical approach to surgery for early gastric carcinoma: a retrospective analysis of the past 16 years in an Austrian general hospital. *Gastroenterol Jpn* 1989; **24**: 732–6.

73. Percivale P, Bertoglio S, Muggianu M *et al.* Long-term postoperative results in 54 cases of early gastric cancer: the choice of surgical procedure. *Eur J Surg Oncol* 1989; **15**: 436–40.

74. Santoro E, Garofalo A, Scutari F, Zanarini T, Carlini M & Santoro E, Jr. Early gastric cancer: total gastrectomy vs. distal resection. Results of a study of 271 cases. The Italian Stomach Cancer Group (A.C.O.I.-I.S.C.G.). *Hepatogastroenterology* 1991; **38**: 427–9.

75. Kitamura K, Yamaguchi T, Okamoto K *et al.* Total gastrectomy for early gastric cancer. *J Surg Oncol* 1995; **60**: 83–8.

76. Siewert JR, Böttcher K, Roder JD, Busch R, Hermanek P & Meyer H. Prognostic relevance of systematic lymph node dissection: results of the German Gastric Carcinoma Study 1992. *Br J Surg* 1993; **80**: 1015–18.

77. Bonenkamp JJ, Songun I, Hermans J *et al.* Randomised comparison of morbidity after D1 and D2 dissection for gastric cancer in 996 Dutch patients. *Lancet* 1995; **345**: 745–8.

78. Hioki K, Nakane Y & Yamamoto M. Surgical strategy for early gastric cancer. *Br J Surg* 1990; **77**: 1330–4.

79. Kim JP, Hur YS & Yang HK. Lymph node metastasis as a significant prognostic factor in early gastric cancer: analysis of 1,136 early gastric cancers. *Ann Surg Oncol* 1995; **2**: 308–13.

80. Suzuki H, Endo M & Suzuki S. A study of the lymph node metastasis of early gastric cancer. *Jpn J Gastroenterol Surg* 1984; **17**: 1517–26.

81. Baba H, Maehara Y, Takeuchi H *et al.* Effect of lymph node dissection on the prognosis in patients with node-negative early gastric cancer. *Surgery* 1995; **117**: 165–9.

82. Maehara Y, Oshiro T, Endo K *et al.* Clinical significance of occult micrometastasis lymph nodes from patients with early gastric cancer who died of recurrence. *Surgery* 1996; **119**: 397–402.

83. Siewert JR, Kestlmeier R, Busch R *et al.* Benefits of D2 lymph node dissection for patients with gastric cancer and pN0 and pN1 lymph node metastases. *Br J Surg* 1996; **83**: 1144–7.

84. Itoh H, Oohata Y, Nakamura K, Nagata T, Mibu R & Nakayama F. Complete ten-year postgastrectomy follow-up of early gastric cancer. *Am J Surg* 1989; **158**: 14–16.

85. Guadagni S, Reed PI, Johnston BJ, De Bernardinis G, Catarci M, Valenti M, di Orio F & Carboni M. Early gastric cancer: follow-up after gastrectomy in 159 patients. *Br J Surg* 1993; **80**: 325–8.

86. Furusawa M, Notsuka T & Tomoda H. Recurrence of early gastric cancer. *Semin Surg Oncol* 1991; **7**: 344–50.

87. Siewert JR & Böttcher K. Ösophago-jejunoplikatio in Stapler-Technik. Ergebnisse einer kontrollierten Studie. *Langenbecks Arch Chir* 1992; **377**: 186–9.

88. Roder JD, Stein HJ, Eckel F *et al.* Vergleich der Lebensqualität nach subtotaler und totaler Gastrektomie beim Magencarcinom. *Dtsch Med Wochenschr* 1996; **121**: 543–9.

89. Hiki Y, Shimao J, Yamao Y *et al.* The concepts procedures and problems related in endoscopic laser therapy of early gastric cancer. A retrospective study on early gastric cancer. *Surg Endosc* 1989; **3**: 1–6.

90. Hiki Y, Shimao H, Mieno H & Sakakibara Y. Laser therapy for early upper gastrointestinal carcinoma. *Surg Clin North Am* 1992; **72**: 571–80.

91. Hiki Y, Shimao H, Mieno H, Sakakibara Y, Kobayashi N & Saigenji K. Modified treatment of early gastric cancer: evaluation of endoscopic treatment of early gastric cancers with respect to treatment indication groups. *World J Surg* 1995; **19**: 517–22.

92. Sano T, Kobori O & Muto T. Lymph node metastasis from early gastric cancer: endoscopic resection of tumor. *Br J Surg* 1992; **79**: 241–4.

93. Tada M, Murakami A, Karita M, Yanai H & Okita K. Endoscopic resection of early gastric cancer. *Endoscopy* 1993; **25**: 445–50.

94. Hiki Y, Shimao H, Mieno H & Sakakibara Y. Laser therapy for early upper gastrointestinal carcinoma. *Surg Clin North Am* 1992; **72**: 571–80.

95. Yasuda K, Mizuma Y, Nakajima M & Kawai K. Endoscopic laser treatment for early gastric cancer. *Endoscopy* 1993; **25**: 451–4.

96. Tada M, Yanai H & Takemoto Z. New technique of gastric biopsy (abstract). *Stomach and Intestine* 1984; **19** 1107.

97. Ohgami M, Kumai K, Wakabayashi G, Otani Y & Katajima M. Innovative treatment for early gastric cancer: laparoscopic wedge resection of the stomach using the lesion-lifting method. *Stomach and Intestine* 1993; **28**: 1461–8.

98. Iriyama K, Asakawa T, Koike H, Nishiwaki H & Suzuki H. Is extensive lymphadenectomy necessary for surgical treatment of intramucosal carcinoma of the stomach? *Arch Surg* 1989; **124**: 309–11.

99. Oleagoitia JM, Echevarria A, Santidrian JI, Ulacia MA & Hernandez Calvo J. Early gastric cancer. *Br J Surg* 1986; **73**: 804–6.

100. Murakimi T. Pathomorphological diagnosis: definition and gross classification of early gastric cancer. *Gann Monogr* 1972; **11**: 53–5.

101. Ichiyoshi Y, Toda T, Minamisono Y, Nagasaki S, Yakeishi Y & Sugimachi K. Recurrence in early gastric cancer. *Surgery* 1990; **107**: 489–95.

102. Folli S, Dente M, Dell'Amore D *et al.* Early gastric cancer: prognostic factors in 223 patients. *Br J Surg* 1995; **82**: 952–6.

103. Ranaldi R, Santinelli A, Verdolini R, Rezai B, Mannello B & Bearzi I. Long-term follow-up in early gastric cancer: evaluation of prognostic factors. *J Pathol* 1995; **177**: 343–51.

104. Friesen G, Dockerty MB & ReMine WH. Superficial carcinoma of the stomach. *Surgery* 1962; **51**: 300–12.

105. Shiu MH, Moore E, Sanders M *et al.* Influence of the extent of resection on survival after curative treatment of gastric carcinoma. A retrospective multivariate analysis. Early gastric carcinoma with special reference to macroscopic classification. *Arch Surg* 1987; **60**: 1099–106.

106. Hattori T, Hosokawa Y, Fukuda M, Sugihara H, Hamada S, Takamatsu T, Nakanishi K, Tsuchihashi Y, Kitamura T & Fujita S. Analysis of DNA ploidy patterns of gastric carcinomas of Japanese. *Cancer* 1984; **54**: 1591–7.

107. Macartney JC, Camplejohn RS, Alder J, Stone MG & Powell G. Prognostic importance of DNA flow cytometry in non-Hodgkin's lymphomas. *J Clin Pathol* 1986; **39**: 542–6.

108. Ohyama S, Yonemura Y & Miyazak I. Proliferative activity and malignancy in human gastric cancers. Significance of the proliferation rate and its clinical application. *Cancer* 1992; **69**: 314–21.

109. Böttcher K, Becker K, Busch R, Roder JD & Siewert JR. Prognosefaktoren beim Magencarcinom: Ergebnisse einer uni- und multivariaten Analyse. *Chirurgie* 1992; **63**: 656–61.

110. De Aretxabala X, Yonemura Y, Sugiyama K *et al.* DNA ploidy in early gastric cancer and its relationship to prognosis. *Br J Cancer* 1988; **58**: 81–4.

111. Fonseca L, Yonemura Y, De Aretxabala X, Yamaguchi A, Miwa K & Miyazaki I. p53 detection as a prognostic factor in early gastric cancer. *Oncology* 1994; **51**: 485–90.

112. Maeda K, Chung YS, Onoda N *et al.* Association of tumor cell proliferation with lymph node metastasis in early gastric cancer. *Oncology* 1996; **53**: 1–5.

113. Kamata T, Yonemura Y, Sugiyama K *et al.* Proliferative activity of early gastric cancer measured by in vitro and in vivo bromodeoxyuridine labeling. *Cancer* 1989; **64**: 1665–8.

114. Sendler A, Dittler HJ, Feussner H *et al.* Preoperative staging in gastric cancer as precondition for multimodal treatment. *World J Surg* 1995; **19**: 501–8.

115. Okamura T, Korenaga D, Baba H, Saito A & Sugimachi K. Postoperative adjuvant chemotherapy inhibits early recurrence of early gastric carcinoma. *Cancer Chemother Pharmacol* 1989; **23**: 319–22.

8
GASTRIC LYMPHOMA

ALEXANDER A. PARIKH
LINDA S. CALLANS
JOHN M. DALY

INTRODUCTION

Primary gastric lymphoma is an uncommon cancer, accounting for <10% of all gastric malignancies. It remains the most common extranodal form of non-Hodgkin's lymphoma, comprising 20–25% of extranodal primary lymphomas and over 50% of gastrointestinal lymphomas. Moreover, its incidence seems to be increasing.

The majority of gastric lymphomas are of B-cell origin, and several different classification schemes have been developed to describe the exact histologic variety. The etiology of the disease is still unclear, but at least a portion of gastric lymphomas may be derived from the accumulation of mucosa-associated lymphoid tissue (MALT) in the gastric submucosa secondary to chronic inflammation.

The diagnosis of gastric lymphoma is usually more difficult to establish than gastric adenocarcinoma. An early and correct diagnosis is important however, since therapeutic approaches differ and gastric lymphoma tends to have a better overall prognosis. Although radiographic studies can suggest the diagnosis in some patients, endoscopic biopsy with histologic and cytologic analysis is always required. With improvements in endoscopic biopsy techniques and imaging studies, a formal laparotomy is not usually necessary for diagnosis and staging.

Gastric lymphoma differs in its clinical behavior and prognosis from nodal malignant lymphoma. The overall prognosis of gastric lymphoma depends primarily on the initial stage of the disease, but histologic grade, wall penetration, size and location of the tumor, and other factors may also be important.

Traditionally, gastric lymphoma has been treated by aggressive surgical resection, especially for local and early stage disease, but some authors have recently advocated primary or adjuvant radiotherapy or chemotherapy alone in managing these lesions with similar survival and complication rates.

The study of gastric lymphoma is hampered by many factors. Prospective data are scanty regarding gastric lymphoma, and series usually include an insufficient number of patients for statistical analysis. Consequently, recommendations regarding treatment, prognosis, and outcome are often conflicting. The rarity of this lesion makes randomized prospective trials difficult to design, and most information is provided from retrospective reviews.

EPIDEMIOLOGY

Most studies report that primary gastric lymphomas represent between 1% and 8% of all gastric tumors, although secondary involvement of the stomach in patients with generalized lymphoma is substantially more common.[1] In Central Europe and North America, between 20–25% of all primary extranodal lymphomas and approximately 60% of all gastrointestinal lymphomas in adults originate in the stomach,[2–4] whereas intestinal malignant lymphomas are rather infrequent.[5] A different pattern is seen in Middle Eastern and Mediterranean countries, where primary intestinal lymphoma accounts for half of all extranodal and 75% of gastrointestinal lymphomas.[6,7]

The incidence of gastric lymphoma in the United States appears to be increasing in men and women equally, and seems more apparent in the elderly population.[8,9] The reasons for this increase is unknown, but may be due to selection bias or improved diagnosis. More recent studies originate in referral centers that may see more cases of gastric lymphoma, and over the past few decades the ability to diagnose this disease has steadily increased with advances in endoscopic biopsy and histopathologic techniques. Furthermore, since the incidence of gastric adenocarcinoma is decreasing,[8] the apparent increase in gastric lymphoma may only represent a change in relative proportion. Despite these explanations, several studies suggest that the true incidence of primary gastric lymphoma has increased.[1,9] In part, this may reflect the increasing incidence of acquired immune deficiency syndrome (AIDS) and lymphomas associated with other immunosuppressive agents, as well as the effect of some environmental, dietary, or occupational exposures.[2,10–12]

PATHOLOGY

Gastric lymphoma originates from the lamina propria and extends laterally along the submucosa. The muscular layer is generally spared until late in the disease, while the mucosa is not primarily involved. There may be diffuse infiltration resulting in rigidity and a linitus plastica appearance, but there is generally no desmoplastic reaction.[2,10,13] This may explain why lymphomas often perforate either spontaneously or during treatment.

On gross inspection, it is often impossible to differentiate lymphomas from carcinomas. Some tumors are polypoid, fungating, or even infiltrating. About 25% are multicentric, while some simulate benign gastric hypertrophy with pronounced mucosal ridges and folds. Ulcers are present in 40–80%, and are often multiple in number. The most common location for the tumor is in the distal two-thirds of the stomach along the posterior wall and lesser curvature, but gastric outlet obstruction is usually rare. The tumor can also involve the entire surface of the stomach.[2,10,14]

Although a small subset of primary gastric lymphomas spontaneously regress, the majority spread locally by submucosal infiltration and then through routes similar to those of gastric adenocarcinoma. The local and regional lymph nodes are initially involved, followed by spread to the para-aortic nodes, omentum, peritoneum, mesentery, and extra-abdominal nodes. Direct extension to adjacent organs such as the liver occurs with bulky disease, and distal tumors may invade the duodenum more commonly than carcinomas. Blood-borne and distant metastases occur later in the disease.[8,10]

Microscopic examination reveals that about 80% of primary gastric lymphomas are of B-cell origin, almost exclusively of the non-Hodgkin's type, although gastric Hodgkin's disease has been reported.[15,16] As with nodal lymphomas, several different histopathologic classifications have been applied to describe gastric lymphomas including the Rappaport, Lukes and Collins, and Kiel classifications (**Table 8.1**). In Rappaport's classification, the diffuse histiocytic lymphomas predominates, while according to the Lukes and Collins classification, the most common type is the follicular center cell type (FCC), particularly small cleaved. Following the Kiel classification, gastric lymphoma is mostly of the diffuse centroblastic–centrocytic (low grade) or of the immunoblastic or centroblastic type (high grade).[17]

Since each of the above classifications has been used to describe gastric lymphoma, comparison between studies is difficult. Controversy continues regarding the influence of histologic type on prognosis, treatment options, and outcome. An attempt to simplify these classification schemes and to make comparisons between systems easier was set forth by the National Cancer Institute in 1982 when a Working Formulation of Non-Hodgkin's Lymphomas was developed for clinical use. According to this scheme, the most common gastric lymphomas are those of the intermediate grade (diffuse large cell-DL) and low-grade (follicular, small, cleaved-FSC).[17]

All of these classifications were originally developed to describe nodal lymphomas, and many authors have since noted that a significant proportion of gastric and other extranodal lymphomas behave quite differently from their nodal counterparts in terms of morphology and clinical course.[18,19] As a result, a new concept for extranodal lymphomas was developed by Isaacson and Wright.[20] They noticed that the histology of certain low-grade, B-cell gastrointestinal lymphomas was similar to that of mucosa-associated

Table 8.1   Comparison among different classification schemes for non-Hodgkin's lymphoma. Adapted from N-HLPC project, 1982[17]

WORKING FORMULATION	KIEL	LUKES–COLLINS	RAPPAPORT
Low-grade			
A. Malignant lymphoma, small lymphocytic (SL)	lymphocytic, CLL lymphoplasmacytic/ lymphoplasmactyoid	small lymphocytic and plasmacytoid lymphocytic	lymphocytic, well-differentiated
B. Malignant lymphoma, follicular, predominantly small cleaved cell (FSC)	centroblastic–centrocytic (small), follicular	small cleaved FCC, follicular or follicular and diffuse	nodular, poorly differentiated lymphocytic
C. Malignant lymphoma, follicular, mixed small cleaved and large cell (FM)	centroblastic–centrocytic (small), follicular	small cleaved FCC, follicular large cleaved FCC, follicular	nodular, mixed lymphocytic–histiocytic
Intermediate grade			
D. Malignant lymphoma, follicular, predominantly large cell (FL)	centroblastic–centrocytic (large), follicular	large cleaved and/or non-cleaved FCC, follicular	nodular histiocytic
E. Malignant lymphoma, diffuse small cleaved cell (DSC)	centrocytic, small	small cleaved FCC, diffuse	diffuse lymphocytic, poorly differentiated
F. Malignant lymphoma, diffuse, mixed small and large cell (DM)	centroblastic–centrocytic, diffuse; lymphoplasma–cytoid, polymorphic diffuse	small cleaved, large cleaved, or large non-cleaved FCC	diffuse mixed lymphocytic–histiocytic
G. Malignant lymphoma, diffuse, large cell (DL)	centroblastic–centrocytic, (large), diffuse; centrocytic (large); centroblastic, diffuse	large cleaved or non-cleaved FCC (diffuse)	diffuse histiocytic
High-grade			
H. Malignant lymphoma, large cell, immunoblastic (IBL)	immunoblastic and T-zone lymphoma	immunoblastic sarcoma, T- or B-cell type	diffuse histiocytic
I. Malignant lymphoma, lymphoblastic (LBL)	lymphoblastic convoluted, or unclassified	convoluted T-cell	lymphoblastic convoluted/non-convoluted
J. Malignant lymphoma, small non-cleaved cell (SNC)	lymphoblastic, Burkitt's type and other B-lymphoblastic	small non-cleaved FCC	undifferentiated, Burkitt's and non-Burkitt's
Miscellaneous composite mycosis fungoides histiocytic extramedullary plasmacytoma unclassifiable other			

lymphoid tissue (MALT) and closely simulated the Peyer's patch rather than the lymph node.[21–23]

In the scheme developed by Isaacson and Wright, B-cell gastric lymphomas are divided into low grade MALToma and high grade lymphoma (**Table 8.2**). In the low-grade MALT lymphoma (**Figure 8.1**), tumor cells infiltrate around and between reactive follicles spreading diffusely into the surrounding mucosa. The small lymphomatous cells disrupt the gastric glands, forming characteristic lymphoepithelial lesions. Although there is considerable variation in cytologic appearance, the cells are often small to medium-sized, with moderately abundant cytoplasm and nuclei that have an irregular outline closely resembling those of centrocytes.[14,22,25] These cells, termed centrocyte-like cells (CCL), are morphologically similar to the follicular center cells seen in nodal lymphomas,[16] but have different immunochemical properties. Low-grade lesions are often multicentric and frequently multifocal.[26]

Some cases of gastric lymphomas previously reported as lymphoplasmacytic/lymphoplasmacytoid, plasmacytic, or centroblastic–centrocytic (follicular center cell) may represent examples of this low-grade MALToma. In addition, "pseudolymphomas," which were originally thought to represent benign reactive lymphoid infiltrates, may also constitute a form of low-grade MALT lymphoma.

Table 8.2 A classification scheme of primary gastrointestinal lymphoma[20,24]

B cell
    MALT type
        Low-grade
        High-grade with or without a low-grade
            component
        Immunoproliferative small intestinal disease
            Low-grade
            High-grade with or without a low-grade
                component
        Mantle cell or malignant lymphoma centrocytic
            (lymphomatous polyposis)
        Burkitt-like
        Other types of low- or high-grade lymphoma
            corresponding to peripheral lymph node
            equivalents
T cell
    Enteropathy-associated T-cell lymphoma (EATL)
    Other types unassociated with enteropathy

Pseudolymphomas are monoclonal lesions demonstrating premalignant potential and invasive properties with their ability to disseminate to regional lymph nodes and beyond.[20,21,27,28]

High-grade gastric lymphomas of larger, transformed blastic cells that are usually thought to be centroblasts, but are often indistinguishable from immunoblasts or plasmablasts (**Figure 8.2**). These lesions are characterized by confluent clusters or sheets of transformed cells outside of colonized follicles.[23] The etiology of high-grade lesions is not clear, but many are thought to have been transformed from the low-grade MALT lymphoma. Foci of high-grade lymphoma may be seen in low-grade MALT lymphoma (and vice versa), and these foci express the same immunoglobulin light chains as the adjacent low-grade lesions.[4,25] The rest of the lesions are thought to be true *de novo* primary high-grade lymphomas, unrelated to MALT. Since the histologic and cytologic features of high-grade lymphoma either arising from MALToma or unrelated to MALT are identical and their clinical behavior similar, the exact etiology of the high-grade lesion may not be clinically important.[25,29] Nevertheless, some authors have suggested that there may be immunologic and molecular differences including the presence of the *bcl-2* onocogene and c-*myc* rearrangements. Moreover, the prognosis of some high-grade MALT-derived lesions may have a better prognosis than their nodal counterparts,[14] although this remains controversial.[18]

ETIOLOGY/PATHOGENESIS

Although the stomach is the most common site of gastrointestinal lymphoma, it is devoid of lymphatic tissue under normal conditions, as is the case in infancy and early childhood. With chronic inflammation, however, lymphocytes can accumulate in the gastric submucosa, resulting in MALT. Several studies indicate that over 80% of cases of gastric lymphoma are associated with achlorhydria, and it has been estimated that 60% of gastric non-Hodgkin's lymphomas evolve from chronic gastritis, a lesion usually caused by infection by *Helicobacter pylori*. Histologic studies have shown that this organism was present in the gastric mucosa in almost all people with gastric lymphoma (**Figure 8.3**).[30] More recently, a large case-control study correlated the presence of *H. pylori* infection with high-grade gastric lymphoma and showed that

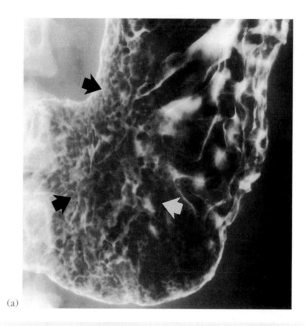

(a)

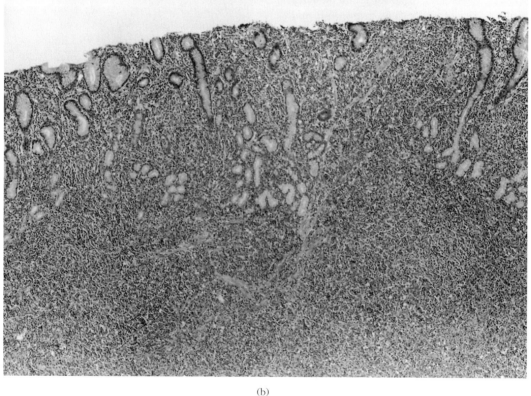

(b)

Figure 8.1 Radiographic and pathologic findings in MALT lymphoma. A. Spot radiograph from a double-contrast upper gastrointestinal examination shows that the normal areae gastricae pattern of the gastric body is disrupted by numerous superficial, round and ovoid elevations of mucosa (black and white arrows). (Illustration courtesy of Stephen E. Rubesin, M.D.) B. Gastric biopsy reveals diffuse infiltration of the mucosa and submucosa by small lymphomatous cells with effacement of germinal centers and displacement of gastric glands (hematoxylin and eosin stain, ×50). (Courtesy of Emma. E. Furth, M.D.)

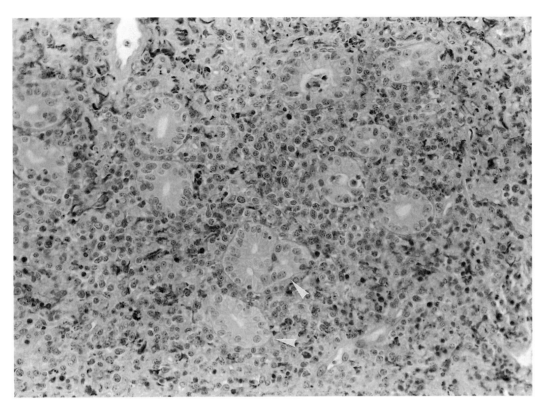

Figure 8.2 High-grade gastric lymphoma. Hematoxylin and eosin stain of a gastric biopsy reveals sheets of large lymphomatous cells infiltrating the submucosa between gastric glands (arrows) (×200). (Courtesy of Emma E. Furth, M.D.)

the infection was present before the lymphoma was diagnosed.[31] Furthermore, eradication of the organism has been associated with histologic regression and tumor remission in patients with low-grade MALT lymphomas.[32–35] Molecular evidence of the neoplastic clone, however, may persist. The significance of molecular evidence of disease in the absence of histologic or clinical evidence is unknown.

Direct evidence of a causal role for *H. pylori* infection, however, was lacking until a series of experiments showed that cells recovered from resection specimens of low-grade gastric MALT lymphoma proliferated and synthesized tumor-specific immunoglobulin when co-cultured with different strains of heat-killed *H. pylori*. Subsequent experiments demonstrated that *H. pylori*-specific helper T cells induced the proliferation of the B-cell lymphoma cells.[23,36] These studies support the concept that *H. pylori* plays a causal role in the development of low-grade gastric MALT lym-

phoma, but most of the cases studied have been early-phase disease. It is unclear whether deeply penetrating lesions or higher-stage disease will respond in a similar fashion.

Other potential causes and associations include occupational exposures to organic solvents, chlorophenols, or phenoxyacetic acids; however, this is based primarily on scattered case reports.[37]

The translocation of the *bcl-2* proto-oncogene from chromosome 18 to chromosome 14 [t(14:18)] adjacent to the immunoglobulin heavy chain locus with subsequent expression of *bcl-2* has been detected by immunohistochemistry in various nodal lymphomas and several epithelial tumors. Using polymerase chain reaction (PCR), this translocation has also been shown in gastrointestinal lymphomas.[38] Recent studies have shown an inverse relationship between *bcl-2* protein expression and *p53* tumor suppressor gene expression in both nodal malignant lymphoma, and primary gastric lymphomas. Furthermore, the frequency of

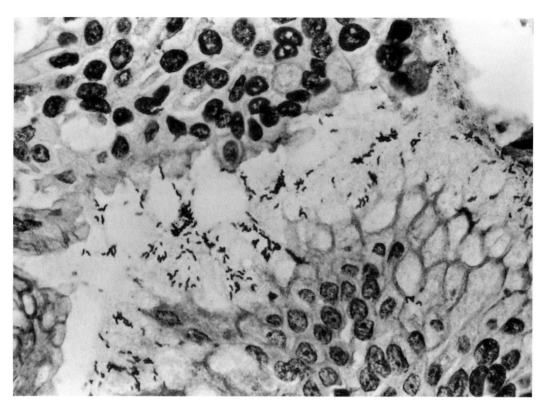

Figure 8.3 Association of *Helicobacter pylori* with MALT lymphoma. *H. pylori* organisms are demonstrated infiltrating between gastric surface mucosal cells. In several studies, *H. pylori* have been documented in nearly all patients with MALToma (silver stain, ×600). (Courtesy of Emma E. Furth, M.D.)

bcl-2 expression decreased and *p53* expression increased with increasing histologic grade, while suggesting that the expression of *bcl-2* and *p53* may be associated with a transition from low-grade to high-grade tumors.[39] Cytogenetic studies of low-grade gastric MALT lymphomas have suggested that trisomy 3 may be characteristic.[40] In addition to the t(14:18) translocation, an unusual translocation, t(1;14), has also been demonstrated in a gastric lymphoma.[23]

CLINICAL PRESENTATION

The presentation of gastric lymphoma is very similar to that of gastric adenocarcinoma or peptic ulcer disease. Most patients present in their mid-fifties or older, but the age at diagnosis ranges from childhood to the nineties. There is a definite sex predilection, with about a 1.7 : 1 male predominance and nearly 90% of patients are caucasian.[4,5,41,42]

The most common presenting symptom is abdominal pain, present in about 70% of patients (**Table 8.3**). The pain is usually of a dull, boring quality, and is often initially attributed to a benign disorder. Nausea, vomiting, and weight loss are also common complaints, while other symptoms include weakness, gastrointestinal bleeding, and

Table 8.3 The most common presenting symptoms in patients with primary gastric lymphoma

SYMPTOM	PROPORTION (%)
Abdominal pain	70
Weight loss	50
Nausea/vomiting	40
Anorexia	25
Bleeding	20
Fatigue/malaise	15
Dysphagia	0–10
Change in bowel habits	0–10

anorexia. Some patients present with gastric per-foration or obstruction. Less than 10% of patients are asymptomatic at the time of diagnosis.[43–46] Several studies have reported a median duration of symptoms of 10 to 30 months before diagnosis and treatment.[8,46] Because of the often vague and insidious onset of symptoms, many patients do not present until after they have developed a large tumor burden.

Common physical findings include cachexia, abdominal tenderness in 39%, and guaiac-positive stools in up to half of the patients. Occasionally, a left upper quadrant abdominal mass may be pal-pated, but most patients have no other abnormal physical findings unless a complication has occurred. Rarely, splenomegaly in patients with direct extension into the spleen, palpable periph-eral adenopathy, or a large retroperitoneal mass may be appreciated.[2,10,11,41,44,46]

DIAGNOSTIC EVALUATION

Plain radiographs are seldom helpful in establish-ing the diagnosis. An upper gastrointestinal con-trast study, however, can suggest an abnormality in over 90% and a malignancy in up to 75% (**Figure 8.4**). It may be difficult to differentiate lym-phoma from carcinoma or sometimes even peptic ulcer disease.[41,44,47,48] Radiologic features that sug-gest gastric lymphoma include: (i) diffuse mucosal hypertrophy with irregular thickening of folds; (ii) innumerable tiny nodules, (iii) single or multiple ulcers associated with diffuse mucosal thickening;[49] and (iv) a mass lesion or a mucosal irregularity extending across the pylorus to the duodenum.[50,51] Lesions >15 cm are usually lym-phomas, and those <5 cm are usually carcinomas.[1] Despite these guidelines, the correct diagnosis of gastric lymphoma from an upper gastrointestinal contrast study is established in less than 20% of cases.[50,52]

Ultrasonography and computerized tomography (CT) have also been reported to be useful. Conventional transabdominal ultrasound may reveal findings consistent with gastric lymphoma, but this is usually only possible with advanced lesions.[52] CT can detect thickening of the gastric wall due to neoplastic infiltration, intra-abdominal extension, and regional or distant lymph node involvement (**Figure 8.5**). However, it cannot dif-ferentiate lymphoma from carcinoma since it can-not discern the specific layers of the gastric wall with intramural versus extramural infiltration, or identify adjacent lymphadenopathy.[53] While neither of these modalities are likely to be used as a primary diagnostic technique, they may help to diagnose equivocal cases of gastric lymphoma and assist in the staging of these lesions, as well as with follow-up.[54]

Endoscopic ultrasonography (EUS) has recently been advocated to help define intramural tumor infiltration as well as spread through the gastric wall. EUS can also identify deep masses or regional lymph node involvement.[55–58] Several studies on gastric cancer and lymphoma show that specific EUS features correlate with histologic findings and allow for correct diagnosis and staging in over 90% of cases.[53,55,57,59] Depending on the echographic pattern of the gastric wall, EUS can differentiate four types of gastric lymphoma: (i) the superficial spreading type; (ii) the diffuse-infiltrating type, which correlates well with low-grade MALT lym-phomas; (iii) the mass-forming or tumorus type, corresponding to intermediate-grade lymphomas without MALT components; and (iv) the mixed-type which most closely resembles diffuse small cleaved type without MALT components.[57,60] EUS is, therefore, considered to be a useful tool for establishing the diagnosis and resectability of the tumor, for preoperative staging, and for follow-up after definitive therapy. Limits of this modality include poor visualization of the antral and pre-pyloric area as well as the proximal part of the lesser curvature.[59]

Upper endoscopy with biopsy is the modality used most commonly to establish the diagnosis, with a specificity ranging from 67% to 96%.[44,61,62] Endoscopy may reveal localized edema, rugal fold hypertrophy, cobblestone-appearing mucosa, mul-tiple tumor nodules, and multiple superficial muco-sal ulcerations overlying a sizable tumor mass.[10] Since the tumor most commonly develops in the submucosal lymphatic tissue and may be covered by normal gastric mucosa, tissue biopsies often show only normal mucosa unless multiple deep samples are taken through the mucosa. As a result, the exophytic type of lymphoma is more easily diagnosed than the infiltrative type.[63] In addition, small biopsies may be inadequate for diagnosis since some of the most common lymphomas rapidly outgrow their blood supply and are asso-ciated with a significant amount of necrotic tissue.

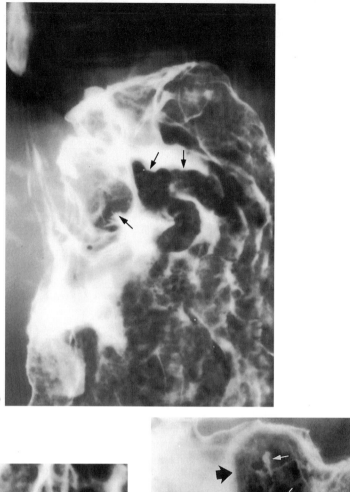

(A)

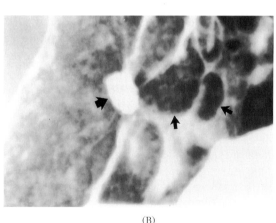

(B)

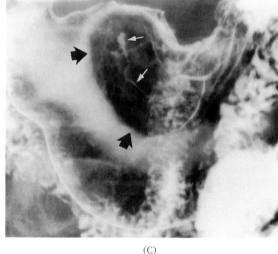

(C)

Figure 8.4 Various upper gastrointestinal findings in non-Hodgkin's lymphoma of the stomach. Among other findings, gastric lymphoma may also be characterized by thickening folds, ulcerations, or polypoid lesions. A. Thickened folds. Radiograph from a double-contrast upper gastrointestinal (GI) examination shows thick, lobulated folds (arrows) in the gastric fundus and upper gastric body. B. Lymphomatous ulcer. This spot radiograph from a double-contrast upper GI examination shows a 1.5-cm ovoid ulcer (large arrow) surrounded by large, lobulated folds (representative folds are indicated by small arrows). C. Polypoid lesion. This double-contrast upper GI study shows a 5-cm, well-circumscribed filling defect (black arrows) in the shallow barium pool. Barium fills a linear ulcer (white arrows) in the center of the tumor. (Courtesy of Stephen E. Rubesin, M.D.)

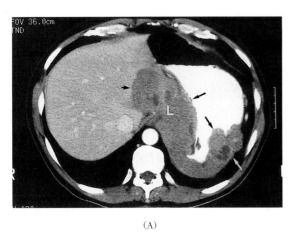 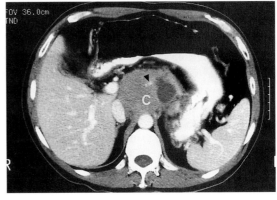

(A)   (B)

Figure 8.5 Computed tomography (CT) findings in advanced gastric lymphoma. A. A CT scan through the gastric body shows marked thickening and lobulation of the posterior and medial gastric wall (long arrows). The gastrohepatic ligament is infiltrated by a large soft tissue mass (L) and the left gastric vessels are encased by tumor. The tumor impresses upon the left lobe of the liver. This scan cannot distinguish liver invasion from extrinsic impression. B. A CT scan caudad to the origin of the celiac axis shows a soft tissue mass (C) surrounding branches of the celiac artery (arrowhead). The mass is clearly separated by a fat plane from the posterior gastric wall. It is difficult to distinguish adenopathy from direct invasion of the retroperitoneum on this scan. (Courtesy of Stephen E. Rubesin, M.D.)

Once satisfactory tissue has been obtained, histologic and cytologic analyses are performed to establish the diagnosis. Monoclonal proliferation is the hallmark in distinguishing malignant lymphoma from a reactive lymphoid infiltrate.[64] Cytology can distinguish abnormal lymphoid cell types, but cannot determine architecture, pattern, or cell type with assurance. Immunohistochemistry with stains for leukocyte common antigen and cytokeratin can help differentiate between lymphoid and epithelial cancers.[65,66] Antibodies for light chain immunoglobulin have been used to facilitate diagnosis,[67] but its use is somewhat restricted to cryostat sections of fresh tissue. *In situ* hybridization techniques have recently been applied to the diagnosis of B-cell lymphomas by detection of monotypic immunoglobulin light-chain mRNA from formalin-fixed, paraffin-embedded sections. The advantage of *in situ* hybridization is that it can localize gene expression within the cell in addition to ensuring cellular accuracy.[68] Confirming monoclonality by demonstrating immunoglobulin gene rearrangement is another strategy for distinguishing neoplastic from reactive lymphocytic disorders.[69]

Both Southern blotting techniques and the PCR have been effective using DNA samples extracted from archival paraffin-embedded tissues.[64,68,69]

Once gastric lymphoma is detected, it must be differentiated from systemic lymphoma with gastric involvement, since the latter is much more common. Most observers have adhered to the modified Dawson's criteria for primary gastric lymphoma which includes: (i) no palpable peripheral adenopathy or mediastinal adenopathy on radiographic examination; (ii) a normal peripheral blood smear; (iii) disease mainly confined to the gastrointestinal tract by diagnostic imaging at laparotomy; (iv) lymphadenopathy limited to regional or retroperitoneal locations; and (v) lack of hepatic or splenic involvement (except via direct spread).[70] Diagnostic modalities to rule out systemic disease include bone marrow biopsy, chest radiogram, and CT scan or magnetic resonance imaging (MRI) of the abdomen. Lymphangiography is rarely used. Largely because of advances in imaging modalities, a formal staging laparotomy is no longer necessary in most cases of gastric lymphoma, though it may be required occasionally to establish tissue diagnosis.

STAGING

Most authors use the Ann Arbor staging system, or one of its modifications such as the Musshoff modification, that were designed to describe extranodal lymphomas. The Musshoff modification, as shown in **Table 8.4**, allows a distinction to be made between stage II patients with regional, or perigastric lymph nodes (IIE_1) and those with distant lymph node involvement at abdominal sites not contiguous with the stomach (IIE_2).

Some authors however, contend that this may not be the most appropriate staging system for gastric lymphoma. The Ann Arbor staging system was developed on the basis of the study of Hodgkin's lymphoma, whereas the most common type of gastric lymphoma is non-Hodgkin's. Furthermore, this system and its modification do not take into account depth of invasion which has been shown to be a prognostic factor in several studies. Thus, TNM staging system with appropriate modifications has been applied to gastric lymphoma (**Table 8.5**).[71,72] The TNM system roughly approximates Musshoff's modification of the Ann Arbor system in that stage I corresponds to stage IE, and stages II and III correspond to stage IIE. In the TNM system, lymph nodes beyond the regional nodes are considered distant metastases or stage IV disease.

A staging system for EUS utilizing the TNM classification has also been developed. According to this scheme, tumors are divided into: EUS-T1, tumors located in the mucosa or submucosa; EUS-T2, tumors in the mucosa and submucosa extending into the muscularis propria or submucosa; EUS-T3, transmural tumors with penetration into the serosa; and EUS-T4, transmural tumors with penetration into adjacent structures.[56,59]

TREATMENT

Until the mid-1900s, the only treatment available for gastric lymphomas was surgical excision. Since that time, the value of radiotherapy and chemotherapy have gradually been realized for nodal lymphoma and, more recently, for extranodal disease. Controversy continues to exist as to the best treatment for primary gastric lymphoma, and the role of surgery in particular. This is especially true for early-stage lymphoma, since successful treatment with surgery, radiation, chemotherapy, and multimodality therapy have all been reported.

This dilemma is compounded by the fact that treatment recommendations have largely been based on the results of empiric treatment and retrospective studies. Most prospective studies consist of a small number of cases and reliable statistical analysis is difficult to perform. Long recruitment periods and varying treatment protocols – sometimes out of date – have led to data that are difficult to compare. Moreover, since gastric lymphomas are classified by a variety of schemes, comparisons among studies are difficult. Finally, several studies group gastric and intestinal lymphomas of various stages together, despite evidence of clinical, biologic and histopathologic differences.

Surgery

Many investigators still favor resection of primary gastric lymphoma for several reasons. First, resection specimens are sometimes needed for accurate

Table 8.4 Staging system used for gastric lymphoma based on Musshoff's modification of the Ann Arbor staging system for non-Hodgkin's lymphoma

Stage IE:	Localized involvement of one or more gastrointestinal sites on the same side of the diaphragm without lymph node involvement
IE_1:	Confined to the mucosa and submucosa
IE_2:	Extending beyond the submucosa
Stage IIE:	Localized involvement of one or more gastrointestinal sites on the same side of the diaphragm with lymph node involvement; penetration of lymphoma through the gut wall
IIE_1:	Regional lymph node involvement
IIE_2:	Lymph node infiltration beyond the regional area
Stage IIIE:	Involvement of the gastrointestinal tract and/or lymph nodes on both sides of the diaphragm
Stage IVE:	Diffuse or disseminated involvement of non-gastrointestinal tract organs or tissues

Table 8.5 Staging system for primary gastric lymphoma according to the TNM system.[71]

T – Primary tumor

T1:	Lymphoma confined to the mucosa
T2:	Involving the mucosa, submucosa, muscularis propria and extending into but not through the serosa
T3:	Penetrating through the serosa with or without involving contiguous structures
TX:	Degree of penetration undetermined

N – Regional lymph nodes

N0:	No involvement of nodes
N1:	Involvement of perigastric nodes
NX:	Nodal involvement undetermined

M – Distant metastasis

M0:	No distant metastasis
M1:	Evidence of distant metastasis including nodes beyond the regional area

Stage 1: No involvement of regional lymph nodes or distant metastasis

A:	T1, N0, M0
B:	T2, N0, M0
C:	T3, N0, M0

Stage 2–3: No involvement of regional lymph nodes
  T1–3, N1, M0

Stage 4: Metastatic disease
  T1–3, N0–1, M1

typing and staging of gastric lymphoma which has therapeutic and prognostic significance. Recent improvements in endoscopic, imaging, and histologic techniques may, however, allow for accurate staging and diagnosis in the absence of surgical resection.

Second, surgical resection alone is curative, especially with localized disease. Overall resectability rates for gastric lymphoma range from 53% to 96%,[6,41,45,47,73–81] and tend to be higher for lower-stage disease.[19,82,83] The overall 5-year survival rate after curative resection ranges from 33% to 66% for all stages,[4,41,45,46,51,73,78,84,85] and from 33% to 84% when considering stages IE and IIE alone.[5,29,48,51,74,86] The 5-year survival rate after resection for localized disease only (stages IE and IIE1) is even higher, ranging from 85% to 100%.[19,79,82,83] Furthermore, as the natural history of low-grade MALT-lymphoma is better understood, suggesting a long period of localized disease, primary surgical therapy for local disease may play an even more important role.

Finally, surgical therapy avoids certain complications of chemotherapy or radiation such as hemorrhage or perforation.[87,88] Surgery is not without risks, however, and the operative mortality rate has been reported to range from 0% to 30%.[29,41,89] Most of the high mortality has been associated with total gastrectomies and palliative resections. With the current practice of subtotal gastrectomies, operative mortality rates have generally fallen below 3%.[82–85,90–92] Perioperative complication rates also vary widely, but have generally been reported to be present in 10–22% of cases.[44,82,85,88]

The type and extent of surgical resection often depends on the stage, grade, and spread of the lesion. Although total gastrectomy with en-bloc resection of adjacent lymph nodes with or without distal pancreatectomy and splenectomy have been used in the past, lesser resections are now more common, especially with the advent of adjuvant therapy. A subtotal gastrectomy with a Billroth I or II reconstruction and regional lymph node dissection is most commonly performed today, particularly with local disease (stage IE–IIE). Proximal spread of the tumor may necessitate total gastrectomy which carries increased morbidity and mortality rates. In general, resection of the distal esophagus or proximal duodenum is not usually warranted, while more extensive resection is recommended when there is direct involvement of the pancreas and/or spleen.[8,41,82,93]

The general goal of curative surgery has been to remove all gross disease and to achieve clear margins. However, several studies have failed to show a significantly poorer prognosis associated with positive margins if the studies controlled for tumor stage, depth of invasion, and grade. With the advent of adjuvant therapy, many feel that clear margins should be achieved if possible, but not at the expense of increased morbidity or mortality. Many authors have reported significantly improved survival in stage IE and IIE lesions when surgical debulking of the tumor results in minimal residual disease.[19,79,94,95]

Radiotherapy

Primary radiotherapy for the treatment of gastric lymphoma, especially for early-stage disease, has been increasingly cited as a successful alternative to surgery. Although prospective trials are lacking, retrospective studies have reported 5-year survival rates (**Table 8.6**) as high as 85% for stage IE disease.[98,102] Studies comparing surgery with primary radiation therapy have shown comparable 5-year survival rates for stage IE and IIE disease.[4,15,101,103] One small study has actually reported an increased median survival for radiotherapy versus surgery for stage IE or IIE disease.[86] Advocates of primary radiotherapy stress the radiosensitivity of lymphoma and the improved quality of life with gastric organ preservation. Many believe that the complications and long-term effects associated with gastric resection are greater than those associated with radiation.

If radiation is to be given, a decision as to the sites and dosing regimens must be made. Although total dosages of 2000–3000 rads (20–30 Gy) have been used with success,[86] most authors recommend total doses in the region of 3000–5000 rads to achieve better outcome.[51,98,100,103,104] The radiation doses are given in several fractions over a period of weeks, and occasionally part of the dose is given to the entire abdomen, and a booster dose to the stomach and para-aortic area.[98,102] Both regional (stomach and adjacent lymph nodes) and total abdominal radiation have been used with similar success and complication rates, although some prefer total abdominal radiation to reduce intra-abdominal tumor recurrence.[15,48,51,86,98,102,103]

Initially severe and life-threatening complications of radiotherapy such as bleeding and perforation were reported in a significant number of patients,[76,88,103,105,106] though more recent studies have not confirmed a high incidence of perforation and hemorrhage.[44,85,98,100] Most authors now believe that these are uncommon com-plications, and quote morbidity and mortality rates comparable with those following surgery.[48,75,82,86,98,100,107,108,123]

Primary chemotherapy

Primary chemotherapy is generally the treatment of choice for high-grade, stage IIIE/IVE gastric lymphoma,[83,109] and the effectiveness against nodal lymphoma is well known.[110] A few studies suggest that chemotherapy alone may be as efficacious as surgery or radiotherapy in the treatment of gastric and gastrointestinal lymphomas, especially in high-grade lesions.[4,5,43,75,81,111,112] The role of primary chemotherapy in early-stage gastric lymphoma is more controversial, though two studies have shown that chemotherapy can eradicate early-stage disease.[113] In contrast, other studies have shown that chemotherapy alone is inferior to the combination of surgery and chemotherapy,[81,94] suggesting that chemotherapy in early-stage disease should be used as an adjuvant to either surgery and/or radiation.[47,48,76,96,97,99,100] Complication rates with primary chemotherapy, including bleeding and perforation, vary widely. Several studies suggest that these complications may be decreased if chemotherapy is used after surgical therapy, even for advanced lesions.[42,44,76,87,88]

The ideal chemotherapeutic regimen for lymphoma of the stomach is also unclear. Cyclophosphamide, doxorubicin, vincristine, and prednisone (CHOP) is very effective in nodal non-Hodgkin's lymphoma and is the primary choice for gastric lymphoma in most studies.[43,75,99,100,113] A variety of other regimens including mBACOD, BACOP, ProMACE-CytaBOM, LNH-84, or MACOP-B have all shown some efficacy.[75,76,109,112]

Multimodality treatment

Surgery plus adjuvant therapy consisting of radiation and/or chemotherapy is the mainstay of therapy, especially in early-stage (IE or IIE) lesions. Although prospective studies are few in number, several large retrospective studies have been published which investigated the role of surgery and adjuvant therapy. The studies of resection followed by radiation compared with surgery alone have been varied. Several studies suggested an improved survival for patients undergoing resection followed by irradiation,[19,41,42,51,73,77,78,86,114] especially in those with positive margins,[115] serosal involvement,[11,83] or regional lymph nodes (stage IIE1).[41,83,85,89] In most of these studies, however, the survival benefit for adjuvant radiation over surgery alone was not statistically significant. While most studies have failed to show any difference in survival, a few studies have reported significantly improved survival with surgery plus radiation.[4,29,46,48,84,96,104]

Several groups have also investigated the role of postoperative chemotherapy in stage IE and IIE gastric lymphoma with or without radiation. Surgical resection was performed for local control and chemotherapy was given for prevention of distant relapse. Again, several authors have suggested that resection followed by chemotherapy is superior to surgery alone in preventing relapses and prolonging survival, but direct comparisons with statistical analysis are lacking.[19,44,52,81,94,96,97,116,117] No benefit to surgery plus adjuvant chemotherapy versus surgery alone was detected in several other studies.[29,42,72,75,82,101]

Radiation/chemotherapy

Several authors have investigated the role of combined radiation and chemotherapy as primary therapy for gastric lymphoma. Radiation is given to treat local disease, while chemotherapy is given for systemic and extra-abdominal spread, thus potentially avoiding the need for surgical resection. In two retrospective studies of stage IE and IIE disease (see **Table 8.6**), Maor and associates were able to achieve a 56–73% overall 5-year survival rate, with one study showing a higher survival rate with stage IE disease (76% versus 42%).[96,100] Other authors have also reported comparable survival rates between combined radiotherapy and chemotherapy and surgical resection with or without adjuvant therapy, but again usually with a small number of patients.[15,75,98,102,108]

Eradication of *Helicobacter pylori*

With the recent suggestion that *H. pylori*-associated gastritis plays a role in the pathogenesis of gastric lymphoma of the MALT-type, eradication of *H. pylori* is at least a theoretical alternative, especially in the early stages of the disease. Although experience is limited, there have been several recent reports that treatment of *H. pylori* infection with antibiotics was associated with histologic regression of lymphomatous tissue in 60–83% of patients

with low-grade B-cell MALT lymphoma.[32–35] The reported follow-ups range from 3 to 12 months, and long-term relapse and survival rates are not known. Thus, eradication of *H. pylori* infection for gastritis and low-grade lymphoma may be an alternative or an adjunct for very early lesions, but direct comparisons with more traditional methods still cannot be made.

Advanced disease

Stage III and stage IV disease is, by definition, locally advanced and systemic disease. Multiple-agent chemotherapy is the mainstay of treatment for these patients, but cure is rarely possible. Surgery may have a role in advanced disease. Improved survival rates in patients with gastric resection with debulking prior to systemic therapy have been reported.[79,88] Part of this improved salvage rate may be due to decreased complication rates with chemotherapy, since gastric resection would preclude life-threatening hemorrhage and or perforation.[76,83,97] Radiation therapy has also been used for local control of bulky disease in patients with advanced, systemic disease.[83]

In summary, surgical resection remains the mainstay for early-stage, low-grade, distally located gastric lymphoma. Chemotherapy and radiation may be a better approach for patients with advanced disease or those requiring total gastrectomy. It remains to be seen whether treatment of *H. pylori* plays a role in the therapy for low-grade MALT lymphoma.

PROGNOSIS AND OUTCOME

Disagreement exists as to the important prognostic indicators for gastric lymphoma, but the stage of the disease at the time of diagnosis seems to be the most important prognostic factor for survival. Although survival varies among different reports and treatment regimens (see **Table 8.6**), overall survival rates correlate well with the stage of disease in essentially all reports. Using the more commonly used Musshoff modification of the Ann Arbor staging scheme, the 5-year survival rate for patients with stage IE disease averages about 80%, and ranges from 57% to 100%. By comparison, stage IIE disease survival ranges from 29% to 78%, with a mean of 50%. There is a higher survival rate for stage IIE1 (63%) than stage IIE2 (35%) in several reports.[5,19,44,46,82,103] Stage III and IV survival

Table 8.6 Results of various treatment modalities for early-stage gastric lymphoma

REFERENCE	YEAR	TOTAL NO. OF PATIENTS	STAGE	TREATMENT MODALITIES	MORTALITY RATE (%)	COMPLICATIONS (%)	FIVE-YEAR SURVIVAL RATE (%)
Bedikian et al.[78]	1980	21	IE, IIE	surgery	–	–	50
				surgery + XRT	–	–	63
Herrmann et al.[86]	1980	25	IE, IIE	surgery	–	–	50
				XRT	–	–	80
				surgery + XRT	–	–	90
Shiu et al.[51]	1982	36	IE, IEE	surgery	9 (operative)	9 (XRT)	33
				surgery + XRT			67
Dworkin et al.[46]	1982	44	IE, IIE	surgery	9 (operative)	–	59
				surgery + XRT			40
Shimm et al.[85]	1983	25	IE, IIE	surgery	–	28 (total)	51
				surgery + XRT			58
Mittal et al.[48]	1983	37	IE, IIE	surgery	10 (operative)	21 (operative)	45
				XRT			37
				surgery + XRT			74
				surgery + XRT + chemo			100
Brooks & Enterline[4]	1983	44	IE, IIE	surgery	8 (operative)	–	65
				surgery + XRT			67
				XRT			67
Maor et al.[96]	1983	77	IE, IIE	surgery	16 (operative)	0 (total, severe)	67
				surgery + XRT			58
				surgery + XRT + chemo			62
				surgery + chemo			100
				XRT	2 (XRT)		21
				XRT + chemo			75
				chemo			40
Sheridan et al.[97]	1985	15	IE, IEE	surgery + chemo	0	–	87
Shiu et al.[83]	1986	24	IE, IIE₁	surgery	0 (operative)	31 (total)	100
				surgery + XRT			73
				surgery + chemo			100
				surgery + XRT + chemo			100
Burgers et al.[98]	1988	24	IE, IIE	surgery + XRT	0	17	85
Shepherd et al.[94]	1988	16	IE, IIE	surgery + chemo	–	–	85
				chemo			67

Table 8.6 Results of various treatment modalities for early-stage gastric lymphoma (contd.)

REFERENCE	YEAR	TOTAL NO. OF PATIENTS	STAGE	TREATMENT MODALITIES	MORTALITY RATE (%)	COMPLICATIONS (%)	FIVE-YEAR SURVIVAL RATE (%)
Sharma et al.[99]	1990	9	IE, IEE	surgery + XRT + chemo XRT + chemo	0 (total)	0 (total)	100 – 1 year 100 – 1 year
Talamonti et al.[88]	1990	20	IE, IEE	surgery ± adjuvant rx XRT or chemo	0 (total)	–	82 50
Maor et al.[100]	1990	34	IE, IIE	XRT ± chemo	6	15	73–79
Schutze & Halpern[74]	1991	35	IE, IIE	surgery + adjuvant rx XRT, chemo or both	0 (operative)	–	84 71
Cogliatti et al.[29]	1991	145	IE, IIE	surgery ± adjuvant rx	5.5 (operative)	–	76
Ben Yosef & Hoppe[15]	1994	24	IE, IIE	surgery + XRT + chemo surgery + XRT XRT + chemo XRT	–	–	53 – 10 year 69 – 10 year 50 – 10 year 0 – 10 year
Bartlett et al.[82]	1996	34	IE, IIE$_1$	surgery surgery + XRT surgery + chemo surgery + XRT + chemo	0 (operative)	26 (total)	100 – 10 year 100 – 10 year 75 – 10 year 60 – 10 year

XRT, radiation therapy

drops significantly to about 22%, with some studies reporting a slightly better survival with stage III disease than stage IV.[52,71] There have been a few reports of survival in advanced stage diseases reaching 50% at 5 years,[79,116] but numbers are limited. Five-year survival also seems to correlate with stage using the TNM staging system, ranging from 100% survival for stages I and IA disease to less than 25% for stage IV disease.[52,71–73,77] Relapse-free survival also decreases with each stage in nearly all reports. Recurrences tend to occur within the first 2 years.[4,41,46,47,71,79,85,86]

While stage correlates well with survival, there is controversy regarding the significance of the prognostic factors. Several authors have reported survival differences based on the histologic grade of the tumor, with high-grade doing poorly compared with low-grade,[5,10,44–46,52,106,118,119] though there is not universal agreement due to differences in classification schemes. Several studies have failed to show a difference once the data are controlled for stage.[73,84,86,93,115,116] Using the newer concept of MALT lymphoma, however, survival differences have been shown between high-grade and low-grade lesions, of similar stages.[19,29,43]

Additional factors that may impact on prognosis include depth of invasion, particularly penetration of the tumor beyond the serosa,[2,4–6,10,19,46,71,84,85,120] size of the tumor,[4,10,46,73,81,101,118] and location of the tumor. Patients with proximal tumors do worse than those with antral or body lesions,[19,52] and tumors along the lesser curvature carry a worse prognosis than those in other locations.[10,85] Male gender and increasing age have been associated with lower survival rates.[42,46,119,121] Poor prognosis has also been associated with the presence of *p53* expression,[39] and increasing levels of Ki-67, a nuclear marker of proliferation.[8]

SUMMARY

Primary gastric lymphoma remains a rare, albeit increasingly common, malignancy, with distinctive features and behavior as compared with nodal lymphomas and other gastric malignancies.[122,124]

The etiology remains unclear, but may relate to chronic gastritis and resultant accumulation of lymphoid tissue in the stomach; *H. pylori* infection may also play a role. Certain chromosomal and molecular abnormalities can be demonstrated. Clinical signs and symptoms are vague, and the diagnosis continues to rely heavily on endoscopic biopsy, although endoscopic ultrasound has shown promise.

The treatment of gastric lymphoma remains a controversial topic, especially early in the disease. Local and early-stage disease are probably best treated with surgical resection and possible adjuvant therapy, though primary radiation and/or chemotherapy may be useful in certain patients. More advanced disease should be treated with systemic chemotherapy, although surgical debulking may decrease complication rates and improve survival. Prospective clinical trials comparing therapetic modalities are still needed to decide on the best treatment regimen for various stages of the disease.

Prognosis depends most on the stage of the tumor, although histologic grade, depth of invasion, and other factors may also affect survival. Overall, patients with gastric lymphoma seem to do better than patients with nodal non-Hodgkins lymphoma or gastric cancer, especially those with early-stage disease.

REFERENCES

1. Hayes J & Dunn E. Has the incidence of primary gastric lymphoma increased? *Cancer* 1989; **63**: 2073–6.
2. Sandler RS. Primary gastric lymphoma: a review. *Am J Gastroenterol* 1984; **79**: 21–5.
3. ReMine SG. Abdominal lymphoma. *Surg Clin North Am* 1985; **65**: 301–13.
4. Brooks JJ & Enterline H. Primary gastric lymphoma: a clinicopathologic study of 58 cases with long-term follow-up and literature review. *Cancer* 1983; **51**: 701–11.
5. Azab MB, Henry-Amar M, Rougier P et al. Prognostic factors in primary gastrointestinal non-Hodgkin's lymphoma. *Cancer* 1989; **64**: 1208–17.
6. Dragosiscs B, Bauer P & Radaszkiewicz T. Primary gastrointestinal non-Hodgkin's lymphomas: a retrospective clinicopathologic study of 150 cases. *Cancer* 1985; **55**: 1060–73.
7. Salem P, El-Hashimi L, Anaissie E et al. Primary small intestinal lymphoma in adults. *Cancer* 1987; **59**: 1670–6.
8. Frazee RC & Roberts J. Gastric lymphoma treatment: medical versus surgical. *Surg Clin North Am* 1992; **72**: 423–31.

9. Severson RK & Davis S. Increasing incidence of primary gastric lymphoma. *Cancer* 1990; **66**: 1283–7.

10. Thomas CR. Update on gastric lymphoma. *J Natl Med Assoc* 1991; **83**: 713–18.

11. Jung SS, Wieman TJ & Lindberg RD. Primary gastric lymphoma and pseudolymphoma. *Am Surg* 1988; **54**: 594–7.

12. Doglioni C, Wotherspoon AC, Moschini A *et al.* High incidence of primary gastric lymphoma in northeastern Italy. *Lancet* 1992; **339**: 834–5.

13. Loehr WS, Mujahed Z, Zahn FD *et al.* Primary lymphoma of the gastrointestinal tract: a review of 100 cases. *Ann Surg* 1969; **170**: 232–8.

14. Isaacson PG. Gastrointestinal lymphoma. *Hum Pathol* 1994; **25**: 1020–9.

15. Ben-Yosef R & Hoppe RT. Treatment of early-stage gastric lymphoma. *J Surg Oncol* 1994; **57**: 78–86.

16. Ishido T, Mori N, Kikuchi M & Nakamura K. Primary gastric malignant lymphoma: a morphological and immunohistochemical study of 38 cases. *Acta Pathol Jpn* 1989; **39**: 229–34.

17. N-HLPC project (The non-Hodgkin's lymphoma pathologic classification project). National Cancer Institute sponsored study of classifications of non-Hodgkin's lymphomas. *Cancer* 1982; **49**: 2112–35.

18. van Krieken JHJM, Otter R, Hermans J *et al.* Malignant lymphoma of the gastrointestinal tract and mesentery: a clinico-pathologic study of the significance of histological classification. *Am J Pathol* 1989; **135**: 281–9.

19. Radaszkiewicz T, Dragosics B & Bauer P. Gastrointestinal malignant lymphomas of the mucosa-associated lymphoid tissue: factors relevant to prognosis. *Gastroenterology* 1992; **102**: 1628–38.

20. Isaacson P & Wright DH. Extranodal malignant lymphoma arising from mucosa-associated lymphoid tissue. *Cancer* 1984; **53**: 2515–24.

21. Moore I & Wright DH. Primary gastric lymphoma – a tumor of mucosa-associated lymphoid tissue. A histological and immunohistochemical study of 36 cases. *Histopathology* 1984; **8**: 1025–39.

22. Isaacson PG & Spencer J. Malignant lymphoma of mucosa-associated lymphoid tissue. *Histopathology* 1987; **11**: 445–62.

23. Isaacson PG. Recent developments in our understanding of gastric lymphomas. *Am J Surg Pathol* 1996; **20**(suppl. 1): S1–7.

24. Isaacson PG, Spencer J & Wright DH. Classifying primary gut lymphomas. *Lancet* 1988; **12**: 1148–9.

25. Chan JKC, Ng CS & Isaacson PG. Relationship between high-grade lymphoma and low-grade B-cell mucosa-associated lymphoid tissue lymphoma (MALToma) of the stomach. *Am J Pathol* 1990; **136**: 1153–64.

26. Wotherspoon AC, Doglioni C & Isaacson PG. Low grade gastric B-cell lymphoma of mucosa-associated lymphoid tissue (MALT) a multifocal disease. *Histopathology* 1992; **20**: 29–34.

27. Schwartz MS, Sherman H, Smith T & Janis R. Gastric psuedolymphoma and its relationship to malignant gastric lymphoma. *Am J Gastroenterol* 1989; **84**: 1555–9.

28. Tokunaga O, Watanabe T & Morimatsu M. Pseudolymphoma of the stomach. *Cancer* 1987; **59**: 1320–7.

29. Cogliatti SB, Schmid U, Schumacher *et al.* Primary B-cell gastric lymphoma: a clinico-pathological study of 145 patients. *Gastroenterology* 1991; **101**: 1159–70.

30. Wotherspoon AC, Ortiz-Hidalgo C, Falzon MR & Isaacson PG. *Helicobacter pylori*-associated gastritis and primary B-cell gastric lymphoma. *Lancet* 1991; **338**: 1175–6.

31. Parsonnet J, Hansen S, Rodriguez L *et al. Helicobacter pylori* infection and gastric lymphoma. *N Engl J Med* 1994; **330**: 1267–71.

32. Wotherspoon AC, Doglioni C, Diss TC *et al.* Regression of primary low-grade B-cell gastric lymphoma of mucosa-associated lymphoid tissue type after eradication of *Helicobacter pylori*. *Lancet* 1993; **342**: 575–7.

33. Bayerdörffer E, Neubauer A, Rudolph B *et al.* Regression of primary gastric lymphoma of mucosa-associated lymphoid tissue type after cure of *Helicobacter pylori* infection. *Lancet* 1995; **345**: 1591–4.

34. Weber DM, Dimopoulos MA, Anandu DP *et al.* Regression of gastric lymphoma of mucosa-associated lymphoid tissue with antibiotic therapy for *Helicobacter pylori*. *Gastroenterology* 1994; **107**: 1835–8.

35. Roggero E, Zucca E, Pinotti G *et al.* Eradication of *Helicobacter pylori* infection in primary low-grade gastric lymphoma of mucosa-associated lymphoid tissue. *Ann Intern Med* 1995; **122**: 767–9.

36. Hussell T, Isaacson PG, Crabtree JE & Spencer J. The response of cells from low-grade B-cell lymphomas of mucosa-associated lymphoid tissue to *Helicobacter pylori*. *Lancet* 1993; **342**: 571–4.

37. Hardell L. Primary gastric lymphoma and occupational exposures. *Lancet* 1992; **340**: 186–7.

38. Shepard NA, McCarthy KP & Hall PA. 14:18 translocation in primary intestinal lymphoma: a detection by polymerase chain reaction in routinely processed tissue. *Histopathology* 1991; **18**: 415–19.

39. Nakamura S, Akazawa K, Kinukawa N *et al*. Inverse correlation between the expression of *bcl-2* and p53 proteins in primary gastric lymphoma. *Hum Pathol* 1996; **27**: 225–33.

40. Wotherspoon AC, Finn T & Isaacson PG. Numerical abnormalities of chromosomes 3 and 7 in lymphomas of mucosa associated lymphoid tissue and the splenic marginal zone. *Lab Invest* 1994; **70**: 124A.

41. Connors J & Wise L. Management of gastric lymphomas. *Am J Surg* 1974; **127**: 102–8.

42. Rackner VL, Thirlby RC & Ryan JA. Role of surgery in multimodality therapy for gastrointestinal lymphoma. *Am J Surg* 1991; **161**: 570–5.

43. Castrillo JM, Montalban C, Obeso G *et al*. Gastric B-cell mucosa associated lymphoid tissue lymphoma: a clinicopathological study in 56 patients. *Gut* 1992; **33**: 1307–11.

44. Schwarz RJ, Connors JM & Schmidt N. Diagnosis and management of stage IE and stage IIE gastric lymphomas. *Am J Surg* 1993; **165**: 561–5.

45. Orlando R, Pastuszak W, Preissler P & Welch JP. Gastric lymphoma: a clinicopathologic reappraisal. *Am J Surg* 1982; **143**: 450–5.

46. Dworkin B, Lightdale CJ, Weingrad DN *et al*. Primary gastric lymphoma: a review of 50 cases. *Dig Dis Sci* 1982; **27**: 986–92.

47. Fleming ID, Mitchell S & Ali Dilawari A. The role of surgery in the management of gastric lymphoma. *Cancer* 1982; **49**: 1135–41.

48. Mittal B, Wasserman TH & Griffith RC. Non-Hodgkin's lymphoma of the stomach. *Am J Gastroenterol* 1983; **78**: 780–7.

49. Levine

50. Sato T, Sakai Y, Ishiguro S & Furukawa H. Radiologic manifestations of early gastric lymphoma. *Am J Roentgenol* 1986; **146**: 513–7.

51. Shiu MH, Karas M, Nisce L *et al*. Management of primary gastric lymphoma. *Ann Surg* 1982; **195**: 196–202.

52. Secco GB, Fardelli R, Campora E *et al*. Primary gastric lymphoma. *J Surg Oncol* 1993; **54**: 157–62.

53. Tio TL, Jager H & Tijtgat BNJ. Endoscopic ultrasonography of non-Hodgkin lymphoma of the stomach. *Gastroenterology* 1986; **91**: 401–8.

54. Francica G, Cozzolino G, Morante *et al*. Gastric lymphoma: diagnosis and follow-up of chemotherapy-induced changes using real time ultrasonography: a report of three cases. *Eur J Radiol* 1990; **11**: 68–72.

55. Bolondi L, Casanova P, Caletti GC *et al*. Primary gastric lymphoma versus gastric carcinoma: endoscopic US evaluation. *Radiology* 1987; **165**: 821–6.

56. Schüder G, Hildebrandt U, Kreissler-Haag D *et al*. Role of endosonography in the surgical management of non-Hodgkin's lymphoma of the stomach. *Endoscopy* 1993; **25**: 509–12.

57. Palazzo L, Roseau G, Ruskone-Fourmestraux A *et al*. Endoscopic ultrasonography in the local staging of primary gastric lymphoma. *Endoscopy* 1993; **25**: 502–8.

58. Fujishima H, Misawa T, Maruoka A *et al*. Staging and follow-up of primary gastric lymphoma by endoscopic ultrasonography. *Am J Gastroenterol* 1991; **86**: 719–24.

59. Caletti G, Ferrari A, Brocchi E & Barbara L. Accuracy of endoscopic ultrasonography in the diagnosis and staging of gastric cancer and lymphoma. *Surgery* 1993; **113**: 14–27.

60. Suekane H, Iida M, Yao T *et al*. Endoscopic ultrasonography in primary gastric lymphoma: correlation with endoscopic and histologic findings. *Gastrointest Endosc* 1993; **39**: 139–45.

61. Arista-Nasr J, Jimenez A, Keirns C *et al*. The role of the endoscopic biopsy in the diagnosis of gastric lymphoma. *Hum Pathol* 1991; **22**: 339–48.

62. Swaroop VS, Mohandas KM, Swaroop VD *et al*. Comparative endoscopic study of primary gastric lymphoma vs. gastric carcinoma. *J Surg Oncol* 1994; **56**: 94–7.

63. Seifert E, Schulte F, Weismüller J *et al*. Endoscopic and bioptic diagnosis of malignant non-Hodgkin's lymphoma of the stomach. *Endoscopy* 1993; **25**: 497–501.

64. Savio A, Franzin G, Wotherspoon AC *et al*. Diagnosis and posttreatment follow-up of *Helicobacter pylori*-positive gastric lymphoma of mucosa-associated lymphoid tissue: histology, polymerase chain reaction, or both? *Blood* 1996; **87**: 1255–60.

65. Dean PJ, Moinuddin SM & Emerson LD. Application of anti-leukocyte common antigen and anti-cytokeratin antibodies to the biopsy diagnosis of gastric cell lymphoma. *Hum Pathol* 1987; **18**: 918–23.

66. de Mascarel A, Merlio JP, Coindre JM *et al*. Gastric large cell lymphoma expressing cytokeratin but no leukocyte common antigen. *Am J Clin Pathol* 1989; **91**: 478–81.

67. Isaacson PG, Spencer J & Finn T. Primary B-cell gastric lymphoma. *Hum Pathol* 1986; **17**: 72–82.

68. Inagaki H, Nonoka M, Nagaya S *et al.* Monoclonality in gastric lymphoma detected in formalin-fixed, paraffin-embedded endoscopic biopsy specimens using immunohistochemistry, in situ hybridization, and polymerase chain reaction. *Diagn Mol Pathol* 1995; **4**: 32–8.

69. Fend F, Schwaiger A, Weyrer K *et al.* Early diagnosis of gastric lymphoma: gene rearrangement analysis of endoscopic biopsy samples. *Leukemia* 1994; **8**: 35–9.

70. Dawson IMP, Cornes JS & Morson BC. Primary malignant lymphoid tumours of the intestinal tract. *Br J Surg* 1961; **121**: 80–9.

71. Lim FE, Hartman AS, Tan EGC *et al.* Factors in the prognosis of gastric lymphoma. *Cancer* 1977; **39**: 1715–20.

72. Shimodaira M, Tsukamoto Y, Niwa Y *et al.* A proposed staging system for primary gastric lymphoma. *Cancer* 1994; **73**: 2709–15.

73. Hockey MS, Powell J, Crocker J & Fielding WL. Primary gastric lymphoma. *Br J Surg* 1987; **74**: 483–7.

74. Shutze WP & Halpern NB. Gastric lymphoma. *Surg Gynecol Obstet* 1991; **172**: 33–8.

75. Gobbi PG, Dionigi P, Barbieri F *et al.* The role of surgery in the multimodal treatment of primary gastric non-Hodgkin's lymphomas. *Cancer* 1990; **65**: 2528–36.

76. Hande KR, Fisher RI, DeVita VT *et al.* Diffuse histocytic lymphoma involving the gastrointestinal tract. *Cancer* 1978; **41**: 1984–9.

77. Jones RE, Willis S, Innes D & Wanebo HJ. Primary gastric lymphoma: problems in staging and management. *Am J Surg* 1988; **155**: 118–23.

78. Bedikian AY, Khankhànian N, Heilburn LK & Valdivieso M. Primary lymphomas and sarcomas of the stomach. *South Med J* 1980; **73**: 21–4.

79. Paulson S, Sheehan RG, Stone MJ & Frenkel EP. Large cell lymphomas of the stomach: improved prognosis with complete resection of all intrinsic gastrointestinal disease. *J Clin Oncol* 1983; **1**: 263–9.

80. Contreary K, Nance FC & Becker WF. Primary lymphoma of the gastrointestinal tract. *Ann Surg* 1980; **191**: 593–8.

81. Economopoulos T, Alexopoulos C, Stathakis N *et al.* Primary gastric lymphoma – the experience of a general hospital. *Br J Cancer* 1985; **52**: 391–7.

82. Bartlett DL, Karpeh MS, Filippa DA & Brennan MF. Long-term follow-up after curative surgery for early gastric lymphoma. *Ann Surg* 1996; **223**: 53–62.

83. Shiu MH, Nisce LZ, Pinna A *et al.* Recent results of multimodal therapy of gastric lymphoma. *Cancer* 1986; **58**: 1389–99.

84. Rosen CB, van Heerden JA, Martin JK *et al.* Is an aggressive surgical approach to the patient with gastric lymphoma warranted? *Ann Surg* 1987; **205**: 634–40.

85. Shimm DS, Dosoretz DE, Anderson T *et al.* Primary gastric lymphoma: an analysis with emphasis on prognostic factors and radiation therapy. *Cancer* 1983; **52**: 2044–8.

86. Herrmann R, Panahon AM, Barcos MP *et al.* Gastrointestinal involvement in non-Hodgkin's lymphoma. *Cancer* 1980; **46**: 215–22.

87. Randall J, Obeid MI & Blackledge GR. Haemorrhage and perforation of gastrointestinal neoplasms during chemotherapy. *Ann Royal Coll Surg Engl* 1986; **68**: 286–9.

88. Talamonti MS, Dawes LG, Joehl RJ & Nahrwold DL. Gastrointestinal lymphoma: a case for primary surgical resection. *Arch Surg* 1990; **125**: 972–7.

89. Bailey R & Laws HL. Lymphoma of the stomach. *Am Surg* 1989; **55**: 665–8.

90. Gouzi JL, Huguier M, Fagniez *et al.* Total vs subtotal gastrectomy for adenocarcinoma of the gastric antrum. *Ann Surg* 1989; **209**: 162–71.

91. Jaehne J, Meyer HJ, Maschek H *et al.* Lymphadenectomy in gastric carcinoma: a prospective and prognostic study. *Arch Surg* 1992; **127**: 290–4.

92. Smith JW, Shiu MH, Kelsey L & Brennan MF. Morbidity of radical lymphadenectomy in the curative resection of gastric carcinoma. *Arch Surg* 1991; **126**: 1469–73.

93. ReMine SG & Braasch JW. Gastric and small bowel lymphoma. *Surg Clin North Am* 1986; **66**: 713–22.

94. Shepherd FA, Evans WK, Kutas G *et al.* Chemotherapy following surgery for stages IE and IIE non-Hodgkin's lymphoma of the gastrointestinal tract. *J Clin Oncol* 1988; **6**: 253–60.

95. Romaguera JE, Velasquez WS & Silvermintz KB. Surgical debulking is associated with improved survival in Stage I–II diffuse large cell lymphoma. *Cancer* 1990; **66**: 267–72.

96. Maor MH, Maddux B, Osborne BM *et al.* Stages IE and IIE non-Hodgkin's lymphomas of the stomach: comparison of treatment modalities. *Cancer* 1984; **54**: 2330–7.

97. Sheridan WP, Medley G & Brodie GN. Non-Hodgkin's lymphoma of the stomach: a prospective pilot study of surgery plus chemotherapy in early and advanced disease. *J Clin Oncol* 1985; **3**: 495–500.

98. Burgers JMV, Taal BG, van Heerde P *et al.* Treatment results of primary stage I and II non-Hodgkin's lymphoma of the stomach. *Radiother Oncol* 1988; **11**: 319–26.

99. Sharma S, Singhal S, De S *et al.* Primary gastric lymphoma: a prospective analysis of 12 cases and a review of the literature. *J Surg Oncol* 1990; **43**: 231–8.

100. Maor MH, Velasquez WS, Fuller LM & Silvermintz KB. Stomach conservation in stages IE and IIE gastric non-Hodgkin's lymphoma. *J Clin Oncol* 1990; **8**: 266–71.

101. Schutze WP & Halpern NB. Gastric lymphoma. *Surg Gynecol Obstet* 1991; **172**: 33–8.

102. Taal BG & Burgers JM. Primary non-Hodgkin's lymphoma of the stomach: endoscopic diagnosis and the role of surgery. *Scand J Gastroenterol* 1991; **188**: 33–7.

103. Weingrad DN, Decosse JJ, Sherlock P *et al.* Primary gastrointestinal lymphoma. *Cancer* 1982; **49**: 1258–65.

104. Bush RS & Ash CL. Primary lymphoma of the gastrointestinal tract. *Radiology* 1969; **92**: 1349–54.

105. Rosenfelt F & Rosenberg SA. Diffuse histiocytic lymphoma presenting with gastrointestinal tract lesions. *Cancer* 1980; **45**: 2188–93.

106. Naqvi MS, Burrows L & Kark AE. Lymphoma of the gastrointestinal tract: prognostic guides based on 162 cases. *Ann Surg* 1969; **170**: 221–31.

107. Roukos D & Encke A. *World J Surg* 1996; **20**: 116–17. (Letter to the Editor.)

108. Swaroop VS, Mohandas KM, Swaroop VD *et al.* Treatment of primary gastric lymphoma. *Gastroenterology* 1993; **105**: 645–6.

109. Fischbach W & Böhm S. Options in the therapy of gastric lymphoma. *Endoscopy* 1993; **25**: 531–3.

110. Laurence J, Coleman M, Allen S *et al.* Combination chemotherapy of advanced diffuse histiocytic lymphoma with the six-drug COP-BLAM regimen. *Ann Intern Med* 1982; **97**: 190–5.

111. Liang R, Todd D, Chan TK *et al.* Gastrointestinal lymphoma in Chinese: a retrospective analysis. *Hematol Oncol* 1987; **5**: 115–26.

112. Salles G, Herbrecht R, Tilly H *et al.* Aggressive primary gastrointestinal lymphomas: review of 91 patients treated with the LNH-84 regimen. A study of the Groupe d'Etude des lymphomes agressifs. *Am J Med* 1991; **90**: 77–84.

113. Tanaka Y, Takao T, Watanabe H *et al.* Early stage gastric lymphoma: is operation essential? *World J Surg* 1994; **18**: 896–9.

114. Skudder PA & Schwartz S. Primary lymphoma of the gastrointestinal tract. *Surg Gynecol Obstet* 1985; **160**: 5–8.

115. Burnett H & Herbert EA. The role of irradiation in the treatment of primary malignant lymphoma of the stomach. *Radiology* 1956; **67**: 723–7.

116. Bellesi G, Alterini R, Messori A *et al.* Combined surgery and chemotherapy for the treatment of primary gastrointestinal intermediate- or high-grade non-Hodgkin's lymphomas. *Br J Cancer* 1989; **60**: 244–8.

117. Mentzer SJ, Osteen RT, Pappas TN *et al.* Surgical therapy of localized abdominal non-Hodgkin's lymphomas. *Surgery* 1988; **103**: 609–14.

118. Filippa DA, Leiberman PH, Weingrad DN *et al.* Primary lymphomas of the gastrointestinal tract. *Am J Surg Pathol* 1983; **7**: 363–72.

119. Aozasa K, Ueda T, Kurata A *et al.* Prognostic value of histologic and clinical factors in 56 patients with gastrointestinal lymphomas. *Cancer* 1988; **61**: 309–15.

120. List AF, Greer JP, Cousar JC *et al.* Non-Hodgkin's lymphoma of the gastrointestinal tract: an analysis of clinical and pathologic features affecting outcome. *J Clin Oncol* 1988; **6**: 1125–33.

121. Valicenti RK, Wasserman TH & Kucik NA. Analysis of prognostic factors in localized gastric lymphoma: the importance of bulk of disease. *Int J Radiat Oncol Biol Phys* 1993; **27**: 591–8.

122. Fischbach W, Kestel W, Kirchner T *et al.* Malignant lymphomas of the upper gastrointestinal tract. *Cancer* 1992; **70**: 1075–80.

123. Hellman S, Chaffey JT, Rosenthal DS *et al.* The place of radiation therapy in the treatment of non-Hodgkin's lymphomas. *Cancer* 1977; **39**: 843–51.

124. Hendricks JC. Malignant tumors of the stomach. *Surg Clin North Am* 1986; **66**: 683–93.

PART

3

Esophageal cancer

9

SURGICAL MANAGEMENT of ESOPHAGEAL CANCER: THE WESTERN EXPERIENCE

GLYN G. JAMIESON
GEORGE MATHEW

INTRODUCTION

The "Western Experience" suggests a clear difference from the Japanese experience, and even a cursory reading of the two chapters in this book will leave little doubt that attitudes and results between these two experiences differ widely in the field of esophageal cancer. This chapter discusses the surgical treatment of esophageal cancer in the West, with particular emphasis on our attitudes to its treatment.

THE NATURE OF ESOPHAGEAL CANCER IN THE WEST

Is cancer of the esophagus in the West fundamentally different from cancer of the esophagus in Japan? The answer to this question is both yes, and no. Yes, because a major proportion of cancers in the West are adenocarcinomas, and there is a very low incidence of such cancers in Japan. However, if we compare like with like, that is squamous cell carcinoma of the esophagus in the West with squamous cell carcinoma of the esophagus in Japan, then on a priori grounds it seems unlikely that there is any fundamental difference between them. Furthermore, it is not at all certain that there is a lot of difference between adenocarcinoma of the esophagus and its course, and squamous cell carcinoma when it presents at a syptomatic stage.[1] Therefore, if there are differences in outcome between Japanese patients and their Western counterparts, it must be because of differences in operative technique, differences of the stage at which the disease is treated, or differences in the methods of reporting results, or some combination of these factors.

Incidence of adenocarcinoma and squamous cell carcinoma of the esophagus

In the West, the incidence of adenocarcinoma of the lower esophagus and cardia is rising.[2,3] Indeed, by some accounts it is rising quite sharply, with one suggestion being at the rate of 10% per year in the USA.[4] The incidence of adenocarcinoma in the first half of this century was reported to be about 0.1 per 100 000, but in the United States it has now reached rates as high or higher than those for squamous cell cancer.[5] Furthermore, as a percentage of cancers involving the esophagus, one report shows that adenocarcinoma has risen from 3.3% during the period 1946–1963, to 39% between 1976 and 1987.[6] In our own unit at the Royal Adelaide Hospital, of 218 esophageal cancers operated on between 1984 and 1994, 56.4% were adenocarcinomas (this excludes sub-cardial cancer).

The reason for this rise in incidence is usually linked to the increased incidence of gastroesophageal reflux disease seen in the West – a disorder which is relatively uncommon in Japan and in the East. Columnar lined change is thought to be the linking factor to the development of adenocarcinoma. However, columnar lined esophagus as an accompaniment to adenocarcinoma is variably reported to occur in only about 50% of cases of adenocarcinoma of the esophagus. In our own series, columnar lined esophagus was either seen by endoscopy or was reported by a pathologist in 55.2% of our cases of adenocarcinoma of the cardia. This may mean that the adenocarcinoma has totally replaced a pre-existent columnar mucosa,[7] or that there is a common factor which promotes adenocarcinoma independent of columnar change, but which also coincidentally promotes columnar change.

Squamous cell carcinoma of the esophagus has been described as an "epidemiologist's delight," as the incidence varies enormously, from 3–5 per 100 000 of population usually seen in the West to >100 per 100 000 population in Linxian county in Northern China. The incidence in the West is currently relatively stable.

SURGICAL TREATMENT OF ESOPHAGEAL CANCER

In the development of surgery for esophageal cancer the major attention has been focused on methods of removing the cancer, and methods of reconstructing the gastrointestinal tract. The removal of lymph nodes associated with the cancer has been seen as of secondary importance. However, the Japanese experience has led some to question this approach, and this will be discussed later.

Selection of patients for treatment

In units which carry out more than 20 esophagectomies per year, the selection of patients is possibly the most important factor in determining operative mortality (see later). Patients who are young, relatively fit, and who have normal cardiac and pulmonary function are at low risk of mortality, and indeed there are now many reported series in the literature with mortality rates of $\leq 2\%$. As a patient's cardiorespiratory function worsens and their age increases, the incidence of complications

and mortality increases.[8] Moreover, in spite of surgeons often taking the view that biological age is more important than chronological age, there would be few, if any, surgeons who would undertake an esophagectomy on a fit patient of 90 years or older. Similarly, few also would reject a fit patient in their seventies. And patients in their eighties? Each patient has to be individualized, but many surgeons would choose non-operative therapies for patients at this age, believing esophagectomy to be too major a procedure to subject a patient to at this time in their life. However, when laparoscopic/thoracoscopic esophagectomy has passed beyond its learning curve these attitudes to age will probably change (see later).

Left thoracotomy (Figure 9.1)

The first successful thoracic resection for esophageal cancer was undertaken by Franz Torek in 1913.[9] He used a left thoracotomy and did not reconstruct the esophagus, but brought out an esophagostomy and gastrostomy in his patient. The patient then fed herself using a tube to bridge between the two stomas, and lived for a further 13 years before dying at the age of 80 of unrelated disease. Most of the early esophagectomies were carried out using this approach, and most were unsuccessful. In 1941 it was reported that of 58 such procedures carried out to that time, only 17 patients had survived the procedure.[10]

This approach, with reconstruction of the gastrointestinal tract using the stomach, was probably the most popular way of dealing with lower esophageal cancer during the 1940s and 1950s, and the procedure was sometimes called eponymously "The Sweet Procedure" after Richard Sweet who described it in 1945.[11] Even though the approach slowly lost popularity it continued to be used on both sides of the Atlantic,[12,13] and is still used successfully by some surgeons.[14]

The approach has been most popular with thoracic surgeons as it allows a completely thoracic approach without the need to alter the patient's position during surgery. However, it has the disadvantages of requiring an incision in the diaphragm for access to the abdomen, and the esophagus is relatively inaccessible behind the aortic arch. This introduces the potential for an inadequate margin of esophagus being taken to allow division of the esophagus to occur distal to the aortic arch. Even if this produces adequate clearance, it means that

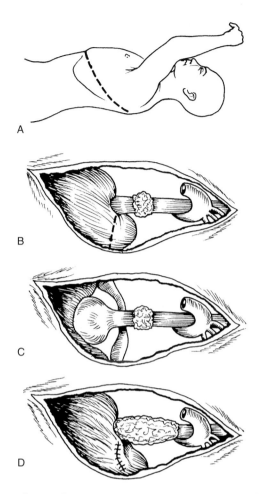

Figure 9.1 Diagrammatic representation of a left thoracotomy approach to esophageal cancer. A. Incision with patient in right lateral position. B. View into left side of the chest with dotted line showing a radial incision of diaphragm. C. View into upper abdominal cavity. D. Reconstruction with anastomosis below the aortic arch.

postoperative reflux is likely to be much worse (see later). Perhaps one other reason for its loss of popularity is the fact that, today, many such operations are carried out for adenocarcinoma of the cardia and there is a high risk of inadequate clearance of this cancer if an anastomosis is carried out distal to the aortic arch.[15,16]

Left thoracoabdominal approach (Figure 9.2)

In 1954, Garlock and Klein stated that "one of the great technical advances in the last decade . . . has

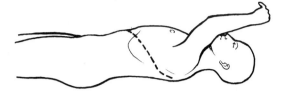

Figure 9.2 Patient in right lateral position for left thoracoabdominal incision.

been the development of the abdomino-thoracic approach."[17]

However, this approach shares the same advantages and disadvantages as the left thoracic approach, except that it provides better access to the abdomen. The approach was particularly popular with general surgeons before the current trend to upper gastrointestinal specialization and the growing use of the approach described next.

Abdominal and right thoracic approach (Figure 9.3)

This approach was first carried out by Ivor Lewis in 1944 and reported in 1946,[18] although in his initial report he advocated the approach only for midesophageal cancers and continued to recommended the thoracoabdominal approach for lower esophageal cancers. The approach had also been undertaken independently by Norman Tanner in 1944,[19] and by Santy in 1947,[20] so the various names attached to the procedure are Ivor Lewis, Lewis–Tanner and Lewis–Santy. There is little doubt that this approach has become the most popular method in the Western world for the treatment of esophageal cancer. For instance, in one study of surgical preferences it accounted for 67% of preferences, while a left-sided approach was preferred in only 21% of cases.[21]

The approach has the advantages of providing the ease of abdominal access for the abdominal procedure, the excellence of access to the thoracic esophagus of a thoracotomy, and the added advantage of excellent access to the thoracic esophagus without the hindrance of the aortic arch as occurs from the left side (the azygos vein is usually divided). This allows an anastomosis to be made high in the apex of the chest in all cases. As usually performed however, it has the disadvantage of having to reposition the patient

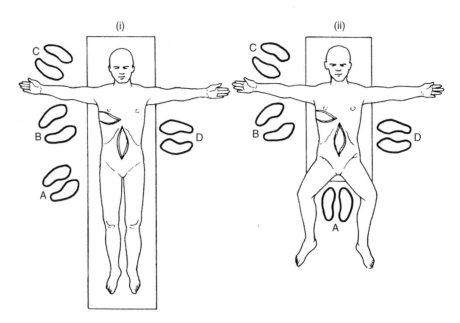

Figure 9.3 Abdominal and right thoracic approach. For the classic Ivor Lewis operation, the patient's position is changed to the left lateral position for a right posterolateral thoracotomy. i. The patient's position for the procedure to be carried out with an abdominal team (A,D) operating synchronously with a thoracic team (B,C). ii. A modification, with the abdominal surgeon (A) standing between the patient's legs.

during the procedure. However it can be undertaken without repositioning the patient using an anterolateral thoracotomy (**Figure 9.3**).[22,23] This has the advantage of allowing the abdominal stage and the thoracic stage of the operation to be performed synchronously. This is facilitated even more if the patient is placed in the lithotomy position with the abdominal surgeon standing between the patient's legs (**Figure 9.3**).[24]

Abdominal and right thoracic and cervical approach

This was first reported by McKeown[25] in 1976 and has the advantage of the esophagogastric anastomosis being made in the neck. Thus, if leakage does occur it is hoped that it will be a less catastrophic event than intrathoracic leakage. The disadvantage is that the gastric tube does not always extend so easily into the neck without compromising its blood supply,[26] so that most observers believe that the leak rate is higher than intrathoracic anastomoses and consequently the stricture rate is also higher (see later).

Transhiatal esophagectomy (Figure 9.4)

Removal of the esophagus without entering the pleural cavity was one of the aims of surgeons in the early part of this century. As performed through the esophageal hiatus, it was probably first undertaken successfully by George Grey Turner who carried it out in a Welsh miner in 1933.[27] The first report of a series of cases was that of LeQuesne and Ranger in 1966.[28] Orringer and his group[29] have probably been the main popularizers of this procedure over the past 20 years after the initial report of Orringer and Sloan in 1978.[30] The main advantage claimed for the technique has been the avoidance of opening the thoracic cavity with projected lower wound morbidity and lower incidence of chest complications. Non-randomized studies have produced conflicting results, however. For instance, Stark *et al.*[31] found a respiratory complication rate of 41% in a group of patients undergoing transhiatal esophagectomy versus 6% in a group undergoing transthoracic esophagectomy. In Robert Guili's overview,[21] the respiratory complication rate was 24% in transhiatal patients versus 23% in transthoracic patients. Tilanus *et al.*[32] found

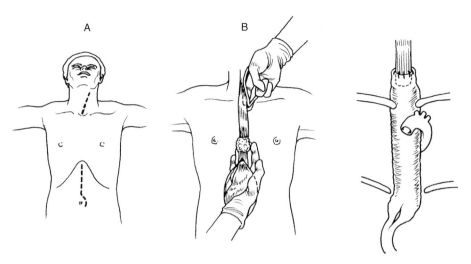

Figure 9.4   Transhiatal esophagectomy. A. The cervical and abdominal incisions. B. How manual dissection is used from both above and below. C. The stomach anastomosed to the esophagus in the neck.

the respiratory complication rate to be 17% for patients having a transhiatal esophagectomy and 34% for patients having a transthoracic approach. In the only randomized study comparing the two operations the incidence of pulmonary complications was about 20% in both groups.[33]

The disadvantages of the technique are the same as for the cervical anastomosis described earlier. Some claim an added disadvantage is that nodal dissection is not so easily achieved, and it is certainly not possible to undertake a radical nodal dissection with this technique. In spite of such reservations this has been a popular procedure in

the past 20 years, and it has been reported with acceptable results from several centers specializing in esophageal surgery.[29,34,35]

The use of esophageal "stripping," either with a ring dissector or an eversion technique, was originally advocated by Akiyama in 1975,[36] and both techniques are variants of the transhiatal technique. Eversion extraction of the esophagus (**Figure 9.5**) has been used successfully and reported in one series which tended to limit its use to specific situations.[37] However, another report has advocated its use more generally in adenocarcinoma of the cardia.[38]

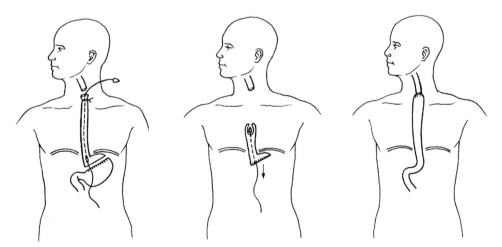

Figure 9.5   Eversion extraction of the esophagus. The vein stripper inverts into the esophagus so that the esophagus emerges everted.

Endoscopic esophagectomy

The popularization of endoscopic surgery during the 1990s has seen it applied to esophageal cancer, with the potential for great benefit to patients. Perhaps more than any other surgical procedure in common use today, esophagectomy is the most traumatic procedure which can be performed on patients. This is reflected not only in the still high death rate associated with the procedure (see later), but also the prolonged morbidity which afflicts many patients. As has been demonstrated in other endoscopic procedures, most morbidity relates in no small measure to the incisions used for access. Thus, it was hoped that endoscopic esophagectomy might be used with great benefit to patients. That such benefits have been a little slow in coming relates to several factors. First, the early techniques were applied mainly to removing the esophagus either transmediastinally[39] or transthoracically,[40] with laparotomy and cervical incisions still being performed. Reports of both the abdominal and thoracic stages being performed laparoscopically/thoracoscopically are beginning to appear,[41] and it is probably only once we are beyond our learning curve for the performance of the procedure *in toto* endoscopically that we will see the potential benefits of this approach emerging. There remains one further problem with endoscopic surgery for malignant disease, and that is the increased incidence of port-site metastases.[42] What the real level of such metastases is, remains to be determined. However, there is some evidence that this problem is more likely to occur in patients with already incurable disease. If this proves to be true, then the trade-off for a relatively painless operation is almost certain to be readily accepted.

METHOD OF RECONSTRUCTION FOLLOWING ESOPHAGECTOMY

The stomach is the most popular substitute for the esophagus when it is removed for cancer. In one review of 709 cases, stomach was used in 88% of cases, colon in 8%, and small bowel in 4%.[21]

The reasons for the popularity of the stomach are obvious and well known. It is relatively straight forward to mobilize it, while maintaining an adequate blood supply, although the latter is sometimes suboptimal once the stomach reaches to the neck.[43] Furthermore, only one anastomosis is required – the esophagogastric anastomosis. One area which, if hardly controversial, provides divided opinion, is whether some form of pyloric destruction should accompany the transposition of the stomach into the chest or neck. Two randomized controlled trials have suggested that pyloroplasty should be added. In both these trials delayed gastric emptying caused problems in a small group of patients who did not have a pyloroplasty performed. Furthermore, in both trials two and three patients respectively died as a result of aspiration problems associated with their delayed gastric emptying.[44,45] However, another randomized prospective study failed to find any difference in delay in gastric emptying between groups with or without a pyloroplasty.[46] Perhaps these studies are not as much at odds as might first appear. In the first two studies, there is no suggestion of the construction of a gastric tube, while the larger study of the two comprised patients undergoing a Lewis–Tanner operation, so that the anastomosis was made in the chest. Under these circumstances the stomach retains a reservoir function and, indeed, it is often easily seen as a fluid-filled bag on a chest radiograph in the early postoperative period. On the other hand, in the last study mentioned above, the authors are explicit that a gastric tube was constructed with anastomosis in the neck. It is possible, even likely, that gastric emptying differs between the two situations so that the conclusions of both trials may be correct. The other technical factor which is worth emphasizing is the height of the esophagogastric anastomosis in the chest or above. In 1978, Borst *et al.*[47] reported a prospectively studied series of patients having esophagectomy, and found that five of 17 patients with apical thoracic anastomosis had endoscopic evidence of esophagitis compared with 19 of 20 patients who had a subhilar anastomosis in the chest. A more recent report also supports the view that the more proximal the anastomosis, the less likely are reflux symptoms. De-Leyn *et al.*[48] found that reflux esophagitis was found in 43% of 30 patients when the anastomosis was intrathoracic, and there was a 13% stricture rate compared with 6% reflux esophagitis and a 2% stricture rate when anastomosis was in the neck.

The jeunum can also be mobilized, but it is more difficult to make it reach the neck and its configuration often has a "gathered" look, which is not ideal for good ingestion.[49] Furthermore, another anastomosis is required, i.e., a jejunojejunal anastomosis.

Colon provides good length, but more extensive dissection is required than with the other two procedures. Furthermore, three anastomoses are required, i.e., esophagocolic, cologastric, and colocolic. Colon also has the reputation of being the most likely of the substitute organs to leak. In one report of a large experience with esophagectomy for cancer, gastric necrosis occurred in seven of 306 cases (2%) and colonic necrosis occurred in three of 32 cases (9.4%).[50] In 1979, Postlethwaite[51] collected 869 patients who had an esophageal replacement by colon, and the necrosis rate was approximately 8%. For this reason, colon tends to be used only when the stomach is not available, or it is wished to retain it as a functioning organ, which is often the case when esophagectomy is being undertaken for benign disease.

INTENSIVE CARE AFTER ESOPHAGECTOMY

At several points during this chapter we mention the fact that the development of intensive care units has played a major role in lowering hospital mortality rates after esophageal resection. We do not believe that anyone would challenge the statement that patients who are extremely ill and who would have died in earlier times, now live because of the expertise of staff in intensive care units. However, there is a perception among many surgeons that patients postoperatively, even after major surgery such as an esophagectomy, do not require intensive care, or perhaps more specifically, prolonged intubation, unless there are specific indications.

In a non-randomized study which nevertheless comprised two groups of closely comparable patients, Caldwell et al.[52] examined 36 patients having overnight postoperative ventilation compared with 45 in whom same-day extubation was practiced routinely. Ten patients in the first group required long ventilation compared with two in the second group. Furthermore, the hospital mortality rate in the first group was 16.7% and in the second group 4.4%. Bartels et al.[53] also investigated the effects of early extubation in a prospective randomized study in 94 patients having esophagectomy. They found no significant difference in either complication rate or mortality rate between those groups extubated early and those who were intubated for 24 h or more. The only significant difference found was in the subgroup of 46 patients undergoing transmediastinal esophagectomy, where the patients having extubation within 6 h of surgery had an average intensive care unit stay of 7 days, while those having ventilation for >24 h had a stay of 12 days. However, the authors also noted some trends in favor of long intubation and so are continuing the trial in order to increase the statistical power of their tests. Therefore, in our cost-conscious times it seems reasonable to assert that, when patients are fit and the operation has been straightforward, then the aim should be to extubate patients once they are fully awake after esophagectomy.

THE RESULTS OF ESOPHAGECTOMY

The results of esophagectomy are discussed here against the background of a survey which was undertaken for this chapter, of all published reports from Western centers of the surgical treatment of esophageal cancer appearing in *Index Medicus* from 1990–1995. A few words of explanation are required in regard to this survey. First, not all data required were available in every paper, and this is the reason why numbers in the patient totals columns vary. Second, it was not always possible to dissect out the relevant data for squamous cell cancers as opposed to adenocarcinoma of the cardia and lower esophagus. In fact, as can be seen from the tables, in the majority of papers the two cancers were treated by the authors as a single entity. Given the results presented here, that may well have been a reasonable position to have taken. Nevertheless, the data for adenocarcinoma of the cardia and lower esophagus and squamous cell carcinoma of the esophagus were sought separately and, where it was possible to obtain such separation, are presented in this manner.

Third, although our initial intention was to examine a greater range of outcomes, it became obvious that only very broad generalities would be obtainable. Thus, eventually we concentrated on leakage rates, operative mortality rates, and survival. In the great majority of papers the leakage rate reported was the clinically important leakage, and in that sense the rates quoted almost certainly underestimate the real leakage rate. Similarly, although we have attempted to report in-hospital mortality rates, it was often not certain whether 30-

day mortality rates or in-hospital mortality rates were being quoted. As hospital mortality rates are almost always higher than 30-day mortality rates, it is likely that the mortality rate figures presented here underestimate the true figures for in-hospital mortality. Although only available in about 12% of the papers surveyed, we have given 1-year mortality rates in an effort to provide a further indication of the important early mortality figures of esophagectomy. After all, it can be argued that if a patient does not survive 12 months from operation, then it really was not worthwhile for that patient having to undergo such a major procedure. The catch is, however, that we do not know in advance which patients are going to do badly. All surgeons have had patients in whom preoperative predictions would have been for a poor outcome, and who subsequently have done well, and vice-versa.

Finally, most – but not all – of these reports come from the era when intensive care units had developed their expertise. Thus, although it could be argued that the results being obtained are likely to be better than the results presented here, it is unlikely that they are much better.

In-hospital mortality (Table 9.1)

In the Western world, intensive care units became common-place in hospitals through the late 1970s and 1980s. With their development, it is not uncommon for patients to survive longer than the 30 days which has often been used in the past for quoting mortality figures after esophagectomy. For example, Smolle-Juettner et al.[54] quoted a series of unselected cases undergoing operations for esophageal cancer with a 1.9% mortality rate at 30 days, but an in-hospital mortality rate of 17.6%. In our own series of 218 unselected cases undergoing operation at the Royal Adelaide Hospital with an in-hospital mortality rate of 13.7%, there were two patients

who died respectively at 82 days and 71 days post-operatively.

Although the mortality rate from operations for esophageal cancer has fallen since the early 20th century, the improvement curve appears to have flattened (**Figure 9.6**). In 1940, Oschner and DeBakey[10] reviewed the world literature and collected reports of 191 esophageal resections with a 72% mortality rate. In 1980, Earlam and Cunha-Melo[55] collected a series from the world literature also of all published cases to that time (83 783 cases) and showed an operative mortality rate of 29%. Muller et al.[56] reviewed published figures from 1980–1990 and, in 43 070 patients resected, identified a mortality rate of 13%. While this is an impressive fall from the 29% quoted by Earlam and Cunha-Melo,[55] it should be remembered that both studies were examining the whole of the world's literature, and thus had included Japanese and Chinese series. These latter series were often not only the largest, but also had the lowest mortality rates. In fact, if only series of >1000 patients resected were extracted from this review, this accounted for 35 922 patients of whom 80.7% were Japanese or Chinese. The hospital mortality rate in these Eastern patients was 4.6%, while that in Western patients was close to 25%.

We reviewed "The Western Experience" from 1990 onwards, and found the overall in-hospital mortality rate in 11 398 patients to be 11%. Thus,

Table 9.1 *Mortality rate after esophagectomy*

TYPE OF CANCER	NO. OF PATIENTS	NO. OF DEATHS (%)
Adenocarcinoma	1232	139 (11.3)
Squamous cell cancer	2235	294 (13.2)
Both types of cancer	7931	817 (10.3)
Total	11 398	1250 (11.0)

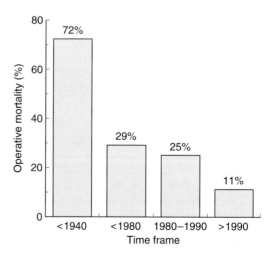

Figure 9.6 Improvement in operative mortality during the 20th century.

the mortality rate for esophagectomy continues to fall.

There are many series in the Western literature with much lower mortality rates than 11%, and some even with 0% mortality. Why is this? Surgeons who quote low mortality figures cannot be blamed for wanting to attribute such figures to the excellence of their surgery, and such excellence cannot be denied in these circumstances. On the other hand, surgeons who quote high mortality rates also understandably cite operating on unselected cases as the primary reason for the higher rates. At least to some degree they are probably right, but it is unquestionable that greater experience brings better results in operations for esophageal cancer. For instance, Andersen et al.[57] surveyed Danish departments of surgery for the period 1985–1988 and in a collected series of 464 patients undergoing surgery for esophageal cancer the hospital mortality rate was 16.6%. However, in those departments performing more than 20 resections a year, the rate was 7%. This also implies that the mortality rate in those departments performing less than 20 per year was considerably higher than 16.6%. Faller[58] reported a similar experience from Hungary, with a nationwide survey of 1197 esophageal resections carried out between 1988 and 1992. The overall mortality rate was 14.7%, but in departments where more than 10 resections per year were carried out it was 12.2%. In contrast, in departments where less than 10 resections per year were performed, the mortality rate was 16.9%.

However, once a certain level of expertise has been reached it seems likely that patient selection is a major factor in causing mortality. If a patient is fit, relatively young and slim, then in experienced hands there is little risk of operative mortality. However, if the patient is unfit, old and obese, there is a much higher risk of operative mortality. It is anecdotal evidence at best, but the senior author operated on a small series of Chinese patients in China and found that operations took about half the time that similar operations take on Western patients. He also found that operating in the fat-free planes of the slim Chinese patients could only be described as a joy! It bought home to us how figures such as 10 464 resections carried out in the period between 1940 and 1980 could have achieved only a 4% operative mortality rate.[59]

As mentioned previously, there seems little point in subjecting a patient to an esophagectomy if they are to die of their disease within a 12-month period. However, the only ways this is likely to change in the future is to operate at an (probably much) earlier stage, or to find effective methods of treating residual disease, which usually is what proves fatal to the patient. In the West, with the exception of surveillance for columnar lined esophagus, there seems little likelihood of detecting esophageal cancer at substantially earlier stages. Therefore, the main hope is that systemic therapy such as immunotherapy and/or chemotherapy will improve in the future.

Anastomotic leakage

Esophageal anastomoses have long had a reputation for higher leakage rates than other gastrointestinal anastomoses. This is usually ascribed to a combination of a poor blood supply, a lack of serosal covering on the esophagus, and a potential for tension on an anastomosis.[60–63] **Table 9.2** shows that this rate remains high. For instance, in the series of cases with squamous cell carcinoma the rate was 17%. Moreover, as some series report rates of 5% or less, it is clear that leakage rates are above 20% in others. There is no doubt that overt leakage and mortality are linked, and it has often been found that there is about a 50% mortality rate when leakage occurs.[64] Nevertheless, this is one area where intensive care units and interventional radiology have contributed to the falling mortality rate.

Percutaneous drainage using such modalities as computed tomography (CT)-guided placement of drainage tubes often establishes an external fistula and avoids the need for a further thoracotomy in a patient who may already be extremely ill. In our own series of 226 patients undergoing surgery at the Royal Adelaide Hospital between 1984 and

Table 9.2 Anastomotic leakage after esophagectomy

TYPE OF CANCER	NO. OF PATIENTS	NO. OF LEAKS (%)
Adenocarcinoma	1191	145 (12.2)
Squamous cell cancer	1691	287 (17.0)
Both types of cancer	6463	662 (10.2)
Total	9345	1094 (11.7)

1994, 33 patients sustained a radiographically demonstrated leak, and of these, 12 died.

Anastomotic techniques would seem to lend themselves to scrutiny by prospective randomized studies, and several such studies have been undertaken to try and improve healing rates. In recent years there has been a trend away from two-layered anastomosis in the gastrointestinal tract. Zieren et al.[65] undertook a randomized comparison of one-layered versus two-layered anastomosis in cervical esophagogastrostomies. Anastomotic leakage rate was the same in both groups (19%), but fibrotic stricture rates were significantly higher in the two-layered group (48% versus 22%). Bardini et al.[66] undertook a prospective randomized study comparing single-layered anastomosis performed either with interrupted sutures or with a continuous suture. They had a low leakage rate overall (1/42 patients), but no significant difference was found between the two groups except for the quicker performance of the continuous suture (10 versus 16 min.). Valverde et al.[67] addressed the question of whether stapled anastomoses were superior to hand-sewn anastomoses in a controlled randomized study, and essentially found no difference between the groups in either leakage rate (15% versus 16%) or stricture formation (13% in both groups).

Although not tested by randomized studies, many surgeons now favor end-to-side over end-to-end anastomosis for esophagogastrotomy. One review of the literature found a substantially lower leakage rate after end-to-side procedures.[68] The bolstering of the posterior wall of the anastomosis with this technique may be one factor in the lower leakage rate, but probably more important is the poorer blood supply of the stomach when the end of a gastric tube or the top most portion of the stomach is used for an anastomosis.

In fact, if one factor seems to be more important than all others in healing of anastomoses, it is the adequacy of the blood supply. This is underlined by the usually reported higher leakage rate with cervical compared with thoracic anastomosis. In a retrospective collected review, the leakage rate was 13% in thoracic anastomoses and 19% in cervical anastomoses.[21] Also, in the Royal Adelaide Hospital series it was 11% and 23%, respectively, for thoracic and cervical anastomoses, while two prospective randomized studies showed similarly higher leakage rates for cervical compared with thoracic anastomoses, e.g., 26% versus 4%[69] and 23% versus 3%.[70]

As might be expected from such figures, postoperative stricture rates are also higher with cervical anastomoses, with 44% versus 14% in our series and 23% versus 14% in Chasseray et al.'s randomized study.[69] Mortality rates were not significantly different in either of the randomized studies; thus, there seems little compelling reason to carry out an anastomosis in the neck as opposed to high in the thorax, unless it is necessary to gain adequate clearance of an esophageal lesion.

Survival figures (Table 9.3)

The 5-year survival figures collected by Earlam and Cuhna-Melo[55] were 5%, while in the large collected Western series reported by Muller et al.[56] this had risen to 15%. Among those papers collected which were reported after 1990, survival had risen further, to 21.4%. One criticism of such figures is that improvements in survival could mean that greater selection is being applied without there being any real overall improvement in survival from this condition. In other words, the denominator, or the whole population, is usually not known. However, in South Australia a state cancer registry for all cases of cancer has been

Table 9.3 Survival rates after esophagectomy

TYPE OF CANCER	NO. OF PATIENTS		NO. OF SURVIVORS (%)	
	1 YEAR	5 YEARS	1 YEAR	5 YEARS
Adenocarcinoma	286	1396	159 (55.6)	407 (29)
Squamous cell cancer	221	1146	119 (53.8)	241 (21)
Both types of cancer	975	4147	436 (44.7)	781 (18.8)
Total	1472	6689	714 (48.5)	1429 (21.4)

in operation since 1977. This has shown a higher age-standardized 5-year survival rate for all cases of esophageal cancer of 16% from 1986 to 1994, compared with 9% for the period 1977–1985.[71] Furthermore, a similar trend has been demonstrated in the United States.[72] Therefore, it does appear that progress is being made, though two factors should be borne in mind. First, a value of 21% for 5-year survival is poor, and it is likely that this figure has increased from the earlier 15% value only because of the lower operative mortality rates today. (These lower rates are probably not due to any improvements in surgical technique, but to better anesthesia, intensive care and interventional radiology.)

Second, it can be seen that the 1-year survival rate is only about 50% and, as mentioned earlier, it seems untenable to subject a patient to esophagectomy if they have less than a year to live. Therefore, it is little wonder that attempts are being made to stage patients more accurately to allow better selection for operation, and either to improve the operation (radical lymph node clearance) or to use additional therapy for an improved outcome (neoadjuvant therapy).

NEOADJUVANT THERAPY

Neoadjuvant therapy is considered in detail elsewhere in this volume, but the development of its use in our hands is presented briefly here.

Adjuvant therapy in the form of preoperative or posteroperative radiotherapy, or preoperative or postoperative chemotherapy, and treatment of esophageal cancer by either modality alone has not led to improvement in survival.[73]

In 1984, when a review of results at the Royal Adelaide Hospital was undertaken, the 5-year survival rate of patients treated surgically was approximately 5%, while that for patients treated by radical radiotherapy alone was 4%. These figures were similar to those published by Earlam and Cuhna-Melo[55] in their extensive review. Also in 1984, Leichmann et al.[74] published their technique involving the use of radiotherapy and chemotherapy concomitantly as preoperative therapy – the form of therapy which has come to be known as neoadjuvant therapy. We have used neoadjuvant therapy for esophageal cancer since that time and found that survival for unse-

lected patients has improved to approximately 23%. We have also found that neoadjuvant therapy seems to have a similar effect on the primary tumor in both adenocarcinoma and squamous cell carcinoma cases. Moreover, complete disappearance of tumor in a resected specimen occurs in about 25% cases, and this has been associated with a 5-year survival rate of 67%.[75–78] During the same period, other groups have also followed the lead of Leichmann et al. with broadly similar results. It is difficult to compare the data between groups because of the variation in drug protocols and doses of radiotherapy, and because of differing criteria in assessing complete response. Furthermore, preoperative staging between the groups has been variable. Most trials have used combinations of 5-fluorouracil and cisplatinum, although there is no agreement on the combination, dosage and duration of therapy. Nevertheless, promising results have been obtained from some of these trials, suggesting that there is significant survival advantage in patients undergoing surgery after neoadjuvant chemotherapy. Other studies have found also that survival is greatly increased for patients who have a complete histologic response.[79,80] Perhaps the most important study published to date is that of Walsh et al.[80] where, for the first time in a controlled and randomized study, a survival advantage has been demonstrated in patients with adenocarcinoma of the esophagus treated with neoadjuvant therapy and surgery compared with those treated by surgery alone. Further similar trials are being undertaken, as well as trials investigating radiotherapy and chemotherapy given synchronously without surgery to see if this is appropriate treatment for some patients.

It is quite likely that an increasing number of patients with advanced esophageal cancer who would previously have been considered fit for palliative surgery, in future will be treated by chemotherapy and radiotherapy alone. It is hoped that such an approach will greatly diminish the number of patients who undergo esophagectomy only to die in the ensuing 12 months. However, the place of chemotherapy and non-radical esophagectomy, vis-a-vis esophagectomy with radical lymph node resections, is a very long way from being resolved.

RADICAL LYMPH NODE RESECTIONS FOR ESOPHAGEAL CANCER

Andrew Logan in Edinburgh is usually credited with introducing the concept of radical lymphadenectomy in esophageal cancer in the West, with a report in 1963 involving 251 patients.[81] Since that time, Skinner and colleagues[82,83] and De Meester and co-workers[84,85] have been the main advocates of this approach. The technique also appears to be gaining favor in certain European centers.[86–88] It is of interest that those surgeons advocating subcarinal two-field lymphadenectomy (**Figure 9.7c**) by and large have not embraced the Japanese three-field lymphadenectomy, although the reasoning for advocating the radicality of the two procedures is essentially the same. No controlled randomized study has been reported comparing less radical esophagectomy procedures with more radical procedures. The closest report to a randomized study is that of Horstmann et al.,[89] who compared prospectively two groups of patients, 46 having a transhiatal esophagectomy and 41 having a transthoracic esophagectomy with systematic two-field en block lymphadenectomy. Statistical methods were used to establish the comparability of data in the two groups. They found no significant difference in either short- or long-term survival. The 3-year survival rate was 21% in the transhiatal group, and 17% in the en bloc lymphadenectomy group. We consider it fair to say that until such time that scientifically sound evidence is produced establishing the superiority of radical lymph node dissections, then they are unlikely to be embraced by the majority of specialist upper gastrointestinal surgeons. This is particularly so since the advent of neoadjuvant therapy seems to produce as good or better results than radical lymph node resection.

Table 9.4 reports survivals and nodal status from well-known groups advocating the procedures listed. Some interesting points emerge from a consideration of these data. The first is that, in the Western series, as the radicality of the procedure increases (**Figure 9.7**) so does the percentage of patients noted to have involved lymph nodes. This makes good sense, for as more nodes are sampled then clearly the greater the chance of finding nodal involvement. It also suggests that the radical procedures will stage patients more accurately. Thus, if a patient has had a three-field lymphadenectomy and a painstaking examination of all nodes removed is undertaken, and no cancer is found, then the statement "node-negative" can be made with some confidence. On the other hand, if the patient has a transhiatal resection and only three or four nodes are removed, and no cancer is found in the nodes, then clearly the term "node-negative" is a relative statement at best. This provides one explanation for the increased survivals reported in the Japanese patients compared with Western patients. That is, Japanese patients who are "node-negative" are actually "N0" patients, while in the Western series many of the patients called "N0" will actually be "N1" or "N2" with a correspondingly worse prognosis. Of course, another explanation for the better survivals in the Japanese series is that three-field lymphadenectomy actually does cure more patients. This has just not been established yet. It is also of interest in the collected series reported by Isono et al.[90] that the incidence of positive lymph nodes recovered from their three-field resection patients

---

Table 9.4 Five-year survival rates reported with different techniques

TECHNIQUE	REFERENCE	PATIENTS WITH POSITIVE LYMPH NODES (%)	5-YEAR SURVIVAL RATE (%)		
			OVERALL	NODE −ve	NODE +ve
Transhiatal esophagectomy	Orringer et al.[29]	52	27	40	13
Ivor Lewis esophagectomy	King et al.[93]	68	23	47	8
Two-field resection	Altorki & Skinner[83]	79	18	40	10
Extended two-field resection	Isono et al.[90]	72	27	46	18
Three-field resection	Isono et al.[90]	61	34	57	23

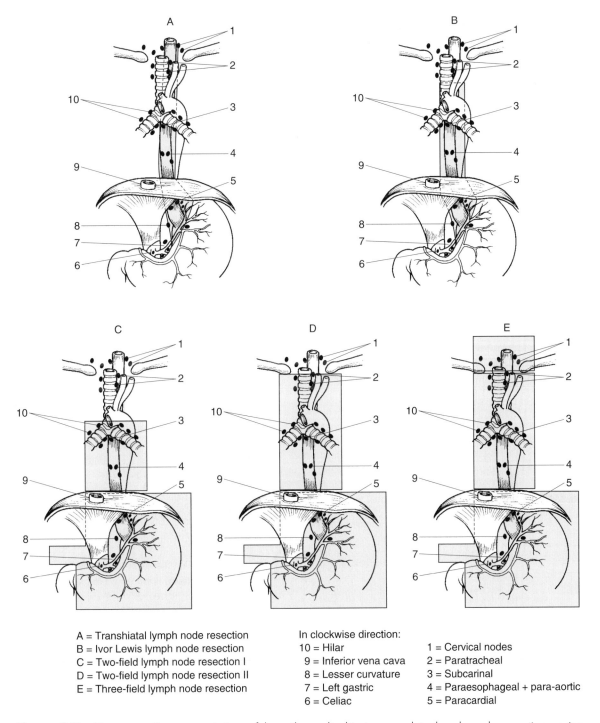

A = Transhiatal lymph node resection
B = Ivor Lewis lymph node resection
C = Two-field lymph node resection I
D = Two-field lymph node resection II
E = Three-field lymph node resection

In clockwise direction:
10 = Hilar
9 = Inferior vena cava
8 = Lesser curvature
7 = Left gastric
6 = Celiac

1 = Cervical nodes
2 = Paratracheal
3 = Subcarinal
4 = Paraesophageal + para-aortic
5 = Paracardial

Figure 9.7 Diagrammatic representation of how the radicality in regard to lymph node resection varies between various procedures. Lymph nodes (1–10) are identified in the lower diagram.

was actually less than recovered from their series of two-field resection patients. When one considers that lower third, middle third and upper third esophageal cancers have incidences of cervical lymph node involvement of 19%, 27.5%, and 42.3% of cases respectively,[90] it seems inconceivable that the node positivity rate should fall in three-field compared with two-field resections, unless the three-field patients were presenting with earlier disease. This seems quite possible, since as surgeons and centers develop expertise in an area, there is often unintended selection which occurs with fitter patients and patients with earlier disease being referred to the center. It is now reasonably well established that the use of historic controls is often fallacious in detecting treatment benefits for a new treatment,[91,92] and this highlights the need for randomized studies in this field.

The other feature of **Table 9.4** is that the overall 5-year survival rates between Orringer's group with the least radical of the operations (27%)[29] is not very different from the 34% quoted by Isono *et al.*[90] for three-field lymphadenectomy. The bald fact is that both survival rates are poor, and new strategies are needed to make an impact in this disease.

REFERENCES

1. Law SY, Fok M, Cheng SW *et al.* A comparison of outcome after resection for squamous cell carcinomas and adenocarcinomas of the esophagus and cardia. *Surg Gynecol Obstet* 1992; **175**: 107–12.
2. Lund O, Hasenkam JM, Aagaard MT *et al.* Time-related changed in characteristics of prognostic significance in carcinomas of the oesophagus and cardia. *Br J Surg* 1989; **76**: 1301–7.
3. Blot WJ, Devesa SS & Fraumeni JFJ. Continuing climb in rates of esophageal adenocarcinoma: an update. *JAMA* 1993; **270**: 1320.
4. Yang PC & Davis S. Incidence of cancer of the esophagus in the US by histologic type. *Cancer* 1988; **61**: 612–17.
5. Blot WJ. Esophageal cancer trends and risk factors. *Semin Oncol* 1994; **21**: 403–10.
6. Alpern HD, Buell C & Olson J. Increasing percentage of adenocarcinoma in primary carcinoma of the esophagus. *Am J Gastroenterol* 1989; **84**: 574.
7. Cameron AJ, Lomboy CT, Pera M *et al.* Adenocarcinoma of the esophagogastric junction and Barrett's esophagus. *Gastroenterology* 1995; **109**: 1541–6.
8. Wong J. Management of carcinoma of oesophagus: art or science? *J R Coll Surg Edinb* 1981; **26**: 138–49.
9. Torek F. The first successful case of resection of the thoracic portion of the oesophagus for carcinoma. *Surg Gynecol Obstet* 1913; **16**: 614–17.
10. Oschner A & DeBakey M. Surgical aspects of carcinoma of the esophagus. *J Thorac Surg* 1941; **10**: 401–45.
11. Sweet RH. Surgical management of carcinoma of the midthoracic esophagus. *N Engl J Med* 1945; **233**: 1.
12. Dark JF, Mousalli H & Vaughan R. Surgical treatment of carcinoma of the oesophagus. *Thorax* 1981; **36**: 891–5.
13. Ellis FHJ. Esophagogastrectomy for carcinoma: technical considerations based on anatomic location of lesion. *Surg Clin North Am* 1980; **60**: 265–79.
14. Jougon J, Velly JF, Clerc F *et al.* Left thoracotomy in the excision of cancers of the cardia and the lower third of the esophagus. Apropos of a series of 210 cases. *Chirurgie* 1994; **120**: 211–14.
15. Molina JE, Lawton BR, Myers WO *et al.* Esophagogastrectomy for adenocarcinoma of the cardia. Ten years' experience and current approach. *Ann Surg* 1982; **195**: 146–51.
16. Papachristou DN, Karas M & Fortner JG. Anastomotic recurrence in the oesophagus complicating gastrectomy for adenocarcinoma of the stomach. *Br J Surg* 1979; **66**: 609–12.
17. Garlock JH & Klein SH. The surgical treatment of carcinoma of the esophagus and cardia: an analysis of 457 cases. *Ann Surg* 1954; **139**: 19–34.
18. Lewis I. Surgical treatment of carcinoma of the oesophagus. *Br J Surg* 1946; **34**: 18–31.
19. Tanner NC. The present position of carcinoma of the oesophagus. *Postgrad Med* 1947; **23**: 109–39.
20. Santy P & Mouchet A. A Traitement chirurgical du cancer de l'oesophage thoracique. *J Chir Paris* 1947; **63**: 505–26.
21. Giuli R. Compte-rendu de la 8eme reunion de l'O.E.S.O. Depart de l'essai therapeutique mondial sur les cancers de l'oesophage. *J Chir Paris* 1986; **123**: 295–9.
22. Jamieson GG, Devitt PG & Britten-Jones R. Combined synchronous oesophageal resections – the two-team approach. In: Jamieson GG (ed.) *Surgery of the Oesophagus*. London: Churchill Livingstone 1988: 687–8.

23. Chung SC, Griffin SM, Wood SD *et al.* Two team synchronous esophagectomy. *Surg Gynecol Obstet* 1990; **170**: 68–9.

24. Baigrie RJ, Watson DI, Devitt PG *et al.* Synchronous combined esophagectomy in the 'French' position. *Dis Esoph* 1996; **9**: 226–7.

25. McKeown KC. Total three-stage oesophagectomy for cancer of the oesophagus. *Br J Surg* 1976; **63**: 259–62.

26. Nabeya K, Hanaoka T, Onozawawa K *et al.* Two-stage esophagogastrostomy for esophageal reconstruction. In: Ferguson MK, Little AG & Skinner DB (eds) *Diseases of the Esophagus, Malignant Diseases*, Vol. 1. Mount Kisko, New York, USA: Futura 1990: 247–52.

27. Turner GG. Excision of thoracic oesophagus for carcinoma. *Lancet* 1933; **2**: 1315–16.

28. Le-Quesne LP & Ranger D. Pharyngo-laryngectomy, with immediate pharyngogastric anastomosis. *Br J Surg* 1996; **53**: 105–9.

29. Orringer MB, Marshall B & Stirling MC. Transhiatal esophagectomy for benign and malignant disease. *J Thorac Cardiovasc Surg* 1993; **105**: 265–76.

30. Orringer MB & Sloan H. Esophagectomy without thoracotomy. *J Thorac Cardiovasc Surg* 1978; **76**: 643–54.

31. Stark SP, Romberg MS, Pierce GE *et al.* Transhiatal versus transthoracic esophagectomy for adenocarcinoma of the distal esophagus and cardia. *Am J Surg* 1996; **172**: 478–81.

32. Tilanus HW, Hop WC, Langenhorst BL *et al.* Esophagectomy with or without thoracotomy. Is there any difference? *J Thorac Cardiovasc Surg* 1993; **105**: 898–903.

33. Goldminc M, Maddern G, Le-Prise E *et al.* Oesophagectomy by a transhiatal approach or thoracotomy: a prospective randomized trial. *Br J Surg* 1993; **80**: 367–70.

34. Peracchia A, Bardini R, Segalin A *et al.* Esophagectomy without thoracotomy as a treatment of esophageal cancer. Indications, technical features and results. *Chirurgie* 1990; **116**: 762–8.

35. Moreno GE, Garcia GI, Pinto GA *et al.* Results of transhiatal esophagectomy in cancer of the eso-phagus and other diseases. *Hepato-gastroenterology* 1992; **39**: 439–42.

36. Akiyama H, Hiyama M & Miyazono H. Total eso-phageal reconstruction after extraction of the esophagus. *Ann Surg* 1975; **182**: 547–52.

37. Jamieson GG, Devitt PG & Game PA. Eversion extraction of the oesophagus. *Aust N Z J Surg* 1989; **59**: 567–70.

38. Bell G, Watt I & Anderson JR. Transhiatal eso-phagectomy using a varicose vein stripper. *Surg Gynecol Obstet* 1992; **175**: 461–3.

39. Buess GF, Becker HD, Naruhn MB *et al.* Endoscopic esophagectomy without thoracot-omy. *Probl Gen Surg* 1991; **8**: 478–86.

40. Cuschieri A. Endoscopic subtotal oesophagectomy for cancer using the right thoracoscopic approach. *Surg Oncol* 1993; **2**(suppl. 1): 3–11.

41. DePaula AL, Hashiba K, Ferreira EA *et al.* Laparoscopic transhiatal esophagectomy with esophagogastroplasty. *Surg Laparosc Endosc* 1995; **5**: 1–5.

42. Dixit AS, Martin CJ & Flynn P. Port-site recur-rence after thoracoscopic resection of oesopha-geal cancer. *Aust N Z J Surg* 1997; **67**: 148–9.

43. Leibermann-Meffert DM, Meier R & Siewert JR. Vascular anatomy of the gastric tube used for esophageal reconstruction. *Ann Thorac Surg* 1992; **54**: 1110–15.

44. Mannell A, McKnight A & Esser JD. Role of pylor-oplasty in the retrosternal stomach: results of a prospective, randomized, controlled trial. *Br J Surg* 1990; **77**: 57–9.

45. Fok M, Cheng SW & Wong J. Pyloroplasty versus no drainage in gastric replacement of the eso-phagus. *Am J Surg* 1991; **162**: 447–52.

46. Fontes P, Nectoux M, Escobar A *et al.* Esophagogastroplasty with and without pyloro-plasty: A Prospective Study. In: Peracchia A, Rosati R, Bonavina L *et al.* (eds) *Recent Advances in Diseases of the Esophagus.* Bologna, Italy: Monduzzi Editore 1996: 241–5.

47. Borst HG, Dragojevic D, Stegmann T *et al.* Anastomotic leakage, stenosis, and reflux after esophageal replacement. *World J Surg* 1978; **2**: 861–4.

48. De-Leyn P, Coosemans W, Van-Raemdonck D *et al.* Functioning of the tube stomach following esophagus resection for carcinoma. *Ned Tijdschr Geneeskd* 1993; **137**: 455–9.

49. Wong J. The use of small bowel for oesophageal replacement following oesophageal resection. In: Jamieson GG (ed.) *Surgery of the Oesophagus.* London: Churchill Livingstone 1988: 749–60.

50. Hanaoka T, Nakata Y, Hamakubo S *et al.* Necrosis in esophagus reconstruction organs after esophageal cancer resection. In: Peracchia A, Rosati R, Bonavina L *et al.* (eds) *Recent Advancies in Diseases of the Esophagus.* Bologna, Italy: Monduzzi Editore 1996: 267–71.

51. Postlethwaite RW. Squamous cell carcinoma of the esophagus. In: Postlethwaite RW (ed.)

Surgery of the Esophagus. Appleton Century Crofts: New York 1979: 341–414.

52. Caldwell MT. Murphy PG, Page R *et al.* Timing of extubation after oesophagectomy (see comments). *Br J Surg* 1993; **80**: 1537–9.

53. Bartels H, Stein HJ & Siewert JR. Early extubation versus prolonged ventilation after esophagectomy: a randomized prospective study. In: Peracchia A, Rosati R, Bonavina L *et al.* (eds) *Recent Advances in Diseases of the Esophagus.* Bologna, Italy: Monduzzi Editore 1996: 537–9.

54. Smolle-Juettner FM, Pinter H, Smolle J *et al.* Surgical and non-surgical treatment of cancer of the oesophagus and the oesophagogastric junction: results of 200 consecutive cases. *Wien Klin Wochenschr* 1992; **104**: 563–9.

55. Earlam R & Cunha-Melo JR. Oesophageal squamous cell carcinoma: I. A critical review of surgery. *Br J Surg* 1980; **67**: 381–90.

56. Muller JM, Erasmi H, Stelzner M *et al.* Surgical therapy of oesophageal carcinoma. *Br J Surg* 1990; **77**: 845–57.

57. Andersen KB, Olsen JB & Pedersen JJ. Esophageal resections in Denmark 1985–1988. A retrospective study of complications and early mortality. *Ugeskr Laeger* 1994; **156**: 473–6.

58. Faller J. Surgery for esophageal and cardia cancer in Hungary: a nationwide retrospective five-year survey. *Surg Today* 1996; **26**: 368–72.

59. Wu YK, Huang GJ, Shao LF *et al.* Honored guest's address: progress in the study and surgical treatment of cancer of the esophagus in China, 1940–1980. *J Thorac Cardiovasc Surg* 1982; **84**: 325–33.

60. Wilson SE, Stone R, Scully M *et al.* Modern management of anastomotic leak after esophagogastrectomy. *Am J Surg* 1982; **144**: 95–101.

61. Hermreck AS & Crawford DG. The esophageal anastomotic leak. *Am J Surg* 1976; **132**: 794–8.

62. Maillard JN, Launois B, Lellouch J *et al.* Cause of leakage at the site of anastomosis after esophagogastric resection for carcinoma. *Surg Gynecol Obstet* 1969; **129**: 1014–18.

63. Cole WR, Petit R & Bernard HR. Factors affecting incidence of anastomotic leak following esophagogastrectomy. An analysis. *Ann Thorac Surg* 1968; **6**: 396–400.

64. Ancona E, Bardini R, Nosadini A *et al.* Esophagogastric anastomotic leakage. *Int Surg* 1982; **67**: 143–5.

65. Zieren HU, Muller JM & Pichlmaier H. Prospective randomized study of one- or two-layer anastomosis following oesophageal resection and cervical oesophagogastrostomy. *Br J Surg* 1993; **80**: 608–11.

66. Bardini R, Bonavina L, Asolati M *et al.* Single-layered cervical esophageal anastomoses: a prospective study of two suturing techniques. *Ann Thorac Surg* 1994; **58**: 1087–9.

67. Valverde A, Hay JM, Fingerhut A *et al.* Manual versus mechanical esophagogastric anastomosis after resection for carcinoma: a controlled trial. French Associations for Surgical Research. *Surgery* 1996; **120**: 476–83.

68. Chassin JL. Esophagogastrectomy: data favoring end-to-side anastomosis. *Ann Surg* 1978; **188**: 22–7.

69. Chasseray VM, Kiroff GK, Buard JL *et al.* Cervical or thoracic anastomosis for esophagectomy for carcinoma. *Surg Gynecol Obstet* 1989; **169**: 55–62.

70. Ribet M, Debrueres B & Lecomte-Houcke M. Resection for advanced cancer of the thoracic esophagus: cervical or thoracic anastomosis? Late results of a prospective randomized study. *J Thorac Cardiovasc Surg* 1992; **103**: 784–9.

71. Luke C & Roder D. *Epidemiology of Cancer in South Australia. Incidence, Mortality and Survival 1977–1995.* Adelaide: South Australian Cancer Registry, 1996.

72. Ries LAG, Miller BA, Hankey BF *et al. SEER Cancer Statistics Review 1973–1991.* Bethesda: NIH Publications, 1994.

73. Ruol A & Panel of experts. Multimodality treatment of non-metastatic cancer of the thoracic esophagus. Results of a Consensus Conference held at the VIth World Congress of the International Society for Diseases of the Esophagus. *Dis Esoph* 1996; **9**(suppl. 1): 39–55.

74. Leichman L, Steiger Z, Seydel HG *et al.* Preoperative chemotherapy and radiation therapy for patients with cancer of the esophagus: a potentially curative approach. *J Clin Oncol* 1984; **2**: 75–9.

75. Denham JW, Gill PG, Jamieson GG *et al.* Preliminary experience with a combined-modality approach to the management of oesophageal cancer. *Med J Aust* 1988; **148**: 9–13.

76. Gill PG, Jamieson GG, Denham J *et al.* Treatment of adenocarcinoma of the cardia with synchronous chemotherapy and radiotherapy. *Br J Surg* 1990; **77**: 1020–3.

77. Gill PG, Denham JW, Jamieson GG *et al.* Patterns of treatment failure and prognostic factors associated with the treatment of esophageal carcinoma with chemotherapy and radiotherapy either as sole treatment or followed by surgery. *J Clin Oncol* 1992; **10**: 1037–43.

78. Bessell JR, Devitt PG, Gill PG *et al.* Prolonged survival follows resection of oesophageal SCC

downstaged by prior chemoradiotherapy. *Aust N Z J Surg* 1996; **66**: 214–17.

79. Vogel SB, Mendenhall WM, Sombeck MD *et al.* Downstaging of esophageal cancer after pre-operative radiation and chemotherapy. *Ann Surg* 1995; **221**: 685–93.

80. Walsh TN, Noonan N, Hollywood D *et al.* A comparison of multimodal therapy and surgery for esophageal adenocarcinoma (see comments). *N Engl J Med* 1996; **335**: 462–7.

81. Logan A. The surgical treatment of carcinoma of the esophagus and cardia. *J Thorac Cardiovasc Surg* 1963; **46**: 150–63.

82. Skinner DB. En bloc resection for neoplasms of the esophagus and cardia. *J Thorac Cardiovasc Surg* 1983; **85**: 59–71.

83. Altorki NK & Skinner DB. En block esophagect-omy: the first 100 patients. *Hepatogastro-enterology* 1990; **37**: 360–3.

84. DeMeester TR, Zaninotto G & Johansson KE. Selective therapeutic approach to cancer of the lower esophagus and cardia. *J Thorac Cardiovasc Surg* 1988; **95**: 42–54.

85. Hagen JA, Peters JH & DeMeester TR. Superiority of extended en bloc esophagogastrectomy for carcinoma of the lower esophagus and cardia. *J Thorac Cardiovasc Surg* 1993; **106**: 850–8.

86. Collard JM, Otte JB, Reynaert M *et al.* Feasibility and effectiveness of en bloc resection of the eso-phagus for esophageal cancer. Results of a prospective study. *Int Surg* 1991; **76**: 209–13.

87. Lerut T, De-Leyn P, Coosemans W *et al.* Surgical strategies in esophageal carcinoma with emphasis on radical lymphadenectomy. *Ann Surg* 1992; **216**: 583–90.

88. Junginger T & Dutkowski P. Selective approach to the treatment of oesophageal cancer. *Br J Surg* 1996; **83**: 1473–7.

89. Horstmann O, Verreet PR, Becker H *et al.* Transhiatal oesophagectomy compared with transthoracic resection and systematic lympha-denectomy for the treatment of oesophageal cancer. *Eur J Surg* 1995; **161**: 557–67.

90. Isono K, Sato H & Nakayama K. Results of a nationwide study on the three-field lymph node dissection of esophageal cancer. *Oncology* 1991; **48**: 411–20.

91. Sacks H, Chalmers TC & Smith H. Randomized versus historical controls for clinical trials. *Br Med J* 1982; **72**: 233–40.

92. Bhansali MS, Patil PK, Badwe RA *et al.* Historical control bias: adjuvant chemotherapy in esopha-geal cancer. *Dis Esoph* 1997; **10**: 51–4.

93. King RM, Pairolero PC, Trastek VF *et al.* Ivor Lewis esophagogastrectomy for carcinoma of the esophagus: early and late functional results. *Ann Thorac Surg* 1987; **44**: 119–22.

10

SURGICAL MANAGEMENT OF ESOPHAGEAL CANCER: THE JAPANESE EXPERIENCE

HIROSHI AKIYAMA
HARUSHI UDAGAWA

INTRODUCTION

The most conspicuous characteristics of esophageal cancer therapy in Japan are the tumor histology and the inclination of Japanese surgeons to perform radical operations. Compared with Western countries, where adenocarcinoma comprises a substantial part of primary esophageal cancer,[1] most esophageal cancer in Japan is squamous cell carcinoma (**Table 10.1**). This fact should be clearly recognized when one compares the results of studies on esophageal cancer in Japan and other countries.

In Japan, complete surgical removal of the tumor has long been regarded as the primary goal of treatment of esophageal carcinoma. The range of lymph node dissection was continually extended until collothoracoabdominal (or three-field) lymph node dissection[2] was developed. However, over a decade has passed since its introduction, so more detailed indications for this procedure and various individualized modifications can now be discussed.

During recent years, rapid and marked advances have been made in many fields of esophageal cancer management in Japan. The new trends include:

- Detection of superficial or very early esophageal cancer.
- Precise preoperative staging of the tumor with endoscopy and newer imaging techniques.
- Development of endoscopic mucosal resection (EMR) and detailed investigation of its indications.
- Introduction of neoadjuvant chemotherapy and chemoradiotherapy.
- Application of autologous blood transfusion to esophagectomy.
- Introduction of video-assisted surgery.
- Investigation of the molecular biology and molecular genetics of esophageal cancer.

In this chapter, each of the above topics is briefly summarized, placing emphasis on the resutls of our 13 years' experience of three-field dissection.

DETECTION OF SUPERFICIAL OR VERY EARLY ESOPHAGEAL CANCER

Needless to say, early detection[3] is one of the keys to improving the results of surgical treatment of esophageal cancer. In order to achieve this aim, close communication, both pre- and postoperatively, between diagnosticians and surgeons is essential. Superficial cancer of the esophagus is increasingly identified in Japan, with 143 institutions having joined the national survey organized

Table 10.1 Histopathologic classification of primary esophageal carcinoma

LOCATION OF MAIN TUMOR	SQUAMOUS CELL	ADENOCARCINOMA	OTHERS	TOTAL
CE	66	0	1	67
UTE	133	1	4	138
MTE	669	2	22	693
LTE	291	12	6	309
AE	63	8	2	73
Total	1222	23	35	1280

Primary esophageal cancers resected in 1972–1996 at Toranomon Hospital.
CE, cervical esophagus; UTE, upper thoracic esophagus; MTE, middle thoracic esophagus; LTE, lower thoracic esophagus; AE, abdominal esophagus.

by Kodama and Kakegawa.[4] Between 1990 and 1995, 2418 patients with superficial esophageal cancer, whose initial symptoms are listed in **Table 10.2**, were evaluated. Of these patients, 55.0% were asymptomatic, while dysphagia or a feeling of esophageal obstruction may have been caused by a particular type of superficial cancer, and soreness and retrosternal pain may have been related to coexisting esophagitis. It should be understood, however, that the disease is usually asymptomatic at this stage, and that the variety of symptoms is not directly related to the lesion. Detection should be carried out early, regardless of symptoms.

How can superficial asymptomatic cancers be found? The main method of early detection is mass screening examinations and annual check-ups. Because of the high incidence of gastric cancer in Japan, mass screening by upper gastrointestinal barium studies is available to many Japanese. The standard annual check-up also includes a barium meal study or endoscopic examination of the upper gastrointestinal tract. Endoscopy is also frequently carried out after barium meal, when even a slight abnormality is suspected. Superficial cancers of the esophagus are thus found during endoscopic examinations not necessarily aimed at esophageal abnormalities. Another factor in early detection is the recognition of high-risk groups,[5] including:

- elderly males who are heavy alcohol drinkers and tobacco smokers;
- those with a strong family history of esophageal cancer;
- the existence of cancer in other organs (multiple cancers), particularly, head and neck or laryngopharyngeal cancers;
- patients with corrosive esophagitis and achalasia; and
- Barrett's esophagus (for adenocarcinoma).

Public enlightenment on the importance of early detection of cancer is basic, while another point which should be emphasized is the quality of examination and diagnosis.

Table 10.2 Initial symptoms of patients with superficial cancer of the esophagus

SYMPTOMS	MALE	FEMALE	TOTAL (%)
None	1191	138	1329 (55.0)
Chest pain, retrosternal pain	146	22	168 (6.9)
Feeling of obstruction	190	46	236 (9.8)
Feeling of foreign body	162	22	184 (7.6)
Dysphagia	72	16	88 (3.6)
Nausea, vomiting	29	6	35 (1.4)
Loss of appetite	36	8	44 (1.8)
Emaciation	12	6	18 (0.7)
Others	235	29	264 (10.9)
Unknown	63	7	70 (2.9)
Total	2136	300	2436 (100.0)

In the General Guidelines for Esophageal Cancer by the Japanese Society for Diseases of the Esophagus,[6] "superficial carcinoma" is defined as a carcinoma in which invasion remains within the submucosa, while "early carcinoma" is defined as superficial carcinoma without lymph node metastasis in pathologic studies on resected specimens. Among gastrointestinal malignancies, early cancer of the esophagus has a worse prognosis than other gastrointestinal cancers with the same extent of mural involvement. Esophageal cancer with submucosal invasion has an approximately 50% incidence of lymph node metastasis. In the Japanese national survey on gastrointestinal malignancies,[7] 5-year survival rates after resection of epithelial (ep) and muscularis mucosae (mm) cancer of the esophagus were 97% and 92%, respectively. These results correspond with those for mucosal and submucosal cancers of the stomach or colon. The five-year survival rate after resection of submucosal cancer of the esophagus was 67%, which was worse than that (80%) after resection of muscularis propria (mp) cancer of the stomach or colon.[8,9]

In recent years, the following endoscopic classification has been widely used for cancer of the esophagus, not only in Japan but also in Western countries.[10] Those cancers in which tumor invasion extends into or beyond the muscularis propria layer are called "advanced type." In the following classification, the superficial cancer is symbolized by "0," and the advanced type by "1 to 4." These are also used for radiographic examination.

0	superficial type
0–I	superficial and protruding type
0–II	superficial and flat type
	0–IIa slightly elevated type
	0–IIb flat type
	0–IIc slightly depressed type
0–III	superficial and distinctly depressed type

1. protruding type
2. ulcerative and localized type
3. ulcerative and infiltrative type
4. diffusely infiltrative type
5. unclassifiable type

Detection of 0–I and 0–III cancers is not difficult, although many problems remain in identifying 0–II cancers. When such lesions contain the component of slight elevation (0–IIa) or slight depression (0–IIc), detection of the disease may be possible. However, it is almost impossible to find the completely flat 0–IIb type cancers using radiography.

Thus, the role of esophagoscopy has become increasingly important in the detection of early cancer, with particular attention being given to the slightest changes in color, elevation, depression, and roughness or erosive changes of the mucosa. Because the main purpose of this chapter is to describe recent Japanese experiences in the surgical management of esophageal cancer, the details of the criteria for depth diagnosis by endoscopy are given elsewhere.[11,12]

Despite the advantage of endoscopic examination over radiographic examination in detecting mucosal pathology, conventional endoscopy still has some limitations for flat lesions in particular. The method of spray dye technique[13–19] may enhance sensitivity, while during the past decade, iodine (Lugol's solution) staining has been the cardinal method among Japanese clinical investigations towards early detection of esophageal cancer and evaluation of dysplastic lesions (**Figure 10.1**). In contrast, in Western countries, this method has often been used to distinguish the esophagogastric junction and to evaluate the results of therapy for reflux esophagitis.

There is no doubt that recent rapid developments in the early diagnosis of cancer of the esophagus have owed much to the dye staining technique and biopsy specimen examinations. Thus, the detection of very early, minute and multicentric cancers is no longer rare in daily clinical practice. Moreover, the results obtained by the comparative analysis of endoscopic findings and the histologic findings of biopsy or resected specimens provide feedback information on promoting the diagnostic quality of endoscopic examination.

PRECISE PREOPERATIVE STAGING OF THE TUMOR WITH ENDOSCOPY AND NEWER IMAGING TECHNIQUES

T staging

In 1972, the present author (H.A.) suggested that radiologic abnormality of the esophageal axis[20] in barium studies may predict local invasion with acceptable accuracy. Although still valid today, the remarkable development of imaging

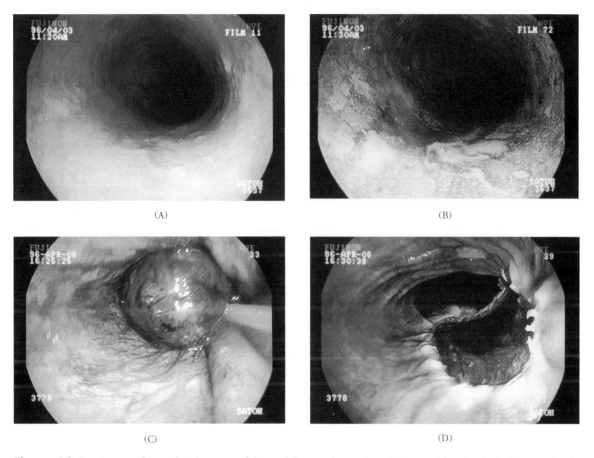

Figure 10.1 A case of superficial cancer of the middle esophagus in a 65-year-old male. A. 0–IIc type; depth: 1pm. B. Lugol staining. Irregular-shaped stained areas are seen in an unstained area, which is due to previous biopsies. C. Endoscopic mucosal resection (EMR). D. Wide shallow ulceration after EMR.

techniques presently offer the capability for much more accurate T staging.

Computed tomography (CT) scanning and endoluminal ultrasound (EUS) are common procedures for preoperative T staging of advanced esophageal carcinoma,[21,22] in addition to magnetic resonance imaging (MRI).[23] Recently developed ultrasound probes can provide more information in patients with stenotic lesions which conventional EUS probes could not pass. For shallower superficial lesions, detailed observation with endoscopy and with ultrasound probes of >15 MHz[24,25] are indispensable examinations (**Figure 10.2**). Preoperative differential diagnosis of early esophageal carcinoma limited to the epithelial layer (carcinoma *in situ*) or lamina propria from lesions reaching the surface of the muscularis mucosae or deeper is now more important than before,

because we know that endoscopic mucosal resection is curative for the former,[26–29] while wide-ranging lymph node involvement can occur with the latter.[30] The accuracy of this very delicate differential diagnosis is acceptable with the examinations listed above,[11,12,24,25] but is not perfect.

Advancement with the use of thin ultrasound probes permitted the development of new devices, including transaortic ultrasonography[31] and transtracheobronchial ultrasonography.[32] These approaches are useful particularly when EUS probes cannot be passed through the stenotic lesion. They provide more convincing evidence of direct tumor invasion than either CT or MRI, because real-time images can display movement or fixation of the tumor and the neighboring organs. Transtracheobronchial ultrasonography can diagnose airway invasion by the tumor more

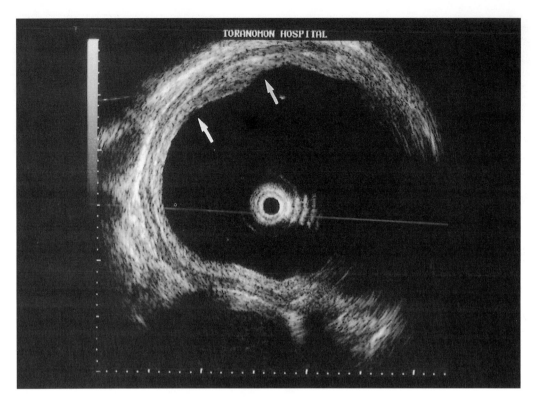

Figure 10.2   Ultrasound image with a high-frequency probe (20 MHz SP-501, Fujinon) applied through the endoscopic channel. A superficial middle esophageal cancer with slight invasion to sm. The tumor (between two arrows) involves the thin 4th hypoechoic layer, but thinning of the 5th echogenic layer (sm) is slight.

accurately than bronchofiberoptic endoscopy (**Figure 10.3**).

N staging

EUS,[22,33] conventional abdominal and cervical ultrasound,[34,35] and CT scanning are common procedures for preoperative N staging. As long as the EUS probe can pass the lesion, EUS is superior to CT in N staging.[36,37] Through the use of detailed histopathologic studies of lymph nodes obtained by three-field lymph node dissection, it is clear that the detection of metastatic lymph nodes based on lymph node size has theoretical limitations because one-fourth of lymph node metastases are microscopic.[38] However, preoperative N staging still has a role in the selection of candidates for preoperative neoadjuvant chemotherapy and in the assessment of its effect.

M staging

Plain chest radiography, CT scanning,[36] conventional abdominal ultrasound,[22] and bone scintigra-

phy are common procedures for preoperative M staging. CT scanning performed for T and N staging can be utilized for M staging if one adjusts the image conditions to view the lung fields.

It is of note that surgeons are themselves in the highly advantageous position of being able to observe directly and ascertain the preoperative imaging, and thus can apply such information to the next step of the examination and eventual surgery.

ENDOSCOPIC MUCOSAL RESECTION AND INVESTIGATION OF ITS INDICATIONS

As mentioned earlier in this chapter, while the number of cases of superficial cancers of the esophagus diagnosed has markedly increased, studies on the postoperative quality of life of esophagectomized patients[39] have revealed the disadvantages and risks of subtotal esophagectomy and reconstruction (**Figure 10.4**).

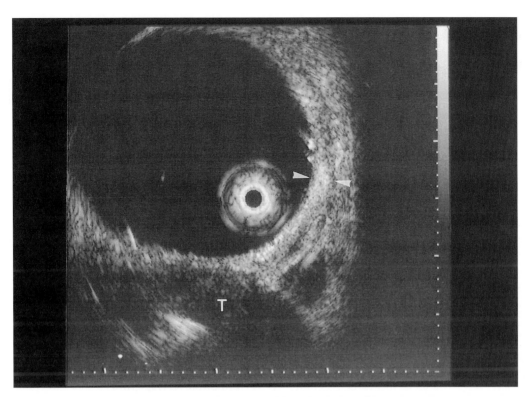

Figure 10.3 Trans-trachael ultrasonography. A 15-MHz ultrasound probe in a water balloon was applied from the tracheal lumen. The tracheal wall (between the arrowheads) is invaded by the esophageal tumor (T), and the two structures are fixed, showing no sliding movement.

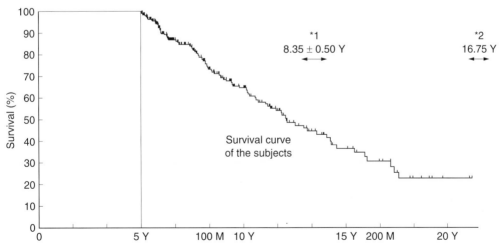

Subjects: 256 cases, survived more than 5 years after operation, excluding patients with tumor recurrence
*1: Average survival time of the subjects after 5-year survival
*2: Average life expectancy of a general population with the same sex and age distribution

Figure 10.4 Comparison of average survival time of postesophagectomy patients without recurrence to average life expectancy of general population.

The indication for endoscopic mucosal resection (EMR) is dependent on the depth of tumor invasion and size and number of lesions.[27–29,40–45] No lymphatic spread was seen in ep (Tis) and lpm cancers, and, as such, these cancers can be cured by local resection such as EMR (see **Figure 10.1**).

Technically, esophageal EMR is more difficult than for the stomach or colon. The esophagus has a narrow lumen, such that endoscopic procedures must be carried out at a tangential angle. There is also a risk of perforation because the wall – especially the adventitia – is thin. Other unfavorable factors include the movement of the esophageal wall with cardiac rhythm, with respiration, and the organ's own peristalsis. Various methods of EMR have been reported, among which the eso phageal endoscopic mucosal resection tube (EEMR-tube) method,[41] double channel method,[42] modification of strip-off biopsy,[43] and EMR-cap method[44] are currently used.

According to the results of the national survey of the Japanese Society for Esophageal Diseases,[4] tumors >3 cm were frequently resected piecemeal. Major complications of EMR are arterial bleeding, perforation, subcutaneous emphysema, and post-EMR stenosis, though in the majority of patients (91.9%), no complications occurred. There were no significant differences in the frequency of complications among the three representative methods. With regard to the manner of EMR (piecemeal or en bloc) and the attendant complications, esophageal perforation occurred more frequently in EMR performed piecemeal, probably because a larger lesion was being resected. The size of lesion is closely related to post-EMR esophageal stenosis, and post-EMR stenosis develops in particular after resection of circumferential mucosa.

Multiple superficial lesions are not a contraindication to EMR, and three or more lesions can be treated simultaneously with EMR as long as each individual lesion fulfills the depth and size criteria. Multi-session EMR for synchronous or metachronous multiple lesions is also not rare. For extensively multifocal or very widespread cancers, however, it is wiser to perform esophagectomy without thoracotomy (**Figure 10.5**).

Accurate pretreatment diagnosis of tumor depth is essential before planning EMR. This can be achieved by endoscopic examination and newer ultrasound methods using endoscopic probes. Naturally, a definite diagnosis of tumor depth is indispensable. Compared with other local approaches such as radiotherapy, laser therapy, high-frequency therapy, ethanol injection, and microwave therapy, EMR has one major advantage in that it is the only method to provide a complete resected specimen for histologic examination. It is important to obtain a good specimen which enables judgment of the adequacy of resection, or the necessity for additional resection. Physical damage to the specimen should be minimized and the *in situ* orientation should be noted. The anatomic relationship of multiple specimens in piecemeal EMR should be clarified. For lesions with a depth that is equivocal in terms of EMR criteria, diagnostic EMR is an acceptable strategy and follow-up examination can be done as necessary. With the increasing early detection of esophageal cancer, EMR is presently – and will be more so in the future – one of the important and common methods of treatment.

NEOADJUVANT CHEMOTHERAPY AND CHEMORADIOTHERAPY

Until recently, the principal adjuvant therapy for esophageal carcinoma was preoperative radiotherapy,[46] although after the negative results seen in controlled prospective studies,[47,48] radiotherapy has been restricted to locally advanced tumors with suspected extraesophageal invasion. After the introduction of cis-diaminedichloroplatinum II (CDDP), many efforts have been made to establish effective regimens of combination postoperative chemotherapy,[49,50] and today, as in Western countries,[51,52] preoperative neoadjuvant chemo- or chemoradiotherapy is attracting attention.[53] However, no clear evidence of the improvement of long-term results have been obtained except for the patients responding to the regimen.[54,55] Another problem is that the postoperative assessment of the initial stage is very difficult when adjuvant therapy is administered preoperatively.[56] The initial high hopes about neoadjuvant chemotherapy have been questioned and the reported increase in mortality and morbidity following surgery is of concern.[57–59]

Therefore, we restrict the application of neoadjuvant chemotherapy to patients with preoperative evidence of extensive lymphatic invasion when:

- five or more definite lymph node metastases are found;

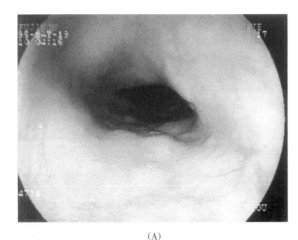

(A)

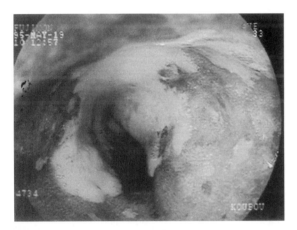

(B)

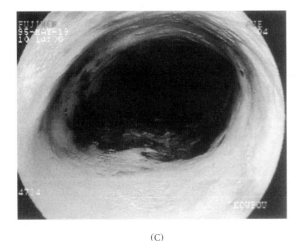

(C)

- three-field lymph node involvement is diagnosed; and
- lymph node metastasis is diagnosed at uncommon sites such as the subaortic arch area and pretracheal area.

We also restrict preoperative chemoradiotherapy to lesions (primary tumor or metastatic lymph nodes) with suspected direct invasion of neighboring structures.

In vitro drug sensitivity tests are expected to become a routine procedure to individualize treatment strategies and improve the response rate of chemotherapy.[60] We still use postoperative chemotherapy and are of the opinion that it should improve the long-term results.[50] The combination of *in vitro* drug sensitivity testing and postoperative chemotherapy, according to results, would be logical in patients with surgically resectable tumors. Because no clear evidence of improved long-term results with chemotherapy has been obtained, and even the promotion of hematogeneous tumor metastases by chemotherapy is suspected,[61] considerable further research is needed in this respect.

THREE-FIELD DISSECTION

Complete surgical extirpation of the tumor has been regarded as the primary goal in the treatment of esophageal carcinoma in Japan. Although many adjuvant therapies have been introduced and developed, this basic concept is still supported by most Japanese surgeons. Collothoracoabdominal lymph node dissection,[2] or three-field lymph node dissection, is the ultimate operative procedure based on this idea.[40,62–64] Despite many doubts and criticisms,[65,66] several institutions outside Japan have reported the superiority of three-field lymph node dissection over the conventional approach.[67,68] The technique has also provided

Figure 10.5 An 80-year-old male with a large superficial cancer of the middle and lower esophagus. A. 0–IIa+IIc type; depth: mm. B. Lugol staining, proximal tumor margin (upper border of unstained area). C. Lugol staining, distal tumor margin (lower border of unstained area). In this case, esophagectomy without thoracotomy was preferred to endoscopic mucosal resection because of the large size of the tumor.

data on the precise distribution of lymph node metastases arising from esophageal carcinoma.[69] Now that more than a decade has passed since we adopted this dissection procedure as our standard treatment, we can summarize the features of lymph node metastases from squamous cell carcinoma of the esophagus and the long-term results of radical lymph node dissection.

Patients

Between October 1972 and December 1996, 1900 patients with esophageal or hypopharyngeal carcinoma were admitted to the Department of Surgery at Toranomon Hospital (**Figure 10.6**). Among these, 1374 underwent surgical resection and 27 had endoscopic mucosal resection. The subjects of the present study were 481 patients with thoracic esophageal squamous cell carcinoma who underwent three-field lymph node dissection, excluding R2 cases (macroscopic residual tumor). As a historical control, we reviewed 284 patients with thoracic esophageal squamous cell carcinoma who underwent esophagectomy with two-field lymph node dissection (excluding R2 cases) before 1984, when we adopted three-field lymph node dissection as our standard procedure. Patients having two-field dissection during the period after we

began three-field dissection were also excluded in order to eliminate bias due to case selection.

Tumor depth (T) in the subjects, according to the main tumor location, is shown in **Table 10.3**. pT1 cases have been increasing owing to the increase of upper gastrointestinal endoscopy.

Table 10.3 Depth of invasion (T category) in lymph node dissection patients

	UPPER TE	MIDDLE TE	LOWER TE	TOTAL
Three-field dissection patients				
pTis	0	3	2	5
pT1	19	79	26	124
pT2	10	44	8	62
pT3	30	145	86	261
pT4	4	15	6	25
pTx	1	3	0	4
Total (*n*)	64	289	128	481
Two-field dissection patients				
pTis	0	3	1	4
pT1	6	32	10	48
pT2	4	27	15	46
pT3	10	98	50	158
pT4	1	10	4	15
pTx	3	5	5	13
Total (*n*)	24	175	85	284

TE, thoracic esophagus.

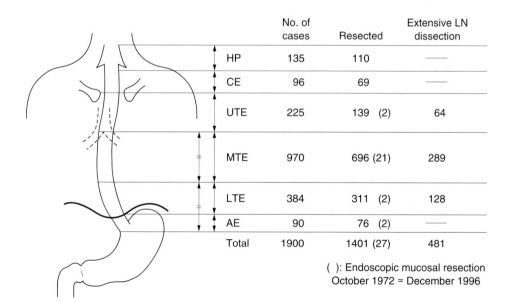

	No. of cases	Resected	Extensive LN dissection
HP	135	110	—
CE	96	69	—
UTE	225	139 (2)	64
MTE	970	696 (21)	289
LTE	384	311 (2)	128
AE	90	76 (2)	—
Total	1900	1401 (27)	481

( ): Endoscopic mucosal resection
October 1972 ≈ December 1996

Figure 10.6 Patients with esophageal carcinoma. AE, abdominal esophagus; CE, cervical esophagus; HP, hypopharynx; LN, lymph node; LTE, lower thoracic esophagus; MTE, middle thoracic esophagus; UTE, upper thoracic esophagus.

Lymph node metastasis

Tumor location and pattern of lymph node metastasis

It is well known that the pattern of lymph node metastasis from intrathoracic esophageal carcinoma varies according to tumor location. **Figure 10.7** shows the relationship between the location of the main tumor and the percentage of patients with metastatic lymph nodes in each region. Tumors in the upper thoracic esophagus have a tendency to produce more metastases in the cervical and superior mediastinal regions, while those in the middle thoracic esophagus cause widespread lymph node metastases in both cranial and caudal directions. Tumors in the lower thoracic esophagus cause more metastases in the middle and inferior mediastinum, as well as in the abdomen. At the same time, cervical lymph node metastasis occurs in 28.1% of these tumors and must not be overlooked.

Lymph node metastasis to the neck

As described above, cervical lymph node metastasis from thoracic esophageal carcinoma is quite frequent. Where in the neck does it occur? **Figure 10.8** shows the distribution of cervical lymph node metastasis. Because we have not experienced any higher cervical metastasis, neck dissection for thoracic esophageal carcinoma has been limited to below the level of the thyroid cartilage, thoroughly covering the point where the recurrent laryngeal nerves enter the larynx. This dissection field was divided into five areas each on the right and left sides, i.e., the cervical paratracheal area (inside the inner border of the carotid sheath) and four areas created by vertical and horizontal lines that run through the center of the dissection field outside the inner border of the carotid sheath. The most frequent site of metastasis was the right cervical paratracheal area (19.3%) and the second most common was the left cervical paratracheal area (9.4%). More than 90% of cervical metastases other than to the paratracheal area occurred in areas lower than the omohyoid muscle. Metastases above omohyoid only occurred in 8.4% of patients with cervical metastasis and 2.7% of all patients.

Depth of tumor invasion and lymph node metastasis

The relationship between the T category and lymph node metastasis is shown in **Table 10.4**. Although no lymph node metastasis was experienced in pTis

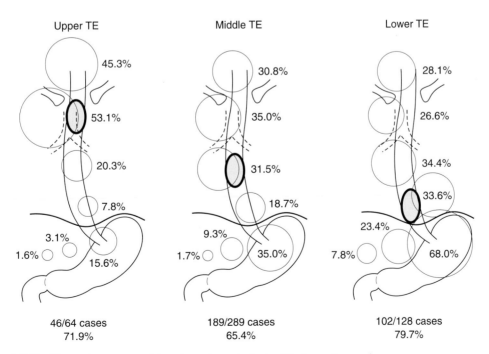

Upper TE	Middle TE	Lower TE
45.3%	30.8%	28.1%
53.1%	35.0%	26.6%
20.3%	31.5%	34.4%
7.8%	18.7%	33.6%
3.1%	9.3%	23.4%
1.6%	1.7%	35.0%	7.8%	68.0%
15.6%		
46/64 cases	189/289 cases	102/128 cases
71.9%	65.4%	79.7%

Figure 10.7 Tumor location and lymph node metastasis. TE, thoracic esophagus.

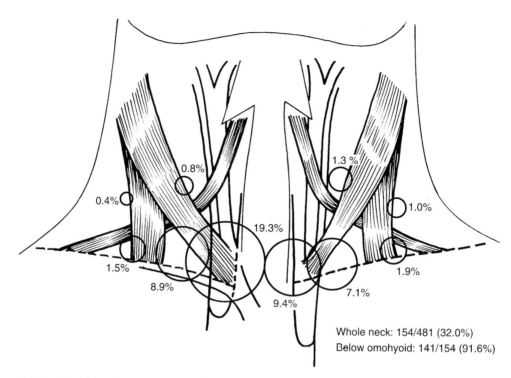

Figure 10.8 Lymph node metastasis to the neck.

(carcinoma *in situ*) patients, nearly 40% of patients with pT1 tumors had lymph node metastasis, while the rate was >70% in pT2 and deeper tumors. When pT1 tumors were divided into 1pm, mm, and sm (**Table 10.5**), the eight patients with 1pm tumors had no lymph node metastasis, while three of 16 patients with mm tumors had lymph node metastasis, as did 44% of those with sm tumors. This indicates that sm tumors should be regarded as advanced lesions which require meticulous and wide-ranging lymph node dissection.

Assessment of the tumor site-specific distribution of lymph node metastasis from pT1 tumors (**Figure 10.9**) showed more site-specific occurrence of lymph node metastasis when compared with all patients (see **Figure 10.7**). In particular, both cervical and superior mediastinal node metastasis from lower thoracic esophageal pT1 tumors were quite rare (one each).

Long-term results

Cumulative survival curves for the three-field and two-field dissection groups are shown in **Figure 10.10**. Survival of the three-field dissection group stratified according to pT category is shown in **Figure 10.11**, and survival according to TNM

Table 10.4 T category and lymph node metastasis

	NO. OF CASES	pN0pM0	pN1pM0	pM1LYM	FREQUENCY OF LN METASTASIS (%)
pTis	5	5	0(0)	0(0)	0
pT1	124	77	26(21)	21(17)	38
pT2	62	16	24(39)	22(35)	74
pT3	261	41	94(36)	126(48)	84.3
pT4	25	4	7(28)	14(56)	84
pTx	4	1	1(33)	2(50)	75
Total	481	144	152(31.6)	185(38.5)	70.1

Table 10.5 Lymph node metastasis in pT1 patients

DEPTH	NO. OF CASES	pN0	pN1	pM1LYM	FREQUENCY OF LN METASTASIS (%)
lpm	8	8	0	0	0
mm	16	13	1	2	19
sm	100	56	25	19	44

lpm, lamina propria mucosae; mm, muscularis mucosae; sm, submucosa.

stage is shown in **Figure 10.12**. It is worth noting that in pT1 patients, 44.4% of whom had lymph node metastasis, a 5-year survival rate of 78.6% was achieved, and even stage IV patients with positive nodes regarded as distant metastases in the TNM system had a 5-year survival rate of 25.5%.

Although this is a retrospective historic study, the improvement of survival in the three-field dissection group over the two-field dissection group was obvious for almost all pN types (pN0, pN1, and pM1 due to distant lymph node metastasis, i.e., lymph node metastasis in the neck or beyond the root of the left gastric artery). In addition, the superiority of three-field dissection was clear in pT3 patients, while pTis patients naturally received no benefit from three-field dissection. Survival of pT4

patients was also not improved by three-field dissection, probably because local factors have a stronger influence on their survival. Among pT1 patients, only those with lesions infiltrating the submucosa showed improved survival, which seems logical based on data obtained from the study of lymph node metastasis. The equivocal result in pT2 patients could be because of an insufficient number of subjects.

A close relationship between the number of metastatic lymph nodes and survival has been well documented.[70,71] Our results support this on the whole, but more than five metastases did not necessarily mean a poor result. Comparison of two-field and three-field dissection revealed the superiority of the three-field approach for almost all metastatic lymph node subgroups.

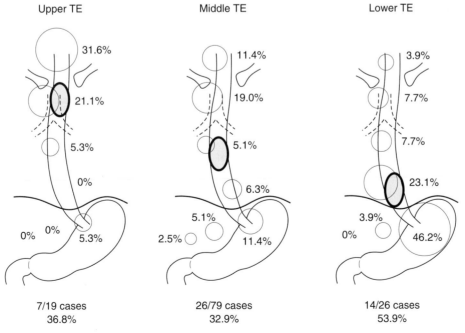

Figure 10.9 Lymph node metastasis in pT1 patients. TE, thoracic esophagus.

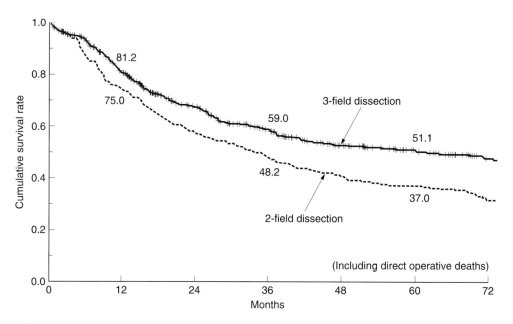

Figure 10.10   Cumulative postoperative survival curves for two- and three-field dissection of lymph node metastases.

Adequacy of three-field lymph node dissection

Tumor location and the distribution of lymph node metastasis are closely related, with this trend being clearer for shallower lesions. Many patients with T1 tumors in the upper thoracic esophagus have a good chance of cure by surgery via the cervical and transmediastinal approaches with median sternotomy, avoiding middle and lower mediastinal dissection. However, when a surgeon wishes to obtain a safe surgical margin during (or) of lymph node dissection, which we believe to be the principle of radical surgery, a right thoracotomy is advisable for thorough

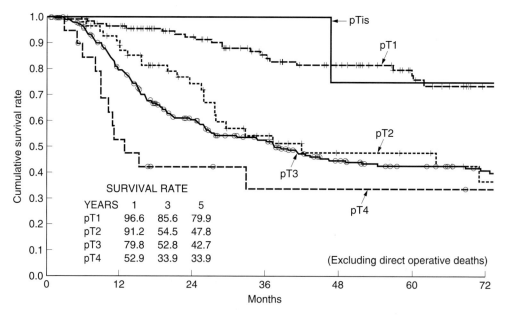

Figure 10.11   pT tumor category and postoperative survival after three-field lymph node dissection.

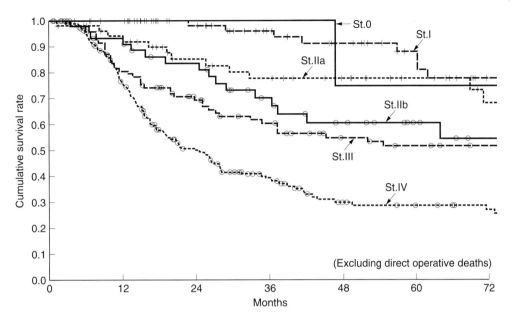

Figure 10.12   TNM stage and postoperative survival after three-field lymph node dissection.

mediastinal dissection if the general condition permits. On the other hand, cervical and superior mediastinal node metastasis is quite rare in patients with pT1 tumors of the lower thoracic esophagus, so cervical and superior mediastinal lymph node dissection can be avoided in such cases. Tis and lpm tumors, in which no lymph node metastasis has been experienced, can be treated curatively by endoscopic mucosal resection or transhiatal esophagectomy without lymph node dissection. No wide neck dissection is necessary for thoracic esophageal carcinoma, since the area defined by the bilateral omohyoid muscles and the subclavian veins is sufficient.

Comparison of the long-term results of three- and two-field lymph node dissection shows the superiority of three-field dissection. This does not simply mean that the addition of cervical lymph node dissection has produced the improved result. The most important point of three-field dissection is thorough continuous dissection of the bilateral paratracheal nodes, particularly nodes in the recurrent laryngeal nerve chain[72] from the superior mediastinum to the neck. Taken together with many other factors such as advances in adjuvant therapy and perioperative care, we feel that this procedure should not be discontinued until other more effective therapeutic measures are developed.[73,74]

ANALYSIS OF POSTOPERATIVE COMPLICATIONS

The improved prognosis with three-field lymph node dissection would be lost if this operation were associated with a higher operative mortality and morbidity. With the extension of lymph node dissection, especially around the tracheo-bronchial tree, three-field dissection is more invasive than two-field dissection. Therefore, many prophylactic and supportive modifications have been made since we first started three-field dissection. We surveyed the postoperative complications of three-field lymph node dissection and clarified the effective countermeasures.

The subjects were 530 consecutive patients in whom radical esophagectomy with three-field lymph node dissection was done between February 1984 and December 1995 (**Tables 10.6–10.8**). Median sternotomy for more aggressive superior mediastinal dissection was added in 46 patients. The right intercostal bronchial artery and the pulmonary branches of the vagus nerves were preserved in 208 patients (**Table 10.7**).

The main postoperative complications are listed in **Table 10.9**. Pulmonary complications accounted for 47.7% of reports, followed by cardiac complications, anastomotic leakage, recurrent laryngeal nerve palsy, and postoperative psychosis.

Table 10.6 Subjects of the analysis of postoperative complications. 530 cases of three-field dissection, February 1984–December 1995

MAIN LESION	NO. PRESENT
CE	2
UTE	70
MTE	311
ITE	130
AE	17

CE, cervical esophagus; UTE, upper thoracic esophagus; MTE, middle thoracic esophagus; ITE, inferior thoracic esophagus; AE, abdominal esophagus.

Table 10.7 Special operative procedures performed in 530 subjects

PROCEDURE	NO. PERFORMED
Median sternotomy*	46
VATS†	3
Respiratory function preservation‡	208

*To improve radicality of superior mediastinal dissection.
†Video-assisted thoracic surgery.
‡Preservation of right intercostal bronchial artery and the pulmonary branches of the vagus nerves.

Pseudomembranous colitis and methicillin-resistant *Staphylococcus aureus* (MRSA) colitis were not rare. When compared with 455 control patients in whom two-field dissection was performed, recurrent laryngeal nerve palsy, pulmonary edema, pulmonary embolism, and arrhythmia were significantly more frequent in the three-field dissection group (**Table 10.10**).

When postoperative pneumonia was divided into severe (requiring ventilation) and mild (not requiring ventilation), severe pneumonia tended to occur earlier (**Figure 10.13**). Thus, when pneu-

Table 10.9 Major postoperative complications of three-field dissection

COMPLICATION	NO. IDENTIFIED (%)
Pulmonary	258 (48.7)
Circulatory	145 (27.4)
Anastomotic leakage	89 (16.8)
Radiologic	56 (10.6)
Clinical	33 (6.2)
Recurrent nerve palsy	88 (16.6)
Delirium	51 (9.6)
Colitis (MRSA, etc.)	20 (3.8)

MRSA, methicillin-resistant *Staphylococcus aureus*.

monia is identified early in the postoperative course, it is likely to become a severe complication. Allogenic blood transfusion was carried out in 20 out of 49 patients with postoperative pneumonia, while only 86 out of 458 patients without postoperative pneumonia received allogenic transfusion (**Table 10.11**). When postoperative recurrent laryngeal nerve palsy occurred, aspiration and pneumonia increased and suction with a bronchofiberscope was needed more frequently (**Figure 10.14**).

Pulmonary edema and acute respiratory distress syndrome (ARDS) occurred in 53 patients. Although all 16 patients with mild disease survived, nine in-hospital deaths occurred among the 37 severe cases.

Pulmonary thromboembolism has long been thought to be a rather rare postoperative complication in Japan. However, in our series of 530 patients of three-field dissection, 18 definite cases of pulmonary thromboembolism were detected through active use of pulmonary perfusion scans to assess postoperative hypoxemia and detailed comparison of the findings with chest radiography. This incidence was higher than that after gastric operations

Table 10.8 Patterns of reconstruction

ROUTE	ORGAN USED AS ESOPHAGEAL SUBSTITUTE		
	STOMACH	COLON	JEJUNUM
Posterior mediastinal	98	1	0
Retrosternal	369	61	1

Table 10.10   Comparison of the incidence of major complications after three- and two-field dissection

MAJOR COMPLICATION	THREE-FIELD DISSECTION (%) ($n = 530$)	TWO-FIELD DISSECTION (%)* ($n = 455$)	P
Major anastomotic leakage	33 (6.2)	31 (6.8)	NS
Recurrent nerve palsy	89 (16.8)	57 (12.5)	0.060
Pneumonia	66 (12.5)	57 (12.5)	NS
Pulmonary edema/ARDS	59 (11.1)	25 (5.5)	0.0015
Pulmonary thromboembolism	17 (3.2)	4 (0.9)	0.0117
Arrythmia	145 (27.4)	81 (17.8)	0.0030

*Historic control.
ARDS, acute respiratory distress syndrome; NS, not significant.

Table 10.11   Allogeneic blood transfusion (BTF) and the incidence of postoperative pneumonia

	BTF (+)	BTF (−)
Pneumonia	7	19
Severe pneumonia	13	10]*
Pneumonia (−)	86	372

*$P = 0.00001$ (chi-square test).

or other operations in our gastroenterologic surgery (**Table 10.12**) department. The treatment and prognosis are shown in **Figure 10.15**. Four patients died, such that the mortality rate was 22.2%. Tissue plasminogen activator, the most

powerful thrombolytic agent, was used in two patients with recurrence of pulmonary embolism, but the effect was temporary and consequentially massive bleeding was lethal. Interventional radiology techniques, such as caval filter insertion and transcatheter aspiration of the thrombus, were not applied to this series of patients, but they should be tried as the next step.

Following this experience, we began routine use of intraoperative heparin and dextran in January 1994 (**Figure 10.16**), though dextran was soon stopped due to poor intraoperative hemostasis. The use of a pneumatic cuff during, and for several days after, surgery was begun in September 1994,

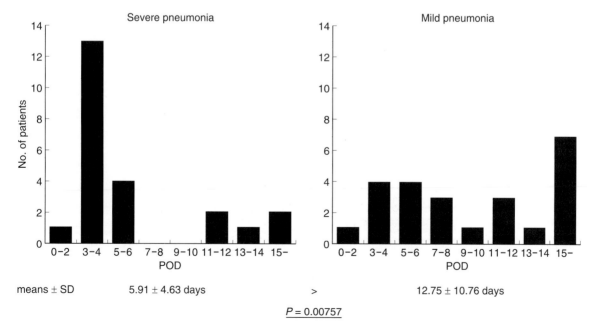

means ± SD   5.91 ± 4.63 days   >   12.75 ± 10.76 days

$P = 0.00757$

Figure 10.13   Postoperative onset of pneumonia and its severity after three-field lymph node dissection. POD, postoperative days.

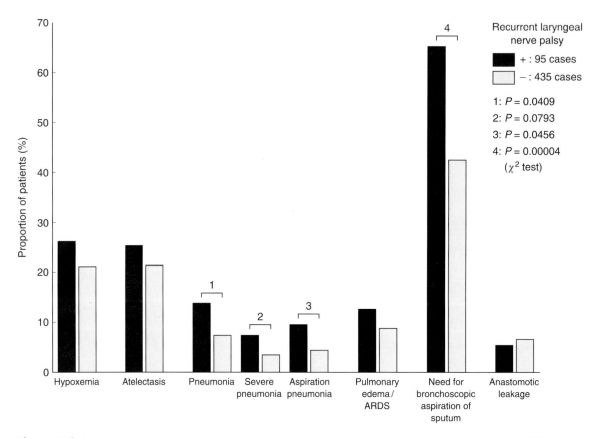

Figure 10.14 Postoperative recurrent largyngeal nerve palsy and postoperative respiratory state. ARDS, acute respiratory distress syndrome.

and consequently postoperative pulmonary thromboembolism was prevented.

Anastomotic leakage occurred in 16.8% of the patients (radiologic leakage in 10.6%, clinical leakage in 6.2%). There were concurrent pulmonary complications in 19.6% of the radiologic group and 36.3% of the clinical group.

Among cardiac complications, arrhythmia occurred most frequently (27% of all patients),

most usually atrial fibrillation and paroxysmal atrial tachycardia. Arrhythmias usually developed on the 2nd–4th postoperative days when excess water and electolytes in the third space re-entered the circulation. Pain, anxiety, hypoxemia, and the effect of superior mediastinal dissection were considered to be accelerating factors. It is important to judge whether the blood volume is excessive or deficient. In another study, it was found that preservation of

Table 10.12 Incidence of postoperative pulmonary thromboembolism

OPERATION	ALL CASES (n)	PTE (n)	INCIDENCE (%)
Esophageal cancer (three-field dissection)	530	18	3.4
Gastric cancer (subtotal, total gastrectomy)	655	11	1.7
Others	1560	4	0.3

$*P < 0.05; †P < 0.001$ (chi-square test).
PTE, pulmonary thromboembolism.

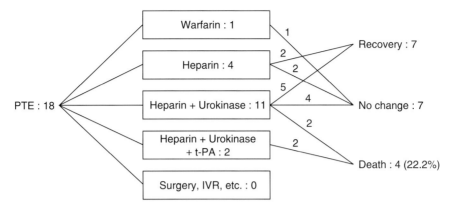

Figure 10.15 Treatment choice and prognosis of postoperative pulmonary thromboembolism. PTE, pulmonary thromboembolism; t-PA, tissue plasminogen activator; IVR, interventional radiology.

the cardiac branches of the right vagus nerve and right bronchial artery, which usually arises from the third right intercostal artery, stabilized heart rate against daily water balance, and lessened the frequency of sputum suction by bronchofiberoscopy.[75] Other authors have suggested the importance of preservation of a thin membrane of connective tissue wrapping the trachea.[76]

Although three-field lymph node dissection applies a major stress to the respiratory and circulatory systems, many technical improvements, aimed at preserving the small nerves to the heart, lungs, and larynx, as well as the blood supply to the tracheobronchial tree, together with advances in

postoperative care, have made this extended operation feasible (**Table 10.13**).

APPLICATION OF AUTOLOGOUS BLOOD TRANSFUSION TO ESOPHAGECTOMY

Allogeneic blood transfusion has many potential risks, including transmission of various viruses such as hepatitis viruses, the AIDS virus, and human T-cell virus (HTLV). Graft-versus-host disease is another grave adverse reaction.[77] It is also claimed that allogeneic blood transfusion suppresses the patient's immune system and thus increases postoperative complications, or leads to

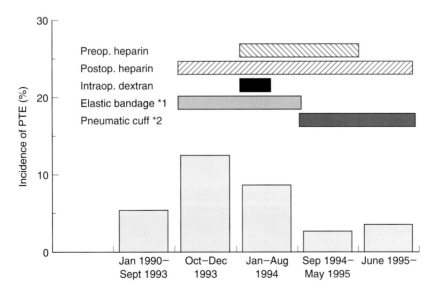

Figure 10.16 Prophylactic measures against pulmonary thromboembolism (PTE). Their change and the incidence of postoperative PTE. *1,*2, for lower extremities.

Table 10.13   Comparison of mortalities of esophagectomy after three- and two-field dissection

OUTCOME	THREE-FIELD DISSECTION (%) ($n = 530$)	TWO-FIELD DISSECTION (%)* ($n = 455$)	P
Death within 30 days	14 (2.6)	7 (1.5)	NS
Hospital death later than 30th POD	15 (2.8)	15 (3.3)	NS

*Historic control.
NS, not significant; POD, postoperative day.

poorer prognosis.[78–80] Autologous blood transfusion is already a common procedure in cardiac surgery and orthopedic surgery. However, the application of this procedure to tumor-bearing patients has not been done so extensively because of several factors. For instance, preparation takes time, tumor-bearing patients are often anemic, and they often have other complications.

On examining our records, we found the mean intraoperative blood loss for standard esophagectomy with three-field lymph node dissection over the past 10 years to be $602 \pm 328\,\mathrm{ml}$. Thus, 800 ml of autologous blood would be sufficient for the operation, and no prolongation of the preoperative hospital stay would occur if 400 ml were collected at the outpatient clinic at the time of the patient's first visit.

We began autologous blood transfusion for esophageal carcinoma surgery in May 1994.[81] The indications for blood collection were defined according to the guidelines of the Japanese Society of Blood Transfusion (**Table 10.14**). The autologous group included 38 patients who underwent esophagectomy with three-field lymph node dissection. A total of 800 ml autologous blood was collected from each patient (**Figure 10.17**) between January and December 1995. The historic control group comprised 50 patients who underwent the same operation from January 1992 to April 1994, and who fulfilled the criteria for autologous blood collection (**Table 10.15**). The results are shown in **Figures 10.18–10.20**. After standard esophagectomy, hemoglobin (Hb) levels were significantly higher in the autologous group than in the control group. The percentage of patients who did not receive allogeneic blood transfusion was significantly greater in the autologous group (36 out of 38 patients, 95%) than in the control group (34 out of 50 patients, 68% $P = 0.002$). Our conclusion is that collection of 800 ml of autologous blood before esophagectomy is useful for maintaining a stable Hb level after surgery, and aids in avoiding allogeneic blood transfusion.

Small operations with minimal blood loss do not benefit from autologous blood transfusion, while a large predicted blood loss makes the program meaningless because we cannot keep patients with malignancy waiting too long for autologous blood collection. Esophagectomy with three-field lymph node dissection fulfills both of these requirements. We know that autologous blood transfusion is expensive, particularly when recombinant human erythropoietin is administered. Therefore, this issue should be examined further from a socioeconomic point of view.

INTRODUCTION OF VIDEO-ASSISTED SURGERY

Along with evolutional and rapid development in endoscopic surgery for many types of organs and diseases, the thoracoscopic approach has also been introduced to esophageal surgery for the aim of minimizing surgical invasiveness.

Animal experiments in thoracoscopic surgery for the esophagus were begun by Kipfmuller et al.[82] and Gossot et al.,[83] and this was followed with clinical use by Cuschieri[84] and Peracchia and

Table 10.14   Indications for autologous blood transfusion of esophagectomy, following Guidelines of the Japanese Society of Blood Transfusion

1. Age ≤ 80 years
2. Bodyweight $\geq 40\,\mathrm{kg}$
3. Hemoglobin $\geq 11.0\,\mathrm{g/dl}$
4. Serum protein $\geq 6.5\,\mathrm{g/dl}$
5. Exception for severe complication

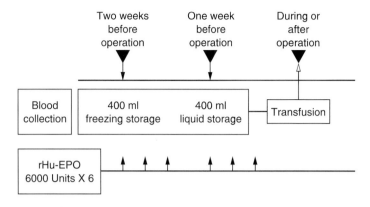

Figure 10.17   Method of autologus blood transfusion. Two units (400ml) of autologus blood were collected before operation. Recombinant human erythropoietin (rHu-EPO) was injected if hemoglobin levels before blood collection were <14.0 g/dl.

colleagues.[85] Since then, numerous reports have been made on endoscopic or video-assisted esophageal surgery. Thoracoscopic or laparoscopic surgery is rightly indicated in almost all benign esophageal diseases.[85–87] With increasing experience, the approach has also begun to be used for cancer of the esophagus. However, in the case of malignancy, the indications for this technique including the extent of resection, and its significance in terms of the patient's general condition, are different

Table 10.15   Comparison of background data between autologous blood transfusion (AuBT) and control groups

	AuBT GROUP ($n = 38$)	CONTROL GROUP ($n = 50$)	P
No. without ALBT	36	34	0.002
Male/female ratio	34/4	45/5	NS
Depth of tumor invasion*			NS
a0	20	22	
a1	10	23	
a2	5	4	
a3	3	1	
Pathological stage*			NS
0	8	9	
1	8	2	
2	1	0	
3	6	14	
4	15	25	
Age (years)	60.5 ± 6.6	63.4 ± 7.2	NS
Bodyweight (kg)	58.3 ± 8.3	56.5 ± 7.6	NS
Hb at admission (g/dl)	13.6 ± 1.2	13.5 ± 1.0	NS
Blood loss during operation (ml)	632 ± 312	529 ± 296	NS
Days from admission to operation	23.4 ± 14.1	20.8 ± 13.2	NS
Type of ALBT (units)†			
Whole blood	0	2	
Packed red blood cells	6	54	

Values are mean ± SD.
*Classification according to *Guide Lines for the Clinical and Pathologic Studies on Carcinoma of the Esophagus.*[6]
†Total administered to each group.
ALBT, allogeneic blood transfusion; Hb, hemoglobin; NS, not significant.

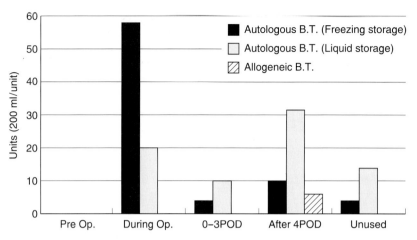

Figure 10.18 Perioperative transfusion for autologous blood transfusion (ABT) group. Of the total autologus blood, 11.8% was not used perioperatively. B.T., blood transfusion; POD, postoperative day.

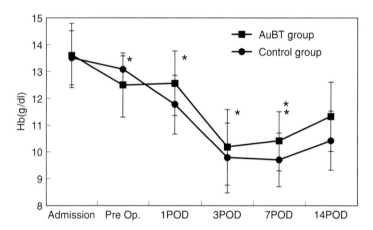

Figure 10.19 Preoperative and postoperative hemoglobin (Hb) concentrations. *P=0.002; **P<0.001. POD, postoperative day; AuBT, autologous blood transfusion.

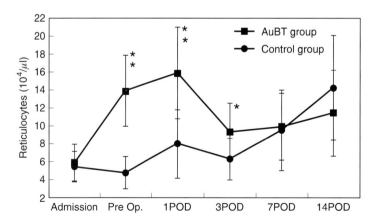

Figure 10.20 Preoperative and postoperative reticulocyte concentrations. *P=0.02; **P<0.001. POD, postoperative day; AuBT, autologous blood transfusion.

depending on the strategy advocated by the surgeons.

If a surgeon considers that lymph nodal dissection is not at all significant and not effective in improving the patients' survival, esophagectomy can be simply done by transhiatal esophagectomy or esophagectomy without thoracotomy, and thoracoscopic surgery has little advantage. However, when an additional procedure such as dissection of selected nodes is needed, thoracoscopic surgery would become useful, although further technical advancement in the near future is necessary. Because most Japanese surgeons have pursued meticulous and thorough lymph node dissection, thoracoscopic esophagectomy for esophageal cancer is not yet widely accepted due to the fear of less extensive lymph node dissection, although some of the technique's advocates claim the opposite.[88]

The disadvantages of thoracoscopic esophagectomy[89–92] are the same as those of video-assisted surgery for other organs. In thoracoscopic esophagectomy, more time and effort is needed in order to maintain a good surgical field, due to the collapse and retraction of the lung, and hence, maintenance of a constant intraoperative PaO_2 level is not always easy. Therefore, in thoracoscopic esophagectomy, the surgical risk is not always small if the operation proceeds for a long time. Accurate and careful operative maneuvers are required, particularly in thoracoscopic esophageal surgery for malignancy, because the esophagus is surrounded by vital organs such as the heart, aorta, lungs and respiratory tract, and vulnerable nerves. However, similar problems more or less also exist in the usual open thoracotomy surgery.

Regarding image quality, thoracoscopic surgery already has some advantages, and soon will have more, over conventional open surgery. Recently developed video camera facilities incorporate compact 3-charged couple devicer (3CCD) image sensor and separate red, green and blue (RGB) outputs to provide endoscopic images with much better resolution. As a result, the images with 3CCD have become clearer and brighter, and its color reproduction has become superb. Furthermore, the introduction of high-definition technology using a three-dimensional system camera will soon make the imaging quality almost perfect. The apparent disadvantages at present are the loss of natural tactile sensation and the discrepancy between optical orientation and the surgeons' body image. Very rapid progress in the technology of "virtual reality" may solve these problems some time in the near future. In addition to these technological advancements, efforts to improve the instruments for thoracoscopic surgery are constantly being made. When these developments are accomplished, thoracoscopic esophagectomy will become much more convenient, more time saving, and safer. It would indeed be a big step forward. That is, the operation could be carried out with better magnification, clarity and with a three-dimensional field. Thus, surgery can be performed with extraordinary accuracy and, therefore, without unnecessary trauma. This will result in a truly minimally invasive esophagectomy. Such advances will be only a question of time, though the enormous cost is still an unsolved problem.

With thorough technical development, video-assisted surgery may become as radical and complete as conventional open surgery. We can then determine which part of surgery is the main cause of invasiveness and risk for the patient, and more precise indications for each procedure will be clarified. Advances of non-surgical therapy in the future might lead to new combinations of adjuvant therapy and surgery for which a video-assisted approach is best indicated.

Only a few of the wide range of advances related to video-assisted surgery, e.g., high-definition video and 3D video systems, will greatly facilitate some surgical procedures. Stereoscopic surgery is not new, being commonly used and almost indispensable among neurosurgeons and ophthalmologists. As such, as in general and other thoracic surgeries, three-dimensional visualization should not be regarded any more as a special technological or as an impractical technical trial, but as a necessary step forward for forthcoming surgical advances.

MOLECULAR BIOLOGY AND MOLECULAR GENETICS OF ESOPHAGEAL CANCER

Recent advances in molecular biology and molecular genetics have been remarkable, and among the vast number of basic investigations, many have been performed on esophageal lesions. These include *bst*-1, *int*-2, *Cyclin D1*, *erb-B*, *MDM2* as oncogenes, *p53*, *Rb*, *APC*, *p16*, *p15*, *p21*, and *p27* as cancer suppressor genes, Ki67, proliferating cell nuclear antigen (PCNA), AgNORs, vascular endothelial growth factor (VEGF) as tumor proliferation-related factors, and E-cadherin, α-catenin, desmoglein I, thrombomodulin, and matrix metalloproteinases (MMPs) as factors related to tumor metastasis and infiltration, DNA ploidy, and so on. Most of the studies have been done in relation to prognosis,[93,94] and assessment of the applications for treatment is quite rare. Recently, a relationship was reported between some of these factors and the sensitivity of various cancers to chemotherapy.[95,96] Experiments on targeted cancer therapy have also been done using some surface markers and receptors.[97] None of these treatments is yet clinically available, but we hope that the zeal of many investigators will bear fruit in the fields of prevention, early tumor detection, treatment, and prognostic information on esophageal cancer.[98]

REFERENCES

1. Casson AG & McKneally MF. Epidemiology. In: Pearson FG, Deslauriers J, Ginsberg RJ et al. (eds) *Esophageal Surgery*. New York: Churchill Livingstone 1995: 551–9.
2. Akiyama H. *Surgery for Cancer of the Esophagus*. Baltimore: Williams & Wilkins 1990: 19–42.
3. Endo M, Takeshita K & Yoshida M. How can we diagnose the early stage of esophageal cancer? Endoscopic diagnoses. *Endoscopy* 1986; **18**: 11–18.
4. Kodama M & Kakegawa T (Japanese Society for Esophageal Diseases) *Report of national survey on superficial carcinoma of the esophagus*. 49th Congress of the Japanese Society for Esophageal Diseases, Otsu, 1995.
5. Yokoyama A, Ohmori T, Makuuchi H et al. Successful screening for early esophageal cancer in alcoholics using endoscopy and mucosa iodine staining. *Cancer* 1995; **76**: 928–34.
6. Japanese Society for Esophageal Diseases. *Guide Lines for the Clinical and Pathologic Studies on Carcinoma of the Esophagus*, 8th edn. Tokyo: Kanehara & Co Ltd, 1992.
7. Endo M. Early esophageal cancers – National survey. *Gastroenterol Endosc* 1990; **32**: 2466–70.
8. Japanese Research Society for Gastric Cancer. *The Report of Treatment Results of Stomach Cancer in Japan* (Cases treated in 1985). No. 44, Tokyo: Miwa Registry Institute for Stomach Cancer, 1996.
9. Japanese Research Society for Cancer of the Colon and Rectum. *Multi-institutional registry of large bowel cancer in Japan*. Vol. 9, Cases treated in 1985. Tokyo: Japanese Research Society for Cancer of the Colon, 1990.
10. Dittler HJ, Pesarini AC & Siewert JR. Endoscopic classification of esophageal cancer: correlation with the T stage. *Gastrointest Endosc* 1992; **38**: 662–8.
11. Makuuchi H, Machimura T, Mizutani K et al. Diagnostic accuracy of endoscopy in estimating the depth of invasion of superficial esophageal carcinoma. *Stomach Intestine* 1992; **27**: 175–84.
12. Momma K, Yoshida M, Yamada Y et al. Endoscopic estimation of depth of invasion in cases with esophageal mucosal cancer. *Stomach Intestine* 1994; **29**: 327–40.
13. Strong MS, Vaughan OW & Incze JS. Toluidine blue in the management of carcinoma of the oral cavity. *Arch Otolaryngol* 1968; **87**: 527–31.
14. Endo M & Ide H. *Endoscopic Staining in Early Diagnoses of Esophageal Cancer*. Tokyo: Japan Scientific Societies Press, 1991.
15. Schiller W. Early diagnosis of carcinoma of the cervix. *Surg Gynecol Obstet* 1933; **59**: 210–22.
16. Voegel R. Die Schillersche Jodprobe im Rahmen der Oesophagus-diagnostik (Vorlaufige Mitterung). *Proct Otorhinolaryngol* 1966; **28**: 230–9.
17. Brodmerkel GJ. Schiller's test: an aid in esophagoscopic diagnosis. *Gastroenterology* 1971; **60**: 813.
18. Toriya S & Akasaka Y. Dye-spraying method in esophagoscopic diagnosis. In: Takemoto T & Kawai K (eds) *Gastrointestinal Endoscopy with Application of Dye*. Tokyo: Igaku Shoin 1972: 34–42.
19. Makuuchi H, Sugihara T & Machimura T. Diagnosis of early stage of superficial esophageal cancer. *Shokaki-ka (Gastroenterology)* 1986; **5**: 520–7.
20. Akiyama H, Kogure T & Itai Y. The esophageal axis and its relationship to the resectability of carcinoma of the esophagus. *Ann Surg* 1972; **176**: 30–6.
21. Picus D, Balfe DM, Koehler RE et al. Computed tomography in the staging of esophageal carcinoma. *Radiology* 1983; **146**: 433.
22. Akiyama H, Tsurumaru M & Udagawa H. Imaging techniques. In: Delarue NC, Wilkins EW, Jr, Wong J (eds) *Esophageal Cancer*. St. Louis: C.V. Mosby 1988: 53–68.
23. Takashima S, Takeuchi N, Shiozaki H et al. Carcinoma of the esophagus: CT vs MR imaging

in determining resectability. *Am J Roentgenol* 1991; **156**: 297–302.

24. Murata Y, Suzuki S, Ohta M *et al.* Small ultrasonic probes for determination of the depth of superficial esophageal cancer. *Gastrointest Endosc* 1996; **44**: 23–8.

25. Hasegawa H, Niwa Y, Arisawa T *et al.* Preoperative staging of superficial esophageal carcinoma: comparison of an ultrasound probe and standard endoscopic ultrasonography. *Gastrointest Endosc* 1996; **44**: 388–93.

26. Goseki N, Koike M & Yoshida M. Histopathologic characteristics of early stage esophageal carcinoma. A comparative study with gastric carcinoma. *Cancer* 1992; **69**: 1088–93.

27. Makuuchi H, Machimura T, Mizutani K *et al.* Controversy in the treatment of superficial esophageal carcinoma – indications and problems of the procedures. *Jpn J Gastroenterol Surg* 1992; **93**: 1059–62.

28. Endo M, Yoshino K, Kawano T *et al.* Clinical evaluation of mucosal cancer of the esophagus: analysis of 1584 cases of superficial esophageal cancer resected in Japan. In: Nabeya K, Hanaoka T, Nogami H (eds) *Recent Advances in Diseases of the Esophagus.* Tokyo: Springer-Verlag 1993: 540–5.

29. Yoshida M, Hanashi T, Momma K *et al.* Endoscopic mucosal resection for radical treatment of esophageal cancer. *Jpn J Cancer Chemother* 1995; **22**: 847–54.

30. Yoshinaka H, Shimazu H, Fukumoto T *et al.* Superficial esophageal carcinoma: a clinico-pathological review of 59 cases. *Am J Gasteroenterol* 1991; **86**: 1413–18.

31. Akiyama S, Kodera Y, Sekiguchi H *et al.* Preoperative intra-aortic ultrasonography to determine resectability in advanced esophageal cancer. *Br J Surg* 1995; **82**: 1971–4.

32. Udagawa H, Matsuda M, Watanabe G *et al.* A new technique for transtracheal ultrasonography. *The Japan Society of Ultrasound in Medicine; Proceedings,* 1992; **61**: 495–6.

33. Murata Y, Hayashi K, Kobayashi A *et al.* Preoperative staging of oesophageal carcinoma by ultrasound. *Asian J Surg* 1994; **17**: 200–7.

34. Udagawa H, Tsurumaru M, Watanabe G *et al.* Preoperative detection of lymph node metastasis in the neck and the superior mediastinum by neck ultrasound examination. *Jpn J Gastroenterol Surg* 1986; **19**: 2176–83.

35. Tachimori Y, Kato H, Watanabe H *et al.* Neck ultrasonography for thoracic esophageal carcinoma. *Ann Thorac Surg* 1994; **57**: 1180–83.

36. Fekete F, Sauvanet A, Zins M *et al.* Imaging of cancer of the esophagus: ultrasound-endoscopy or computed tomography? *Ann Chir* 1995; **49**: 573–8.

37. Botet JF, Lightdale CJ, Zauber AG *et al.* Preoperative staging of esophageal cancer: comparison of endoscopic US and dynamic CT. *Radiology* 1991; **181**: 419–25.

38. Udagawa H, Watanabe G, Ono Y *et al.* Role of ultrasound in management of esophageal carcinoma. *Diagnostic Imaging of the Abdomen* 1990; **10**: 310–18.

39. Udagawa H, Tsurumaru M, Kajiyama Y *et al.* Problems related to radical esophagectomy and reconstruction – study of postoperative patients without tumor recurrence. *Jpn J Gastroenterol Surg* 1995; **28**: 2052–56.

40. Akiyama H, Tsurumaru M, Udagawa H *et al.* Radical lymph node dissection for cancer of the thoracic esophagus. *Ann Surg* 1994; **220**: 364–73.

41. Makuuchi H, Shimada H, Mizutani K *et al.* Endoscopic mucosal resection in early esophageal cancer. *J Jpn Bronchoesophagol Soc* 1996; **47**: 150–4.

42. Momma K, Sakaki N & Yoshida M. Endoscopic treatment for mucosal cancer of the esophagus: endoscopic mucosectomy. *Gastroenterol Endosc* 1990; **2**: 501–6.

43. Tada M, Murata M, Murakami F *et al.* Development of the strip-off biopsy. *Gastroenterol Endosc* 1984; **26**: 833–9.

44. Inoue H & Endo M. Endoscopic esophageal mucosal resection using a transparent tube. *Surg Endosc* 1990; **4**: 198–201.

45. Kawano T, Inoue H, Izumi Y *et al.* Indications and techniques of endoscopic surgery for esophageal diseases. *J Jpn Bronchoesophagol Soc* 1996; **47**: 155–9.

46. Nakayama K. Yanagisawa F, Nabeya K *et al.* Concentrated preoperative irradiation therapy. *Arch Surg* 1963; **87**: 1003–18.

47. Launois B, Delarue D, Compion JP *et al.* Preoperative radiotherapy for carcinoma of the esophagus. *Surg Gynecol Obstet* 1981; **153**: 690–2.

48. Iizuka T, Ide H, Kakegawa T *et al.* Preoperative radioactive therapy for esophageal carcinoma, randomized evaluation trial in eight institutions. *Chest* 1988; **93**: 1054–8.

49. Japanese Esophageal Oncology Group. A comparison of chemotherapy and radiotherapy as adjuvant treatment to surgery for esophageal carcinoma. *Chest* 1993; **104**: 203–7.

50. Udagawa H. Tsurumaru M, Akiyama H *et al.* Evaluation of adjuvant therapy for esophagectomy with collo-thoraco-abdominal lymph node dissection. In: Nabeya K, Hanaoka T, Nogami H (eds) *Recent Advances in Diseases of the Esophagus.* Tokyo: Springer-Verlag 1993: 884–90.

51. Kelsen PK & Ilson DH. Chemotherapy and combined-modality therapy for esophageal cancer. *Chest* 1995; **107**: 224s–232s.

52. Fink U, Stein HJ, Wilke H *et al.* Multimodal treatment for squamous cell esophageal cancer. *World J Surg* 1995; **19**: 198–204.

53. Ando N, Ozawa S, Miki H *et al.* Neoadjuvant chemotherapy and chemoradiotherapy in the treatment of esophageal cancer. *Jpn J Cancer Chemother* 1995; **22**: 1878–85.

54. Lackey VL, Reagan MT, Smith RA *et al.* Neoadjuvant therapy of squamous cell carcinoma of the esophagus: role of resection and benefit in partial responders. *Ann Thorac Surg* 1989; **48**: 218–21.

55. Gill PG, Denham JW, Jamieson GG *et al.* Patterns of treatment failure and prognostic factors associated with the treatment of esophageal carcinoma with chemotherapy and radiotherapy either as sole treatment or followed by surgery. *J Clin Oncol* 1992; **10**: 1037–43.

56. Minamiide J, Koizumi H, Ozawa Y *et al.* Case report of an advanced esophageal carcinoma treated by neoadjuvant chemotherapy (CDDP+5-FU) and evaluation of effect on metastatic lymph nodes. *Jpn J Cancer Chemother* 1993; **20**: 1849–53.

57. Schlag PM. Randomised trial of preoperative chemotherapy for squamous cell cancer of the esophagus. The Chirurgische Arbeitsgemeinschaft Fuer Onkologie der Deutschen Gesellschaft Fuer Chirurgie Study Group. *Arch Surg* 1992; **127**: 1446–50.

58. Le Prise E, Etienne PL, Meunier B *et al.* A randomized study of chemotherapy, radiation therapy, and surgery versus surgery for localized squamous cell carcinoma of the esophagus. *Cancer* 1994; **73**: 1779–84.

59. Roth JA, Pass HI, Flanagan MM *et al.* Randomized clinical trial of preoperative and postoperative adjuvant chemotherapy with cisplatin, vindesine, and bleomycin for carcinoma of the esophagus. *J Thorac Cardiovasc Surg* 1988; **96**: 242–8.

60. Okuma T, Yoshioka M, Isechi S *et al.* Preoperative chemotherapy for esophageal cancer based on chemosensitivity testing. *J Thorac Cardiovasc Surg* 1994; **108**: 823–9.

61. Nakashio T, Akiyama S, Kasai Y *et al.* Effects of carcinostatic agents in the hematogeneous metastasis of cancer. *Jpn J Cancer Chemother* 1997; **24**: 591–6.

62. Sannohe Y. Cervical lymph nodes metastases in carcinoma of the esophagus. *Jpn J Gastroenterol Surg* 1981; **14**: 1016–22.

63. Tsurumaru M, Udagawa H, Ono Y *et al.* Surgical treatment of intrathoracic esophageal carcinoma: analysis of 481 cases of resected squamous cell carcinoma. In: Nabeya K, Hanaoka T, Nogami H (eds) *Recent Advances in Diseases of the Esophagus.* Tokyo: Springer-Verlag 1993: 697–702.

64. Isono K, Sato H & Nakayama K. Results of a nationwide study on the three-field lymph node dissection of esophageal cancer. *Oncology* 1991; **48**: 411–20.

65. Peracchia A, Ruol A, Bardini R *et al.* Lymph node dissection for cancer of the thoracic esophagus: how extended should it be? Analysis of personal data and review of the literature. *Dis Esoph* 1992; **5**: 69.

66. Law SYK, Fok M & Wong J. Cervical lymphadenectomy is of limited value in resection of oesophageal carcinoma. Implications from study of recurrence patterns. In: Peracchia A, Bonavina L, Fumagalli U *et al.* (eds) *Recent Advances in Diseases of the Esophagus.* Bologna: Monduzzi Editore S.p.A 1996: 307–313.

67. Lerut T, Deleyn P, Coosemans W *et al.* Surgical strategies in esophageal carcinoma with emphasis on radical lymphadenectomy. *Ann Surg* 1992; **216**: 583–590.

68. Altorki NK. Extended resections in the management of esophageal carcinoma. *Curr Opin Gen Surg* 1994; 113–16.

69. Kato H, Tachimori Y, Watanabe H *et al.* Lymph node metastasis in thoracic esophageal carcinoma. *J Surg Oncol* 1991; **48**: 106–11.

70. Skinner DB, Ferguson MK, Soriano A *et al.* Selection of operation for esophageal cancer based on staging. *Ann Surg* 1986; **204**: 391–401.

71. Ellis FH, Jr, Watkins E, Jr, Krasna MJ, Heatly GJ & Balogh K. Staging of carcinoma of the esophagus and cardia: a comparison of different staging criteria. *J Surg Oncol* 1993; **52**: 231–5.

72. Haagensen CD. *The Lymphatics in Cancer.* Philadelpha: Saunders 1972: 60–84.

73. Akiyama H. For the debate on the significance of lymphadenectomy in esophageal cancer. In: Nabeya K, Hanaoka T, Nogami H (eds) *Recent Advances in Diseases of the Esophagus.* Tokyo: Springer-Verlag, 1993: 600–5.

74. Fujita H, Kakegawa T, Yamana H *et al.* Mortality and morbidity rates, postoperative course, quality of life, and prognosis after extended radical lymphadenectomy for esophageal cancer. Comparison of three-field lymphadenectomy with two-field lymphadenectomy. *Ann Surg* 1995; **222**: 654–62.

75. Kajiyama Y, Tsurumaru M, Ono Y *et al.* Clinical effect of cardiac branch of the right vagal nerve on the postoperative condition after the resection of esophageal cancer with 3-regional lymph node dissection. *Jpn J Gastroenterol Surg* 1992; **25**: 2446.

76. Kusano C, Baba M, Yoshinaka H *et al.* Significance of preservation of tracheal proper sheath at the time of cervical and upper mediastinal lymph node dissection for thoracic esophageal cancer. *J Jpn Surg Soc* 1994; **95**: 154–61.

77. Takahashi K, Juji T, Miyamoto M *et al.* Analysis of risk factors for posttransfusion graft-versus-host disease in Japan. *Lancet* 1994; **343**: 700–2.

78. Tartter PI, Burrow L, Kirschner P *et al.* Perioperative blood transfusion adversely affects prognosis after resection of Stage I (sub-set N0) non-oat cell lung cancer. *J Thorac Cardiovasc Surg* 1984; **88**: 659–62.

79. Foster RS, Costanza MC, Foster JC *et al.* Adverse relationship between blood transfusions and survival after colectomy for colon cancer. *Cancer* 1985; **55**: 1195–201.

80. Creasy T, Veitch P, Bell PRF *et al.* A relationship between perioperative blood transfusion and recurrence of carcinoma of the sigmoid colon following potentially curative surgery. *Ann R Col Surg Engl* 1987; **69**: 100–3.

81. Kinoshita Y, Tsurumaru M, Udagawa H *et al.* Autologous blood transfusion for resection of esophageal carcinoma. *Jpn J Gastroenterol Surg* 1996; **29**: 2227–32.

82. Kipfmuller K, Naruhn M, Melzer A *et al.* Endoscopic microsurgical dissection of the esophagus. Results in an animal model. *Surg Endosc* 1989; **3**: 63–9.

83. Gossot D, Ghnassia MD, Debiolles H *et al.* Thoracoscopic dissection of the esophagus: an experimental study. *Surg Endosc* 1992; **6**: 59–61.

84. Cuschieri A. Endoscopic subtotal oesophagectomy for cancer using the right thoracoscopic approach. *Surg Oncol* 1993; **2**: 3–11.

85. Peracchia A, Ancona E, Ruol A *et al.* Use of mini-invasive procedures in esophageal surgery. *Chirurgie* 1992; **118**: 305–9.

86. Bardini R, Segalin A, Ruol A *et al.* Video-thoracoscopic enucleation of esophageal leiomyoma. *Ann Thorac Surg* 1992; **54**: 576–7.

87. Pinotti HW, Domene CE, Nasi A *et al.* Management of megaesophagus by video-laparoscopy. (Technical Standardization) *Arq Bras Cir Dig* 1994; **9**: 17–19.

88. Akashi T, Kaneda I, Higuchi N *et al.* Thoracoscopic en bloc total esophagectomy with radical mediastinal lymphadenectomy. *J Thorac Cardiovasc Surg* 1996; **112**: 1533–40.

89. Peracchia A, Rosati R, Fumagalli U *et al.* Thoracoscopic esophagectomy: are there benefits? Personal experience and review of literature. *Semin Surg Oncol* 1997; **13**: 259–62.

90. Dexter SP, Martin IG & McMahon MJ. Radical thoracoscopic esophagectomy for cancer. *Surg Endosc* 1996; **10**: 147–51.

91. Robertson GS, Lloyd DM, Wicks AC *et al.* No obvious advantages for thoracoscopic two-stage oesophagectomy. *Br J Surg* 1996; **83**: 675–8.

92. Gossot D, Cattan P, Fritsch S *et al.* Can the morbidity of esophagectomy be reduced by the thoracoscopic approach? *Surg Endosc* 1995; **9**: 1113–15.

93. Ito H & Tahara E. Oncogene and patient prognosis. *Jpn J Cancer Chemother* 1991; **18**: 1075–83.

94. Shimada Y & Imamura M. Prognostic factors for esophageal cancer – from the viewpoint of molecular biology. *Jpn J Cancer Chemother* 1996; **23**: 972–81.

95. Bergh J, Norberg T, Sjogren S *et al.* Complete sequencing of the p53 gene provides prognostic information in breast cancer patients, particularly in relation to adjuvant systemic therapy and radiotherapy. *Nature Med* 1995; **1**: 1029–34.

96. Nakamura T, Ide H, Eguchi K *et al.* Expression of bcl-2 protein and metallothionein predicts resistance of esophageal squamous cell carcinoma to chemotherapy. In: Peracchia A, Bonavina L, Fumagalli U *et al.* (eds) *Recent Advances in Diseases of the Esophagus*. Bologna: Monduzzi Editore S.p.A., 1996: 437–42.

97. Ozawa S, Ueda M, Hirota N *et al.* New strategy of treatment for esophageal squamous cell carcinoma using immunotoxin which reacts to epidermal growth factor receptor. In: Nabeya K, Hanaoka T, Nogami H (eds) *Recent Advances in Diseases of the Esophagus*. Tokyo: Springer-Verlag, 1993: 417–20.

98. Roth JA. Molecular surgery for cancer. *Arch Surg* 1992; **127**: 1298–302.

11
COMBINED MODALITY THERAPY: ESOPHAGEAL ADENOCARCINOMA

THOMAS P.J. HENNESSY

INTRODUCTION

The comprehensive review of the literature on the surgical treatment of carcinoma of the esophagus published by Earlam and Cunha-Melo[1] in 1980 called attention to the low resectability rate, the high perioperative mortality, and the poor long-term survival of patients undergoing treatment for cancer of the esophagus. A subsequent review of the literature for the succeeding decade by Müller et al.[2] demonstrated a decline in mortality and an improvement in resectability rate, but long-term survival remained essentially unchanged with only 18% of patients who underwent surgery surviving for 5 years. It is evident from Müller's review that developments in pre- and postoperative care had greatly improved resectability rates and significantly lowered perioperative mortality. Surgical morbidity had also improved because of increasing experience, even though the actual techniques had changed very little. Although some surgeons had adopted McKeown's three-phase esophagectomy, most series employed the Lewis–Tanner approach for mid-thoracic tumors and a left-sided thoraco-abdominal approach for tumors of the cardia and lower esophagus.

The extent of the lymph node dissection was very variable. One-third of surgeons carried out a detailed abdominal lymphadenectomy and about 50% of authors resected the intrathoracic nodes. However, the extent of the mediastinal node dis-

section is not clear, and it is probable that in most cases dissection of lymph glands did not proceed proximal to the carina. Few surgeons performed a cervical lymph node dissection, and fewer than 25% of surgeons employed adjuvant therapy. While most reports on esophageal cancer now make a clear distinction between squamous cell carcinoma and adenocarcinoma and report them separately, the distinction was often blurred in the earlier literature, including some of the papers included in Earlam and Cunha-Melo's review.[1]

Most cancers of the esophagus are either squamous cell tumors or adenocarcinomas, and while both tumors have many clinical features in common, they differ completely in their etiology and, to some extent, in their prognosis. A few decades ago the majority of esophageal tumors were squamous, but adenocarcinomas are now seen with increasing frequency and their incidence is rising at an unprecedented rate (10% per annum) in most Western countries.

Adenocarcinomas of the lower esophagus and cardia are a group of tumors of which three types are clearly identified: (i) tumors having their origin in the ectopic epithelium of Barrett's esophagus; (ii) tumors arising from the epithelium of the gastric cardia; and (iii) carcinomas of the upper end of the stomach involving the fundus and proximal third and invading the lower esophagus. These latter are a separate entity and are essentially gastric cancers. Most adenocarcinomas of the lower esophagus arise from dysplastic Barrett's epithelium, but all have a common clinical presentation although the prognosis and management are somewhat different for the gastric cancers.

Adenocarcinoma of the cardia has had a consistently poor prognosis. Webb and Busuttil[3] were of the opinion that these tumors possessed an intrinsic biologic aggressiveness which, in combination with their extensive lymphatic drainage above and below the diaphragm, made long-term survival an unlikely prospect. They noted that 79% of patients operated on for tumors of the gastroesophageal junction were dead within 2 years. Giuli and Lortat-Jacob,[4] in reviewing the late results of surgery for carcinoma of the esophagus and cardia, observed that no patient with adenocarcinoma had survived 5 years.[2] A bad prognosis is also reported by Skinner[5] and Griffith and Davies.[6] In an extensive review of their experience with tumors of the esophagus and cardia over a 25-year period, Lund et al.[7] found that the outlook for patients with adenocarcinoma of the upper two-thirds of the esophagus, the lower third and adenocarcinoma of the cardia were different. While the latter had a 5-year survival rate of 9%, the 5-year survival rate for adenocarcinoma of the lower third of the esophagus was only 2%, and no patient with adenocarcinoma of the upper two-thirds of the esophagus survived 5 years. Despite the different prognosis, the degree of histologic differentiation, lymph node involvement and tumor stage did not differ between the three groups. In our own experience, the 5-year survival rate of patients with adenocarcinoma, in general, has fallen from a level of 18% reported in 1987[8] to 8% in 1995.[9] This dramatic fall reflects the increased incidence of stage 3 and 4 tumors also noted by Lund et al.[7] Our 5-year survival rate for adenocarcinomas where an associated Barrett's epithelium could be identified was 13%.[10]

Despite the poor long-term prognosis, the immediate outcome following resection for adenocarcinoma is good. Ellis and Maggs[11] reported a 1.7% mortality rate for resection of tumors of the gastroesophageal junction, and McKeown[12] reported a mortality rate of 5.6%. Although our current mortality rate is 6%, low mortality rates are not consistently reported and mortality rates ranging as high as 20% have been noted.[13] There is a correlation between mortality rate and resectability rate and the incidence of advanced stage tumors.

The rising incidence of adenocarcinoma of the esophagus and cardia has been confirmed by numerous clinical and epidemiologic studies. Blot et al.[14] have shown that during the period 1976–1987 in the United States, while the incidence of squamous cell carcinoma remained stable there was an increase of more than 100% in the incidence of adenocarcinoma in men. The rising incidence is apparent in all age groups. Adenocarcinoma of the esophagus and cardia is a disease of white males which accounts for 34% of all esophageal tumors in that group. By contrast, only 3% of esophageal tumors in black males are adenocarcinomas. Similar upward trends in the incidence of adenocarcinoma of the esophagus and cardia have been noted in Europe.[15]

Although no clearly identifiable cause of the increased incidence of this tumor has emerged, the increasing incidence of gastroesophageal reflux disease (GERD) and the subsequent development of Barrett's esophagus has been implicated by clinicians. Barrett's esophagus is a premalignant condition known to be associated with adenocarcinoma of the cardia and lower esophagus. The condition is more common in men than in women, and is found more in white than in black populations. However, the percentage of adenocarcinomas arising from the metaplastic epithelium of Barrett's esophagus is not known. In our own series of patients, carcinomas arising in Barrett's epithelium accounted for 23.7% of all adenocarcinomas of the esophagus resected during the period 1971–1990.[10] However, this depends on identifying Barrett's esophagus on the periphery of the tumor, and the aberrant epithelium may be entirely replaced by tumor. A Canadian study[16] found an increased prevalence of duodenal ulcer and hiatal hernia in patients with adenocarcinoma of the esophagus and cardia when compared with other stomach cancers. Since Barrett's esophagus is an acquired condition associated with GERD, this provides a further link in the etiologic chain. Although there is no evidence that alcohol consumption or the use of tobacco plays any part in the etiology of adenocarcinoma, abuse of these substances cannot be positively excluded from the etiology.

The occurrence of dysplastic change in Barrett's metaplastic epithelium is of ominous significance. Low-grade dysplasia is associated with inflammation and is probably reversible with suppression of the inflammatory process. High-grade dysplasia is associated with irreversible genetic damage. High-grade dysplasia which is really indistinguishable from carcinoma in-situ is an indication that frank invasive carcinoma is either imminent, or already present. Severe dysplasia is, therefore, considered to be an indication for surgical resection. The prevention of dysplastic progression would obviously provide valuable prophylaxis and early surgical intervention or intensive medical treatment with omeprazole might go some way towards achieving that goal. The induction of regression in the metaplastic epithelium would be more effective as a prophylactic measure, but there is no convincing evidence that either anti-reflux surgery or medical treatment has ever achieved significant regression.

The experiments of Gillen[17] in our laboratory demonstrated that a metaplastic change in columnar epithelium could be induced in a canine reflux model, and that this columnar epithelium developed from the esophageal glands. Subsequent studies by Li et al.[18] showed that if this metaplastic epithelium was ablated and the reflux suppressed, the totipotent cells of the esophageal gland ducts progressed to a squamous epithelial lining. Such ablation of metaplastic epithelium and restoration of normal squamous lining has proved successful in clinical practice using either lazer or heat probe, and may prove valuable as prophylaxis against the development of high-grade dysplasia and adenocarcinoma of the lower esophagus and cardia.

SURGICAL RESECTION

The conventional approach to tumors around the gastroesophageal junction has been through a left thoracoabdominal incision with resection of the eighth rib. It includes radial division of the left hemidiaphragm, and division of the costal margin and the left rectus muscle. This approach provides excellent access but may give rise to postoperative problems such as herniation of abdominal contents through the repaired diaphragm and necrosis of the costal cartilage. For these reasons, many surgeons preserve both costal margin and diaphragm. The abdominal and thoracic dissections can be carried out without difficulty on either side of the intact diaphragm. Preservation of the diaphragm provides better postoperative pulmonary function.[19] An alternative is to carry out the abdominal dissection through a midline epigastric incision with a separate left thoracotomy for the thoracic dissec-

tion. If the tumor is wholly within the lower esophagus, the Lewis–Tanner approach may facilitate a more adequate proximal clearance.

McKeown[12] recommended that tumors in the supradiaphragmatic portion of the esophagus should have en bloc resection of the lower esophagus, spleen, and distal pancreas with the body of the stomach to the level of the antrum and the associated lymphatic fields which would include lymph glands around the celiac axis, hepatic artery, and left gastric artery. Paracardial glands are also dissected. For tumors involving the infradiaphragmatic portion of the esophagus, McKeown[12] recommended that a similar dissection should be carried out including total gastrectomy. Our view is that if the tumor extends beyond the cardia to the lesser curvature, a total gastrectomy is necessary.

The failure of conventional surgical techniques to achieve long-term survival can be attributed to a number of factors, the most important of which is late presentation. Shao et al.[20] have demonstrated the excellent outcome which can be anticipated with early-stage tumors and comparable results for early tumors are found in the literature generally. However, the incidence of early-stage tumors is depressingly low, particularly in Western countries. In our own experience, < 5% of patients present with a stage 1 tumor. While it is impractical to establish screening programs in countries with an incidence of esophageal carcinoma of 7 per 100 000, some effort towards earlier diagnosis has been made by increasing public awareness of symptoms and by setting up immediate-access endoscopy units. It is unlikely, however, that these measures will greatly affect the problem of late presentation.

Long-term survival is also significantly affected by the failure of conventional surgery to control locoregional disease in carcinoma of the esophagus. In a review of 2400 patients, Giuli and Gignoux[21] demonstrated that 50% of early deaths after surgery were due to mediastinal or anastomotic recurrence rather than to distant metastases. Residual tumor may be the result of extension of the tumor laterally through the full thickness of the esophageal wall, extensive involvement of local regional nodes, and extensive microscopic mucosal and submucosal spread beyond the visible and palpable margins of the tumor. Skinner[22] has indicated that the two most important prognostic factors in esophageal carcinoma are wall penetration and lymph node involvement. When wall penetration is incomplete and lymph nodes are not involved, the 5-year survival rate is 55%, but if the tumor has breached the wall and more than five nodes are involved, then 5-year survival rate is reduced to < 12%.

Involvement of resection margins with microscopic tumor extension has been a persistent problem. With conventional resection techniques which generally provide a 5-cm vertical clearance, marginal involvement in squamous cancers has been as much as 20%. Proximal mucosal and submucosal spread regularly extends for a distance of 3 cm and has been recorded as having spread a distance of 9 cm in 11% of cases in a study by Miller.[23] Distal spread is less extensive and rarely exceeds 5 cm. In Watson's[24] view, a proximal clearance of 10 cm and a distal clearance of 5 cm will avoid involved margins in 97% of cases. However, adenocarcinoma extending below the diaphragm and involving the lesser curvature is an exception to this and warrants total gastrectomy. Skinner advises 10 cm proximal and distal clearance in en bloc resection.

Surgical techniques involving more extensive resection have contributed to the improved control of locoregional disease. McKeown's three-phase resection provides a 10-cm proximal margin in the majority of patients, and using this technique in a modified form[25] we have reduced proximal margin involvement from 19% to 7%. The advantages of the modified technique are that the operating time is shortened considerably, and the problem of extracting a bulky tumor through the thoracic inlet is avoided. In addition, if the tumor has been understaged preoperatively and is inoperable, this becomes apparent at an early stage of the operation. The operation is begun via a right thoracotomy and the thoracic esophagus is fully mobilized and the mediastinal lymph nodes dissected. The patient is then placed in the supine position and the cervical and abdominal dissections are carried out simultaneously by two surgeons. The cervical esophagus is divided above the thoracic inlet, a length of Penrose drain is attached to the distal cut end, and the thoracic esophagus can then be withdrawn from the mediastinum into the abdominal cavity. After resection of the esophagus and cardia, the stomach is reconstructed as a tube, attached to the Penrose drain, and then drawn up through the mediastinum into

the neck. Anastomosis is then carried out between posterior gastric fundus and cervical esophagus. The normal cervical incision is along the anterior border of the left sternomastoid. If bilateral cervical adenectomy is to be carried out, a U-shaped incision from one border of sternomastoid to the other is the most appropriate.

Skinner's en bloc resection provides 10 cm proximal and distal margins and wide lateral clearance of tumor. Lateral clearance involves resection of a block of tissue which includes the thoracic esophagus with both pleural surfaces, the azygos vein, the thoracic duct, the posterior pericardium, and all adjacent lymphatic and fibro-fatty tissue. A significant advantage of this operation is that local or mediastinal recurrence is reduced to 5%. Long-term survival, however, is dependent on staging. With incomplete wall involvement and negative lymph nodes, the 5-year survival rate was > 50%, but when the esophageal wall was penetrated and more than five lymph nodes were involved, this figure was reduced to < 12%. A further point to note is that although local recurrence in the chest was rare, recurrence in the cervical nodes was found to be 20% in a small series of adenocarcinomas arising in Barrett's esophagus.[26]

LYMPH NODE DISSECTION

Lymph flow in the thoracic cavity is preferentially longitudinal rather than circumferential.[27] The pattern of drainage from the middle and upper esophagus is mainly to the upper mediastinal and cervical glands, while the lower esophagus tends to drain to the abdominal lymph nodes. While such a drainage pattern is regularly seen with tumors of the esophagus, the location of the primary tumor does not always determine the distribution of the involved lymph nodes, and Akiyama[28] has reported widespread involvement of superior mediastinal and celiac glands irrespective of primary tumor site. Fekete et al.[29] noted a progressive involvement of nodes in 52% of patients with proximal nodes first becoming involved followed by more distal nodes. In the remaining 48%, the node distribution was much more unpredictable, with N2 and N3 node involvement occurring in the absence of N1 spread. A further anomaly is the small but regular number of stage 2B patients in whom nodes are involved, although wall penetration is incomplete. While both three-stage esophagectomy and en bloc resection of the eso-phagus were mainly designed for squamous cell lesions, they are also used for adenocarcinomas in the middle and lower esophagus.

Cervical node involvement has been noted in 27% of patients in the large nationwide study car-ried out in Japan.[30] Both this study and the report by Tsurumaru et al.[31] found a correlation between the frequency of cervical node involvement and the position of the primary tumor, with upper esopha-geal tumors yielding almost twice as many patients with distal esophageal involvement. Nevertheless, even in these latter patients the incidence of posi-tive cervical nodes remained around 20%.

A detailed consideration of the advantages and disadvantages of three-field dissection is provided in Chapter 10. For our purposes it is sufficient to note that a number of reports[30–33] have documen-ted a long-term survival advantage following eso-phageal resection with three-field node dissection. Only one study was conducted as a prospective controlled trial, and there were some queries about the validity of the randomization in that par-ticular study. There is also a diversity of view on whether survival advantage is maintained if cervi-cal nodes are involved. One study suggests that survival advantage is confined to patients with negative cervical nodes; another study claims that advantage occurs only with positive cervical nodes; a third reports an advantage for all patients.[30,33,34] Conventional mediastinal node dissection tends to be confined to the area below the carina, and few studies have been made on the outcome of conven-tional abdominal lymphadenectomy plus complete mediastinal lymphadenectomy including the superior mediastinum. Ide et al.[35] have reported a 60% actuarial survival for this limited lymph node dissection when preoperative studies have excluded the presence of involved cervical lymph nodes. Such an incomplete lymph node dissection would be less demanding on both patient and sur-geon, but would not eliminate the risk of recurrent laryngeal nerve injury as these nerves would be at risk on the left side in the paratracheal dissection proximal to the arch of the aorta and the right side in relation to the right subclavian artery at the apex of the pleural cavity.

It should be noted that the Japanese data on lymph node involvement relate to squamous cell carcinoma. However, as already mentioned, Skinner's group reported 20% cervical node recur-rence after en bloc resection of adenocarcinoma arising in Barrett's esophagus. Isono's extensive study suggested that 27% of patients with tumors around the cardia may have cervical lymph node metastases.[30] Three-field lymph node dissection may, therefore, be a reasonable option for patients with adenocarcinoma of the lower esophagus and cardia, but may be less relevant for tumors of the upper stomach.

It is evident from the poor prognosis and the high incidence of local recurrence that conven-tional surgery not only does not cure the patient but also does not control locoregional disease. The distribution of lymph node metastases outlined above illustrated the need for more extensive lym-phadenectomy, and the results obtained with this technique suggest that total thoracic esophagect-omy and three-field lymph node dissection may improve the prospect of long-term survival in patients with carcinoma of the cardia and lower esophagus as well as those with carcinoma of the body of the esophagus.

Despite the remarkably low mortality rate reported from the Japanese multicenter study[30] and the experience of Peracchia et al.,[36] whose mortality rate was also low, there is an alternative view that because of the older age range and higher incidence of concurrent disease – particularly pul-monary pathology – an operation of such duration and magnitude would not be well tolerated by Western patients.

It is evident from the data presented above that a great deal can be done to increase the scope of surgical resection and to reduce the incidence of locoregional recurrence. However, the problem of systemic spread remains and, as Orringer has pointed out, this may occur at a relatively early stage of the disease. This raises the question of the role of adjuvant therapy in the treatment of carcinoma of the esophagus.

MULTIMODALITY THERAPY

Radiotherapy is seldom used alone nowadays, and when patients with curable cancer of the esopha-gus were treated with radiotherapy alone, the 2-year survival rate was only 10%. By contrast, when chemotherapy was added to the irradiation, the 2-year survival rate rose to 38%.[37] Neither pre-operative or postoperative radiotherapy offers any survival advantage over surgery alone. Single drug or multi-drug chemotherapy rarely induces a complete pathologic response, and does not improve survival.

Multimodality therapy is predicated on the hypothesis that the radiosensitizing capacity of the chemotherapeutic drugs will enhance the local effects of radiotherapy when given concurrently, and the cytotoxic properties of the chemotherapy will also exert a systemic effect. Such therapy given as neoadjuvant therapy before surgery may reduce the incidence of micrometastases, control systemic disease, and increase resectability. Despite suggestions to the contrary, surgical resection is necessary even when a complete pathologic response appears to have occurred, as resection is the only satisfactory method of ensuring that residual tumor is not present. If residual tumor is present, the need for surgery is obvious. In our own experience, 75% of patients with adenocarcinoma would have been left with residual tumor if neoadjuvant therapy had not been followed by surgery.[38]

Multimodality regimens incorporating 5-fluorouracil (5-FU) and radiotherapy have been used effectively in patients with both squamous cell carcinoma and adenocarcinoma of the esophagus and have been shown to be successful when compared with historic controls. To date, there have been few prospective randomized controlled trials, but such trial reports are now emerging and will provide more information on the results which can be anticipated from multimodality treatment. Multimodality therapy is inevitably associated with toxic side effects to a greater or lesser degree, though this depends on the choice of chemotherapeutic agents and also on the dose of radiotherapy. The inclusion of extended rather than conventional surgery may impose an additional burden on the patient. Nevertheless, this is something which should be considered in view of the incidence of cervical lymph node recurrence in spite of apparently adequate abdominal and mediastinal lymphadenectomy. The addition of hyperthermia to radiochemotherapy has been shown to enhance the cytotoxic effect of therapy and to improve survival rate when combined with resection.[39] However, this is still a controversial matter, and needs further validation. Conventional combined therapy usually lasts about 6 weeks with a further 2-week interval before surgery. Initial reaction to therapy may cause significant dysphagia, and this may require at least one (if not more)

dilatations. It is also important to ensure that adequate nutrition is maintained during neoadjuvant therapy. In most cases this can be achieved by judicious supervision of oral diet, but in more difficult circumstances tube feeding or parenteral nutrition may be necessary. Feeding by jejunostomy is usually reserved for the postoperative period.

COMBINED THERAPY

Neoadjuvant therapy combining chemotherapy and radiation was employed initially to improve the results of surgical resection for squamous cell carcinoma of the esophagus. The regimen chosen by Leichman et al.[40] was a combination of 5-FU and cisplatin with external beam radiation. Cisplatin was selected in preference to mitomycin C which had previously been used, because of its activity as a single agent against esophageal carcinoma. Cisplatin also has the advantage of having less bone marrow toxicity, thus enabling higher doses to be used. Both 5-FU and cisplatin possess radiosensitizing properties. In Leichman's pilot study, a complete response was obtained in five of 15 patients, and this coincided with an improved median survival for these patients.

The response of adenocarcinoma to radiation historically was unclear, as few patients were treated by radiation alone. However, reports by Danoff et al.[41] and Smithers[42] indicated that adenocarcinomas were responsive to irradiation.

The inclusion of some patients with adenocarcinoma in reports of combined treatment of esophageal cancer with chemotherapy and radiation provided anecdotal evidence of response in adenocarcinoma to a protocol that included 5-FU and radiotherapy.[43,44] A subsequent report by Coia et al.[45] indicated a high percentage of complete responders in adenocarcinoma to a regimen of 5-FU and mitomycin C with 60 Gy radiotherapy. Good palliation was also achieved in patients with disseminated disease.

In a retrospective study of adenocarcinoma of the esophagus and esophagogastric junction, Whittington et al.[46] found that chemotherapy and radiotherapy used as single-treatment modalities had a recurrence rate of 100%. Surgery and postoperative radiotherapy reduced local recurrence to 24%, while chemosensitized radiation alone reduced local recurrence to 48%. A combination of chemotherapy and radiation added to surgery reduced the local recurrence rate to 15%. Similarly chemotherapy, radiation, and surgery had the longest median survival of 21 months, whereas median survival for surgery alone was 15 months, for chemosensitized radiation alone it was 10 months, and for radiation alone it was 5 months.

Gill et al.[47] treated 29 patients with adenocarcinoma of the cardia with a regimen of 5-FU, cisplatin, and radiotherapy and observed complete regression of the tumor endoscopically in 19 patients. In 14 patients, the chemoradiotherapy was followed by resection and in six patients no microscopic tumor was found in the resected specimen. However, tumor cells persisted in the remaining eight, indicating the need to include surgery in any combined therapy regimen.

A study by Urba et al.[48] employing chemoradiotherapy and transhiatal resection in 24 patients with adenocarcinoma failed to show any improvement in survival when compared with historic controls. The chemotherapy regimen consisted of 5-FU infusion only, administered concurrently with radiotherapy. The total radiation dosage was 49 Gy, and toxicity was reflected in marked pleural and pericardial effusions.

Hoff et al.[49] treated 68 patients with adenocarcinoma ($n = 39$) and squamous cell carcinoma ($n = 29$) with a complex protocol of two cycles of cisplatin, 5-FU, etoposide, and leucovorin with 30 Gy of radiation followed by resection. Twelve patients did not proceed to operation because of death during chemotherapy ($n = 4$) or deterioration in clinical status ($n = 7$). One patient was awaiting resection at the time of the report. A complete histologic response was noted in 19% of adenocarcinomas and 25% of squamous cell carcinomas. Although an improved median and actuarial survival could be demonstrated when compared with historic controls, it is of interest that survival advantage did not correlate with complete response to preoperative treatment. However, the numbers of complete responders were relatively small and this may have affected the findings.

A regimen of cisplatin, 5-FU, and leucovorin with and without etoposide plus concomitant irradiation with 30 Gy also showed an improved median survival rate when compared with historic controls. Toxicity was minimal.[50]

The findings from these last three studies would seem to suggest that a combination of chemotherapeutic agents is more effective than a single agent, even if the latter is accompanied by a higher dose of radiation. Also, it seems evident that radiation doses in the region of 50 Gy are significantly toxic. Cisplatin and 5-FU appear to be the most effective drugs, although good results have also been obtained with the inclusion of doxorubicin and mitomycin C. The effect of 5-FU may be enhanced by leucovorin, and higher response rates have been obtained with adenocarcinoma of the stomach and colon with this combination than with 5-FU alone. Consensus has not been reached on the most appropriate dosage for 5-FU, though most regimens favor dosage in the region of 1000 mg/m^2/day. It is perhaps worth noting that in Urba's trial, which failed to show a survival improvement against historic controls, not only was 5-FU employed singly, but was also at the low dosage of 300 mg/m^2/day.

Despite the use of two courses of intensive preoperative chemotherapy and three conventional dose courses postoperatively, Ajani et al.[51] did not record a survival advantage in their 26 patients, the median survival duration being 12.5 months. The agents employed were etoposide, doxorubicin, and cisplatin. Hematologic toxicity was significant and was treated with granulocyte macrophage colony-stimulating factors (GM-CSF). Non-hematologic toxicity was also significant with this regimen. The lack of complete pathologic response, the short median survival duration, and a curative resection rate of < 70% despite repeated courses of allegedly effective chemotherapeutic agents all suggest that chemotherapy on its own has little impact on the status of adenocarcinoma, and a combination of chemotherapy and radiotherapy may be a more fruitful option.

Further evidence on the inadequacy of preoperative chemotherapy alone consisting of two courses of etoposide, doxorubicin, and cisplatin was offered by Adelstein et al.[52] A symptomatic improvement was noted in 77% of patients with endoscopic improvement evident in 69%. However, only two of the 13 patients (15%) showed reduction in T or N staging with endoscopic ultrasound. Clinical evidence of disease progression was observed in four patients during treatment. The overall survival at 31 months follow-up was 31%, and the authors rightly concluded that there was limited, if any, value in this regimen and its further study could not be recommended.

TOXICITY

Radiotherapy

Complications of radiotherapy include radiation myelitis which may give rise to paraplegia. This is a rare complication and modern techniques provide adequate protection for the spinal cord. Radiation pneumonitis and pulmonary fibrosis may also occur. The risk of injury to the lung can be substantially reduced by employing a three-field technique with oblique, rather than opposing, fields. Pleural effusion was recorded as a frequent late complication 3 to 14 months after treatment by Urba et al.[48] In our own experience, pleural effusion is a very common acute complication which usually appears in the postoperative period and is presumably due to the cumulative effects of irradiation, chemotherapy, and surgery.

Cardiotoxicity is a not uncommon sequel to neoadjuvant therapy, and may be due to radiation-induced pericarditis or toxicity from the chemotherapy regimen where either 5-FU or cisplatin may be implicated. Fatalities from cardiac tamponade following pericardial effusion have been recorded.[48]

Radiation esophagitis is a frequent complication and varies considerably in severity, the principal symptom being local pain which is exacerbated by eating. Symptoms may be severe enough to warrant temporary suspension of treatment. Treatment may involve the use of antibiotics and corticosteriods, and the maintenance of nutrition by the parenteral route.

Chemotherapy

Toxicity from chemotherapy includes respiratory, renal, and cardiac complications, gastrointestinal problems, leucopenia, and thrombocytopenia. Urba et al.[48] have suggested that the pulmonary toxicity induced by radiotherapy may be exacerbated by the use of 5-FU. Respiratory problems may be precipitated by other cytotoxic agents, and the pulmonary fibrosis following the use of bleomycin is well recognized. A significant degree of nephrotoxicity is a hazard when using cisplatin, but vigorous pre- and post-administration hydration reduces the risk to an acceptable level.

It is now generally agreed that 5-FU is more cardiotoxic than was previously appreciated.

Ensley et al.[53] described seven patients who developed cardiac complications while undergoing chemotherapy with 5-FU, the range of problems including dysrrhythmias, ischemic changes, and myocardial infarction. Sudden death may also occur. These authors also observed an increased frequency and greater prolongation of ischemic episodes on Holter monitoring in a group of patients receiving 5-FU when compared with reactions during administration of saline solution. There was also an increase in cardiac enzyme levels. In our own series of patients, angina was a not uncommon complaint which we attributed to administration of cisplatin, but it may well have been related to the course of 5-FU. In our own experience, one patient died of myocardial infarction after treatment, though of course it is not possible to establish a cause-and-effect relationship.

Nausea and vomiting are common during chemotherapy and these symptoms need vigorous treatment. Gastrointestinal symptoms are much more marked during the administration of cisplatin. Our practice has been to administer the serotonin antagonist ondansetron prophylactically both before and during treatment with cisplatin, and this has been very effective in controlling symptoms. Nausea and vomiting is experienced to a lesser extent in some patients during treatment with 5-FU, but the concurrent radiotherapy may in large part be accountable.

Myelosuppression is a major complication of chemotherapy, and severe neutropenia renders the patient susceptible to infection and may cause undesirable delays between the end of the neoadjuvant therapy and surgery. GM-CSF is a hematopoietic factor that has been shown to stimulate granulocytosis, and Ajani et al.[51] reported a beneficial response to the drug in a study involving preoperative chemotherapy. Intravenous administration of GM-CSF produced a variety of symptoms including fever, chills, weakness, and anorexia. Hypotension was also noted in some patients. However, these problems were eliminated by changing to subcutaneous injection. We have found GM-CSF valuable in treating chemotherapy-induced leucopenia, and have been able to reduce operative delay after chemotherapy to a minimum by using GM-CSF to restore the granulocyte count.

OUTCOME OF SURGERY

Over the past several decades surgical resection has offered the best prospect of eradicating early esophageal cancer and achieving permanent cure, and has probably provided the best palliation for advanced lesions. However, as already indicated, early presentation is rare and for most published series – including the meta-analyses of Earlam and Cunha-Melo,[1] and Müller et al.[2] – the 5-year survival rate has remained at around the 20% level and in many instances significantly below that.

The experience in our unit spans the period between 1971 and 1997, and figures are available for the 24-year period between October, 1971 and November, 1995. The data were collected retrospectively on 398 patients up to 1989, and subsequently compiled prospectively on 302 patients.[9] Data from November, 1995 have still to be analyzed in detail. When resections for pharyngeal or high esophageal carcinoma which require pharyngolaryngectomy are excluded, 600 resections are available for analysis.

Interim analysis of the outcome of resection in adenocarcinoma of the esophagus in our unit in 1987 demonstrated 5-year survival rate of 18%.[8] There were 108 resections for adenocarcinoma, and 104 squamous cell cancers.

The 5-year survival rate for resected squamous cell carcinomas at that time was 18.7%. Paradoxically, survival figures compiled in 1994 from a database of 362 resections carried out more than 5 years previously showed that the 5-year survival rate for adenocarcinoma had fallen to 8%, while that for squamous cell carcinoma had dropped to 10%. It is noteworthy that all 5-year survivors in the adenocarcinoma group had stage 1 tumors, and all but one of the 5-year survivors in the squamous cell carcinoma group had a stage 1 tumor also. In the data from 1994, node-negative tumors continued to have a survival advantage with both adenocarcinoma and squamous cell cancers, but there had been a significant fall in the percentage of tumors at the stage 1 level.

During the 24-year period under review, operability and resectability rates remained high at 84% resectability for adenocarcinoma and 94% for squamous cell carcinoma. Towards the end of the series the resectability rate was adjusted downwards after recording an unacceptably high mortality rate for patients over 80 years of age. However, there was a gratifying fall in the mortality rate over the study period with current mortality rates of 6% for adenocarcinoma and 10% for squamous cell carcinoma. The cause of death in 50% of cases was either a respiratory or cardiac complication. Some 85% of perioperative fatalities were directly due to failure of technique, viz. hemorrhage, chylothorax, anastomotic leak, etc.

The conclusions we drew from this retrospective analysis of 600 resections for carcinoma of the esophagus and cardia were:

- In keeping with experience in Europe and the USA, the incidence of adenocarcinoma had increased while that of squamous cell carcinoma had remained static.
- There had been a continuous fall in perioperative mortality rate for both adenocarcinoma and squamous cell carcinoma during the period of observation.
- The mortality rate could be reduced further by a more selective policy for resection with stricter criteria for old patients (80+ years) and those at risk from previous cardiac or respiratory complications.
- There had been no improvement, and probably a disimprovement, because of increased numbers of late-stage tumors in the incidence of long-term (5-year) survivors. This required a reappraisal of surgical techniques, with the possibility of more extensive surgery including three-field lymphadenectomy and also a consideration of the potential of multimodality therapy.

CLINICAL TRIAL OF MULTIMODALITY THERAPY

Because of the rapidly increasing numbers and the changes in tumor biology which gave rise to poorer differentiation and fewer stage 1 tumors leading to a diminished 5-year survival rate, our first priority was to devise a new protocol for the treatment of adenocarcinoma of the esophagus. The fall in perioperative mortality rate to 6% indicated that current surgical techniques were safe, and that the reduction in margin involvement indicated probable adequate clearance of the primary tumor. The benefits of three-field lymphadenectomy for adenocarcinoma remain unproven. We, therefore, felt that multimodality therapy might be the best opportunity for improved survival.

Since a number of trials had already demonstrated the effectiveness of 5-FU-based chemotherapy and radiotherapy for adenocarcinoma of the esophagus, we undertook to investigate the outcome of multimodality therapy in the context of a prospective randomized controlled clinical trial using this combination, with the addition of cisplatin. The trial was begun in May, 1990.[38] Patients in the multimodality arm received two courses of chemotherapy and a total of 40 Gy of radiotherapy. The latter was commenced on the same day as the first course of chemotherapy and was fractionated to 5 days per week for three weeks.

The chemotherapy consisted of 5-FU given as an infusion over 16 h on days 1–5 and days 36–40 in a daily dose of 15 mg/kg bodyweight. On days 6 and 41, patients were hydrated with 2 l of 0.9% NaCl. Cisplatin was infused over 8 h on days 7 and 42 in a daily dose of 75 mg/m^2 body surface.

Surgical resection was carried out 8 weeks from the beginning of treatment, provided that the leucocyte count was > 2500/mm^3, and the platelet count was > 100 000 mm^3 (**Figure 11.1**).

Patients in the control arm underwent surgical resection only. Surgical technique was not standardized, and location of the tumor was the deciding factor. Since the majority of tumors were located at the cardia or in the lower esophagus, the procedures most frequently employed were abdominal and left chest approach ($n = 32$) and the Lewis–Tanner approach ($n = 43$). Sixteen patients with tumors located in the mid third of the esophagus had a three-stage resection performed with anastomosis in the neck. There was no significant difference between the numbers of patients having a particular operative approach in either arm of the trial.

Neoadjuvant therapy was well tolerated and had no adverse effect on the subsequent surgery. There were no significant differences in postoperative complications between patients receiving preoperative treatment and those undergoing surgery only. There were two anastomotic leaks in each group. Twenty-eight multimodality and 32 surgery-only patients developed respiratory complications, while cardiac problems occurred in 14 multimodality patients and 13 surgery-only patients. One patient in each group developed chylothorax and one in each group sustained recurrent laryngeal nerve palsy. One surgery-only patient had a postoperative hemorrhage which required reoperation (**Table 11.1**).

Toxicity with this particular regimen was low, but nine patients had significant treatment-related toxicity. Six patients had grade III toxic reactions, three of which were gastrointestinal, two hematologic, and one cardiac. There were two grade IV reactions, one gastrointestinal, and one cardiac, and one patient had a fatal hemorrhage from the tumor bed which was probably treatment-related.

Three patients died during the perioperative period after multimodality treatment, and one patient died perioperatively in the surgery-only group, giving an overall mortality rate of 4%. There were three deaths in patients who did not complete the assigned protocol. One died preoperatively of hemorrhage from the tumor bed, one died postoperatively following early intervention because of complete dysphagia, and a further postoperative death occurred after emergency surgery following perforation of the esophagus with a dilator.

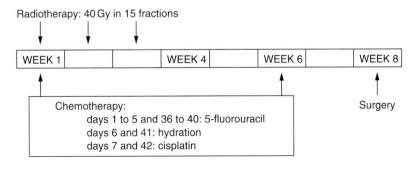

Figure 11.1 Multimodality therapy schedule.

Table 11.1   Postoperative complications

	MULTIMODALITY GROUP	SURGERY-ONLY GROUP
Respiratory	28	32
Cardiac	14	13
Anastomotic leak	2	2
Recurrent nerve paralysis	1	1
Chylothorax	1	1
Postoperative pancreatitis	1	–
Postoperative hemorrhage	1 (fatal)	1

There was a complete pathologic response to treatment in 25% ($n = 13$) of patients in the multimodality group. Lymph node metastases in the resected specimen were observed in only 42% of patients randomized to the multimodality arm, in contrast to 82% of patients in the group who had surgery only. Tumor progression was observed in two patients in the chemoradiation group.

Survival was evaluated as median survival and also as a percentage at 1, 2, and 3 years. Using the intention-to-treat principle, median survival was 16 months in the multimodality group versus 11 months in the surgery-only group ($P = 0.01$). Based on treatment actually received, the multimodality group had a median survival of 32 months versus 11 months for surgery-only ($P = 0.001$). At 3 years, survival on the basis of intention-to-treat was 32% in the multimodality group and 6% in the surgery-alone group. Based on treatment actually received, survival at 3 years was 37% in the multimodality group and 7% for surgery-only. Despite the limitations of this trial with regard to numbers and duration of follow-up, it provides significant evidence that multimodality therapy is superior to surgery alone in patients with resectable adenocarcinoma of the esophagus (**Figures 11.2 and 11.3**).

Optimal treatment for the future would appear to be a combination of neoadjuvant therapy (as outlined above) in combination with more extensive surgical resection involving at least 10 cm of proximal clearance and total gastrectomy when the upper stomach is involved in tumor. While

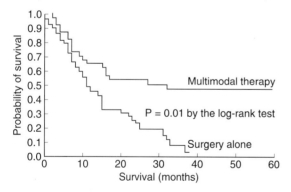

Figure 11.2 Kaplan–Meier plot of survival on patients with esophageal adenocarcinoma, according to the intention-to-treat analysis. Reproduced from: A comparison of multimodal therapy and surgery for esophageal adenocarcinoma. Walsh TN, Noonan N, Hollywood D, Kelly A, Keeling N, Hennessy TPJ. *N Engl J Med* 1996; **335**(7): 462–7. Copyright © 1996 Massachusetts Medical Society. All rights reserved.

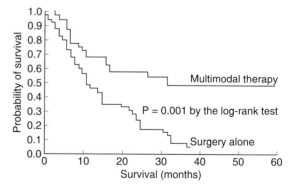

Figure 11.3 Kaplan–Meier plot of survival on patients with esophageal adenocarcinoma, according to the treatment actually received. Reproduced from: A comparison of multimodal therapy and surgery for esophageal adenocarcinoma. Walsh TN, Noonan N, Hollywood D, Kelly A, Keeling N, Hennessy TPJ. *N Engl J Med* 1996; **335**(7): 462–7. Copyright © 1996 Massachusetts Medical Society. All rights reserved.

three-field lymphadenectomy may not be indicated for adenocarcinoma, there is sufficient evidence of benefit to encourage more complete mediastinal and upper abdominal lymphadenectomy.

The ability to predict which patients would respond to chemoradiotherapy would be of enormous advantage in selecting patients for treatment. Patients categorized as non-responders could proceed directly to surgery, thus avoiding the toxicity and expense of neoadjuvant treatment, while responders could undergo the full multimodality protocol. Regrettably, no reliable method of prediction of response has yet emerged. Experience in our unit using immunohistochemical staining of pretreatment biopsies to determine the expression of epidermal growth factor receptor (EGFR) and proliferating cell nuclear antigen (PCNA) in patients with squamous cell carcinoma showed promise initially,[54] but further evaluation with larger numbers demonstrated that its predictive value was not sufficiently reliable. Further research in this area may reveal more reliable predictive markers.

REFERENCES

1. Earlam R & Cunha-Melo JR. Oesophageal squamous cell carcinoma: a critical review of surgery. *Br J Surg* 1980; **67**: 381–91.
2. Müller JM, Erasmi H, Stelznet M, Zieren U & Pichlmaier H. Surgical therapy of oesophageal carcinoma. *Br J Surg* 1990; **77**: 845–57.
3. Webb JN & Busuttil A. Adenocarcinoma of the oesophagus and of the oesophago-gastric junction. *Br J Surg* 1978; **65**: 475–9.
4. Giuli R & Lortat-Jacob JL. Long term results in surgical treatment of oesophageal carcinoma. In: Silber W (ed.) *Carcinoma of the Oesophagus*. Rotterdam, Capetown: Balkema, 1978: 390–412.
5. Skinner DB. Esophageal malignancies: experience with 110 cases. *Surg Clin North Am* 1976; **65**: 137–47.
6. Griffith JL & Davis JT. A twenty year experience with surgical management of carcinoma of the esophagus and gastric cardia. *J Thorac Cardiovasc Surg* 1980; **79**: 447–52.
7. Lund O, Hasenkam JM, Aagaard MT & Kimose HH. Time-related changes in characteristics of prosnostic significance in carcinomas of the oesophagus and cardia. *Br J Surg* 1989; **76**: 1301–7.
8. Hennessy TPJ & Keeling P. Adenocarcinoma of the esophagus and cardia. *J Thorac Cardiovasc Surg* 1987; **94**: 64–8.
9. Walsh TN. Surgery for oesophageal carcinoma. Studies on predicting and improving outcome. MD Thesis 1995.
10. Li H, Walsh TN & Hennessy TPJ. Carcinoma arising in Barrett's esophagus. *Surg Gynecol Obstet* 1992; **175**: 167–72.
11. Ellis FH, Jr & Maggs PR. Surgery for carcinoma of the lower oesophagus and cardia. *World J Surg* 1981; **5**: 527–33.
12. McKeown KC. Total three-stage oesophagectomy for cancer of the oesophagus. *Br J Surg* 1976; **63**: 259–62.
13. Van Andel JG, Dees J & Dijkhins CM. Carcinoma of the esophagus: results of treatment. *Ann Surg* 1979; **190**: 684–9.
14. Blot WJ, Devesa SS, Kneller RW & Fraumeni JF Jr. Rising incidence of adenocarcinoma of the esophagus and gastric cardia. *JAMA* 1991; **265**: 1287–9.
15. Husemann B. Cardia carcinoma considered as a distinct clinical entity. *Br J Surg* 1989; **76**: 136–9.
16. MacDonald WC & MacDonald JB. Adenocarcinoma of the esophagus and/or gastric cardia. *Cancer* 1987; **60**: 1094–8.
17. Gillen P & Hennessy TPJ. Barrett's oesophagus. In: Hennessy TPJ, Cuschieri A & Bennett JR (eds) *Reflux Oesophagitis*, Vol. 4, London, Boston: Butterworths 1989: 87–111.
18. Li H, Walsh TN, O'Dowd G, Gillen P, Byrne PJ & Hennessy TPJ. Mechanisms of columnar metaplasia and squamous regeneration in experimental Barrett's oesophagus. *Surgery* 1994; **115**: 176–81.
19. Carey JS, Plested WG & Hughes RK. Esophagogastrectomy. Superiority of the combined abdominal right thoracic approach (Lewis operation). *Ann Thorac Surg* 1972; **14**: 59–68.
20. Shao LF, Li ZC, Liu SX *et al.* Surgical treatment of 210 cases of early carcinoma of the esophagus and gastric cardia. *Chinese J Surg* 1981; **19**: 259–61 (in Chinese).
21. Giuli R & Gignoux M. Treatment of cancer of the oesophagus. *Ann Surg* 1980; **192**: 44–52.
22. Skinner DB. En bloc resection for neoplasms of the esophagus and cardia. *J Thorac Cardiovasc Surg* 1983; **85**: 59–69.
23. Miller C. Carcinoma of the thoracic esophagus and cardia: a review of 40 cases. *Br J Surg* 1962; **49**: 507.
24. Watson A. Pathologic changes affecting survival in esophageal cancer. In: Delarue NC, Wilkins EW Jr & Wong J (eds) *International Trends in*

General Thoracic Surgery: Esophageal Cancer. St. Louis: Mosby 1988: 90–7.

25. Hennessy TPJ. Three-stage esophagectomy. In: Donohue JH, van Heerden JA & Monson JRT (eds) *Atlas of Surgical Oncology.* Oxford: Blackwell Science 1995: 131–41.

26. Altorki NK, Skinner DB, Ferguson MK & Little AG. Barrett's adenocarcinoma: long-term survival and recurrence patterns. In: Fergus MK, Little AG & Skinner DB (eds) *Diseases of the Esophagus: Malignant Diseases.* New York: Futura, 1990: 229–38.

27. Haagensen CD. *The Lymphatics in Cancer.* Philadelphia: Saunders 1972; 245–9.

28. Akiyama H. Squamous cell carcinoma of the thoracic esophagus. In: Akiyama H (ed.) *Surgery for Cancer of the Esophagus.* Baltimore: Williams & Wilkins 1990: 19–49.

29. Fekete F, Gayet B & Molas GJM. Prophylactic operative techniques: thoracic esophageal squamous cell cancer surgery, with special reference to lymph node removal. In: Delarue NC, Wilkins EW Jr & Wong J (eds) *Esophageal Cancer: International Trends in General Thoracic Surgery.* St. Louis: Mosby 1988: 133.

30. Isono K, Sato H & Nakayama K. Result of a nationwide study on the three-field lymph node dissection of esophageal cancer. *Oncology* 1991; **48**: 411.

31. Tsurumaru M, Akiyama H, Udagawa H, Ono Y, Suzuki M & Watanabe F. Cervical-thoracic-abdominal lymph node dissection for intrathoracic esophageal carcinoma. In: Ferguson MK, Little AG & Skinner DB (eds) *Diseases of the Esophagus: Malignant Diseases.* New York: Futura Publishing 1990: 187–96.

32. Kato H, Hiroshi W, Tachimori Y & Iizuka T. Evaluation of neck lymph node dissection for thoracic esophageal carcinoma. *Ann Thor Surg* 1991; **51**: 931–5.

33. Abe SI, Tachibana M, Shiraishi M & Nakamura T. Lymph node metastasis in resectable esophageal cancer. *J Thorac Cardiovasc Surg* 1990; **100**: 287–91.

34. Kakegawa TN & Fujita H. Arguments for extended three-field esophagectomy for thoracic esophageal cancer. Reported at the 13th Postgraduate Course of the Technical University of Munich, 1992 (unpublished report).

35. Ide H, Hanyu F, Murata Y, Kobayashi A, Yamada A & Kobayashi S. Extended dissection of thoracic esophageal cancer based on pre-operative staging. In: Ferguson MK, Little AG & Skinner DB (eds) *Diseases of the Esophagus:* *Malignant Diseases.* New York: Futura Publishing 1990: 177–86.

36. Peracchia A, Ruol A, Bardini R, Segalin A, Castoro C & Asolati M. Lymph node dissection for cancer of the thoracic esophagus: how extended should it be? Analysis of personal data and review of the literature. *Dis Esoph* 1992: **5**: 69.

37. Herskovic A, Martz K, Muhyi AS *et al.* Combined chemotherapy and radiotherapy compared with radiotherapy alone in patients with cancer of the esophagus. *N Engl J Med* 1992; **326**: 1593–7.

38. Walsh TN, Noonan N, Hollywood D, Kelly A, Keeling N & Hennessy TPJ. A comparison of multimodal therapy and surgery for esophageal adenocarcinoma. *N Engl J Med* 1996; **335**: 462–7.

39. Matsuda H, Tsutsui S, Nagamatsu M *et al.* Histopathologic and long term effects of hyperthermia combined with chemotherapy and irradiation for esophageal carcinoma. In: Ferguson MK, Little AG & Skinner DB (eds) *Diseases of the Esophagus: Malignant Diseases.* New York: Futura Publishing 1990: 311–15.

40. Leichman L, Steiger Z, Seydel HG *et al.* Preoperative chemotherapy and radiation therapy for patients with cancer of the esophagus: a potentially curative approach. *J Clin Oncol* 1984; **2**: 75–9.

41. Danoff B, Cooper J & Klein M. Primary adenocarcinoma of the upper esophagus. *Clin Radiol* 1978; **29**: 519–22.

42. Smithers D. Adenocarcinoma of the oesophagus. *Thorax* 1956; **11**: 257–67.

43. Abitbol A, Straus MJ & Franklin G. Infusional chemotherapy and cyclic radiation therapy in inoperable esophageal and gastric cardia carcinoma. *Am J Clin Oncol* 1983; **6**: 195–201.

44. Lokich JJ, Shea M & Chaffey J. Sequential infusion 5-fluorouracil followed by concomitant radiation for tumours of the esophagus and gastroesophageal junction. *Cancer* 1987; **60**: 275–9.

45. Coia LR, Paul AR & Engstrom PF. Combined radiation and chemotherapy as primary management of adenocarcinoma of the esophagus and gastroesophageal junction. *Cancer* 1988; **61**: 643–9.

46. Whittington R, Coia LR, Haller DG, Rubenstein JH & Rosato EF. Adenocarcinoma of the esophagus and esophago-gastric junction: the effects of single and combined modalities on the survival and patterns of failure following treatment. *Int J Radiat Oncol Biol Phys* 1990; **19**: 593–603.

47. Gill PG, Jamieson GG, Denham J *et al.* Treatment of adenocarcinoma of the cardia with

synchronous chemotherapy and radiotherapy. *Br J Surg* 1990; **77**: 1020–3.

48. Urba SG, Orringer MB, Perez-Tamayo C, Bromberg J & Forastiere A. Concurrent preoperative chemotherapy and radiation therapy in localized esophageal adenocarcinoma. *Cancer* 1992; **69**: 285–91.

49. Hoff SJ, Stewart JR, Sawyers JL *et al.* Preliminary results with neoadjuvant therapy and resection for esophageal carcinoma. *Ann Thorac Surg* 1993; **56**: 282–7.

50. Stewart JR, Hoff SJ, Johnson DH *et al.* Improved survival with neoadjuvant therapy and resection for adenocarcinoma of the esophagus. *Ann Surg* 1993; **218**: 571–8.

51. Ajani JA, Roth JA, Ryan MB *et al.* Intensive preoperative chemotherapy with colony stimulating factor for resectable adenocarcinoma of the esophagus or gastro-esophageal junction. *J Clin Oncol* 1993; **11**: 22–8.

52. Adelstein DJ, Rice TW, Boyce GA *et al.* Adenocarcinoma of the esophagus and gastroesophageal junction. *Am J Clin Oncol* 1994; **17**: 14–18.

53. Ensley JF, Patel B, Kloner R *et al.* The clinical syndrome of 5-fluorouracil cardiotoxicity. *Invest New Drugs* 1989; **7**: 101–9.

54. Hickey K, Grehan D, Reid I, O'Briain S, Walsh TN & Hennessy TPJ. Expression of epidermal growth factor receptor and proliferating cell nuclear antigen predicts response of esophageal squamous cell carcinoma to chemoradiotherapy. *Cancer* 1994; **74**: 1693–8.

12

COMPLICATIONS: PREVENTION AND MANAGEMENT

SIMON Y.K. LAW
JOHN WONG

INTRODUCTION

Despite advances in the various therapeutic modalities for carcinoma of the esophagus, surgery has remained the mainstay of treatment. Surgery is, however, associated with substantial morbidity and mortality. In a selective review by Earlam and Cunha-Melo in 1980,[1] the mean mortality rate of 122 series over a 25-year period from 1953 to 1978 was 29%. Surgical results have improved since. Muller reviewed 130 reports from 1980–1988, and showed the average hospital mortality rate following resection to be 13%.[2] In recent reports, operative mortality rates of <10% and even as low as 1.7% in selected patients managed by specialized centers were reported.[3–7]

From a global perspective, esophageal resection remains a formidable procedure. Most patients with esophageal cancer are elderly, and present with an advanced stage of disease. Most are chronic smokers and drinkers, malnourished, and with co-morbid diseases. Esophagectomy is a complex procedure with many pitfalls. Cardiopulmonary complications and sepsis from anastomotic leakage remain the main causes of medical and surgical mortality, respectively, worldwide.

In the absence of a cost-effective screening program, age at presentation and disease stage cannot be altered. The improvement in surgical outcome should therefore be achieved first, by identifying patients with prohibitively high risk and excluding them from surgery; second, optimizing patients' physiologic status before surgery; and third, refinement of operative technique and perioperative care. Although, for ease of discussion, we will approach these factors in sequence, this division is arbitrary as the phases are closely related to each other. While postoperative complications may clearly lead to mortality, such events may arise from poor patient selection, intraoperative mishaps, and suboptimal perioperative care. Special emphases will be placed on the genesis and prevention of pulmonary complications and anastomotic leakage, since these are the two most common causes of mortality in esophageal cancer surgery. Other surgical complications are also discussed individually.

RISK ANALYSIS AND PATIENT SELECTION

The outcome of surgery appears to relate primarily to patient selection, operative skills, and experience of the surgeon. Stringent selective criteria in choosing only the fittest patient with early-stage disease will lead to good surgical results. Thus, a low resectability rate may imply a more selective approach. It is however difficult to make hasty conclusions based on reported resectability rates alone, since such figures are dependent on many factors, for instance the referral pattern of individual centers, the treatment philosophy of the surgeons, and the possible mortality that the surgeon is prepared to accept. A referral center which only received patients with early-stage disease already screened by the gastroenterologist will automatically have a high resectability rate and correspondingly good results. In Muller's review, the mean resectability rates among centers was 56% (range 24–95%), while mean hospital mortality was 13% (range 1–40%).[2] In the West, in patients not preselected by the referral physicians to surgeons, the resectability rate is in the range of 40%.[8] There is no doubt that the lowest mortality rates were found by surgeons having large personal experience with a great number of resections.

Selecting the appropriate patients for esophagectomy goes a long way to avoiding complications and mortality. In a consensus conference of the International Society for Diseases of the Esophagus held in Milan, 1995, all participating experts agreed that objective evaluation of operative risk was mandatory for patients undergoing esophagectomy.[9] Some of the factors often implicated are reviewed in the discussion to follow.

Advanced age

Advanced age has been identified as a significant risk factor after major surgery. In esophagectomy, poorer outcome is also shown in the aged.[10–15] As a risk factor, advanced age reflects the deterioration of physiologic reserve and the presence of co-morbid diseases. This is especially true in esophageal cancer patients, who are frequently heavy smokers and drinkers. With advancing age, critical airway closing volumes increase and approach functional residual capacity, and atelectasis develops easily. Together with retained bronchial secretion and poor cough effort, infection becomes likely. The incidence of cardiac diseases is also higher. It was shown that elderly patients (over 70 years of age) have a reduction in the maximum response of the stress hormones to esophagectomy, with significantly more multiorgan dysfunction which correlated with postoperative complications.[16] If this increased risk in the aged is carefully identified and optimal perioperative care undertaken, morbidity and mortality rates are comparable with those of the patients' younger counterparts.[17]

In a recent study at the authors' institute comparing patients over 70 with those younger, the resect-ability rate in the older patients was 48% compared with 65% in those under 70. Chronic pulmonary disease or abnormal function was present in 43% of the over-70 group compared with only 26% in the younger group. This was similar for cardiac disease (21% and 12%, respectively). Patients in the over-70 group underwent more transhiatal resections without thoracotomy, and postoperative tracheostomy and bronchoscopic aspiration of sputum was needed more frequently. The older age group developed more cardiopulmonary complications, but no difference in mortality rate was found. This shows that with appropriate selection of patient, operative procedure, and active perioperative care, similar results can be obtained in the elderly patients compared with their younger counterparts. In addition, the resectability rates in the over-70 group increased from 44% during 1982–1989 to 54% during 1990–1996. In spite of this, hospital deaths decreased from 24% to 12% for the two periods. Surgical experience and better perioperative care allow less stringent patient selection, with improved outcome.[18]

Pulmonary functional assessment

Pulmonary disease is an obvious risk factor. Patients for esophagectomy, especially smokers, should have history and signs of chronic lung disease carefully evaluated. Abnormal chest radiography is a risk factor and should prompt further detailed investigations.[13] Objective pulmonary function tests are obtained to guide treatment, especially where a thoracotomy is considered, though which test and what parameters are most accurate remain controversial.

A low preoperative PaO_2 was found to be of poor prognostic value.[15] Spirometric parameters have not been consistently useful.[14,19] Simple parameters such as peak flow rate, forced expiratory volume in one second (FEV_1) and forced vital capacity (FVC) are commonly used to predict pulmonary complications.[10,15,20] An FEV_1 of <90% of predicted value for age and height carried a three-fold (20% versus 6.5%) risk of fatal pulmonary complications,[21] while our own data with the same cut-off point showed a relative risk of 1.9 in developing pulmonary complications.[13] Obstructive pattern on spirometric tests, clinical, and spirometric improvement with bronchodilators should prompt optimal treatment before surgery. More elaborate parameter like "Diffusing Capacity correlated for volume and hemoglobin" is also found to be predictive, although it is questionable if it is superior to simple spirometry.[12] While pulmonary function tests are the best way to define chronic lung disease, their utility seems to lie in the ability to identify patients who will not have complications rather than those who will (their negative predictive value is high). Incentive spirometry, a form of maximum inspiratory technique to prevent atelectasis, also reflects the patients' respiratory muscle strength, coordination and mental cooperation, and was also predictive of outcome.[13]

Nutritional status

Cancer patients have the highest incidence of protein-energy malnutrition (PEM) seen in hospitalized patients, with a significant degree occurring in more than 30% of patients undergoing major upper gastrointestinal procedures.[22] Weight loss is common in such patients, and has been associated with poor outcome. In a review of more than 3000 patients, significantly improved survival in those patients without weight loss was found compared with those who had lost 6% or more of their bodyweight.[23] Poor wound healing, depressed immunocompetence, wound infection, prolonged postoperative ileus, and hospital stay and mortality have been linked to PEM. Direct measurement of protein depletion by *in vivo* neutron activation analysis correlates with poorer respiratory muscle strength and spirometric parameters, and in turn with significantly higher incidence of postoperative respiratory complications.[24]

Etiologically, the development of PEM is multifactorial. Tumors may be obstructive in the gastrointestinal tract, as in esophageal cancer, leading to a reduction in oral intake. Alteration in taste perception, malabsorption, a raised metabolic rate, and psychologic factors all may contribute. In the short term, cytokines serve to promote an acute phase response by re-routing nutrients from the periphery to the liver. In the long term, they result in anorexia and abnormalities in metabolism.

Much work has been done to evaluate nutritional parameters in risk prediction for esophageal cancer. Significant PEM has been found in 50% of patients at presentation,[25] and those with abnormal nutritional status had higher mortality rates.[26]

In one study, assessing anthropometric, biochemical, immunologic data and using the prognostic nutritional index (PNI), it was not possible to assess the risk of esophagectomy preoperatively on nutritional parameters solely. Even though clear loss of weight was evident in two-thirds of the patients studied, the nutritional status was still within the normal range in most cases, and hence the risk burden was low.[27] In another report, various biochemical and anthropometric parameters in combination, reflecting a "host defense index" against sepsis, were found to be nearly 90% predictive of pulmonary complications.[28]

Serum albumin level was shown by many to be related to adverse outcome.[13,19,28,29] While not solely dependent on nutrition (also affected by liver cirrhosis, sepsis, abnormal metabolism), a normal serum albumin maintains plasma oncotic pressure and in theory reduces pulmonary transudate of fluid and so helps prevent pulmonary edema.[13,19,29] In animal studies, esophagectomy was found to increase the amount of extravascular lung water, especially when vagotomy was performed, and may be aggravated by decrease in plasma oncotic pressure.[30] In addition, low plasma oncotic pressure may increase bowel edema, and hence increase the risk of anastomotic leakage. Since low albumin level is related to the two major complications after esophagectomy, its poor prognostic significance is not unexpected.

The problem in evaluating studies on nutritional assessment is the inadequacy of existing methods in defining PEM. In general, the parameters used lack specificity in identifying the patient at risk. A detailed clinical assessment was shown to be as good as standard anthropometric, biochemical, derived nutritional indices and skin testing to recalled antigen, in predicting complications. However, overall, an adverse outcome could only be identified accurately in two-thirds of patients.[31]

Cirrhosis

Liver cirrhosis is associated with a marked increase in postoperative mortality.[20,32,33] Ruol et al.[34] observed a 21% mortality rate, 23% anastomotic leakage rate, and 4% necrosis of the esophageal substitute even in Child's class A cirrhosis. In many centers, patients with decompensated cirrhosis are excluded from esophagectomy. In the absence of frank cirrhosis, the aminopyrine breath test, which measures hepatic cytochrome P_{450} function, may help in identification of the high-risk patient (H. Bartels *et al.*, personal communication, 1997).

Disease stage

Predictably, patients who had early tumors fared better when compared with those who had advanced tumors. Thus, we found that patients with curative resections fared better when compared with those with palliative resections (the clinical correlate of stage of disease), with mortality rates of 9% and 20%, respectively. Death related to advancing malignancy accounted for 25% of hospital deaths in our experience,[13] a point which reflected our high resectability rates in a group of unselected patients with advanced tumors. Our in-hospital mortality also included death up to 6 months after surgery, a time at which many patients had recovered from their operation but stayed in hospital for socioeconomic reasons. Among a group of patients in whom we performed surgical bypass, 25% had stage IV disease, and bypass carried a 30-day mortality rate of 27%. A review of bypass procedures in 10 reports showed an average mortality of 18%, with morbidity rates of 35% to 71%.[35] With the myriad of new and effective palliative modalities available, a bypass procedure is perhaps not justified unless in the situation where unexpected advanced disease is encountered at attempted resection and a lesser procedure of bypass is performed. There is no doubt, however, that after a successful bypass procedure, the quality of food that the patient can ingest is superior, and require less re-intervention compared with other modalities of palliation.

In the collective review by Muller *et al.*,[2] mortality rates were 11% and 18% in resections performed with curative intent in 13 061 patients compared with that in 16 024 patients with palliative intent. The favorable outcome in early-stage disease was also reported by others.[20] In the West, most patients present at an advanced stage of disease; however, if only early-stage tumors are operated on, the outcome is also excellent with low mortality and good long-term survival. Moghissi[36] reported a mortality rate of 1.6% in patients with stage I cancer, while a collective review by the Groupe Europeen pour l'Etude des Maladies de l'Oesophage (GEEMO) of early cancer treatment in 17 European centers stated a mortality rate of 9%.[37]

Advanced stage of disease may be related to other adverse factors which contribute to poor outcome. Nutrition and exercise tolerance are likely to be worse for those with advanced disease because of more tumor burden and more complete dysphagia. Blood loss is more likely to be in excess if a difficult resection is encountered, and this is most likely with locally advanced tumors when surrounding structures are infiltrated. Our analysis of risk factors showed that blood loss was a risk factor in both pulmonary complications and death after surgery.[13] Patients with very advanced tumors are thus at high risk and alternative therapies should be considered.

Value of risk models in risk prediction

One main criticism of risk prediction is that the parameters used for assessment often lack objectivity. The "general status," American Society of Anesthesiologists (ASA) grading, Karnofsky index, ECOG score, "mental co-operation" are just some of these subjective predictors.[10,13] However, these parameters reflect the general status of the patient as a whole and may be superior to an isolated criterion which examines only an isolated body system in predicting overall functional performance. Assessment of exercise tolerance by stair climbing, and bicycle test are useful adjuncts in risk assessment.[10,13]

Instead of expensive and sophisticated tests, simple bedside assessment by an experienced surgeon is invaluable and has been shown to be accurate in nutritional evaluation.[38] These tests have the advantage of being simple and less costly. In our experience, a detailed clinical assessment with basic hematologic and biochemical tests, chest radiograph, electrocardiogram, grip strength, incentive spirometry and pulmonary spirometric tests, and exercise tolerance evaluation are adequate for the majority of patients. More sophisticated tests, e.g., echocardiography for those with ischemic heart disease, are only requested if specially indicated.

Many authors have utilized statistical techniques to generate risk models in order to make risk analysis more objective. The number of inter-related factors is reduced by multivariate analysis and so would ease their clinical application. Risk stratification to different degrees of risk is also possible.[9,12,13,20,28,39–41] With risk models so generated, the accuracy is in the region of 75–80%. Using a model incorporating vital capacity, presence of liver cirrhosis, and stage of tumor, Nagawa et al. could predict pulmonary complications with 75% accuracy, 79% sensitivity, and 73% specificity.[20] Our own analyses in predicting pulmonary complications and hospital death were accurate in about 75% of cases.[13] These models are usually generated by retrospective studies, but rarely validated through prospective evaluation. In some instances, the use of such validated risk models to select appropriate patients for surgery has been shown to improve outcome (H. Bartels et al., personal communication, 1997).

Ideally, one aims at accurate risk prediction with preoperative factors alone. However, it is unlikely that a higher degree of precision could be derived from these assessments since intraoperative events and postoperative care cannot be predicted before surgery. Some deaths are due to technical faults or mishaps, or unexpected medical or surgical complications developed after surgery. In one study, perioperative variables including blood loss, New York Heart Association (NYHA) class, and the type of operative procedure were found to be more predictive than preoperative factors in predicting pulmonary complications.[12] In a detailed analysis of causes of death at the authors' institute, the inclusion of intraoperative factors could add about 10% accuracy to preoperative factors alone.[13] Surgical complications accounted for 21% of deaths. If the causes of surgical failure can be identified and reduced, one may expect the predictive accuracy of preoperative physiologic assessment to improve further.

OPTIMIZATION OF PHYSIOLOGIC STATUS

Identification of risk factors goes a fair way to prevent complications, since all efforts should be channeled to improve the physiologic systems that are found to be suboptimal. Smoking should be stopped, and active physiotherapy instituted. As a therapeutic measure, incentive spirometry trains respiratory muscles, in terms of both coordination and cooperation, and was shown to be comparable with chest physiotherapy in preventing pulmonary complications after abdominal surgery.[42] Bronchodilator therapy is indicated in those who demonstrate clinical response, or by peak flow measurements and spirometry. These should all be continued in the postoperative phase.

The impact of perioperative nutritional repletion and intervention on morbidity and mortality of esophagectomy has been controversial. Reduced anastomotic leakage rate and mortality was shown in patients with esophageal cancer fed parenterally, when compared with those who were not.[43,44] Other studies have found weight gain or improved nitrogen balance by total parenteral nutrition (TPN) without clinical benefit.[29,45,46] The benefit of TPN in esophageal cancer patients undergoing surgery is unproven. In a large multicenter trial conducted by the Veterans Affairs Total Parenteral Nutrition Co-operative Group, the benefit of TPN during major surgery was only shown in patients with severe malnutrition,[47] a fact which may explain the lack of clinical benefit shown in most trials in esophageal cancer with small number of patients. Most patients did not meet the criteria of severe malnourishment and the effect would not be apparent.

Recent advances in the understanding of the gut barrier to bacterial translocation suggest that enteral feeding may be superior to parenteral nutritional support.[48] This finding is particularly important since TPN is not without complications. A recent randomized trial comparing enteral and parenteral nutrition after esophagectomy showed that 45% of the parenteral group developed serious complications (catheter sepsis and axillary vein thrombosis), while enteral nutrition was safe although improved outcome was not demonstrated.[49] Early enteral feeding is no doubt possible after esophagectomy, as a review of 523 patients who were fed by a feeding jejunostomy placed at the time of esophagogastrectomy reported only a 2.1% complication rate related to the feeding tube.[50] One study comparing jejunostomy feeding after esophagectomy with conventional diet advancement showed that caloric needs could be met much earlier in the former group, as 77% of the patients received their full nutritional needs within 3–5 days of initiation of feeding. A "trend" for shorter hospital stay was also found, a clinical benefit was much more difficult to demonstrate.[51] The reasons why nutritional interventions have not been shown to improve clinical outcome in esophagectomy are that first, the incidence of truly severely malnourished patients is low; second, significant clinical outcome difference would require a large number of patients to demonstrate; and third, the genesis of complications are multifactorial and poor nutrition is only one of many facets. The impact of nutritional status on outcome following esophageal surgery will not be apparent unless these problems are isolated.

Although hyperalimentation by whatever route has not been proven to alter postoperative outcome, it is unethical to leave severely dysphagic patients without adequate nutrition. Supplementary nutrition with high calorie and protein contents is given in soft or liquid form in those who can still swallow. In those with severe dysphagia, enteral nutrition is given via a feeding tube. In our experience, it is nearly always possible to place a fine-bore tube beyond the tumor in the stomach. In tumors of high-grade stenosis, endoscopic placement with a guidewire and the Seldinger technique may be required; a radiologic screening facility aids accurate placement. Enteral nutrition involves minimal cost and has the advantage of maintaining intestinal function compared with parenteral nutrition. Only rarely is TPN required. The period of preoperative nutritional supplement depends on the length of time required for patient assessment and investigation, and local scheduling of the operation. Prolonged preparation and full repletion of body protein and cell mass is neither practical nor desirable in cancer patients, as even a few days of nutritional/metabolic repair has demonstrable improvement. It was shown that biochemical improvement (transferrin and prealbumin), physiologic improvement (including grip strength, respiratory muscle strength and spirometric parameters) occurred soon after commencement of TPN (averaging 12% as early as 4 days), without any demonstrable increase in total body protein.[52]

Plasma albumin level should be normalized to restore plasma oncotic pressure. Electrolytes disturbances are corrected and trace elements and vitamins supplied. Patients should also be prepared psychologically for surgery. In most patients, the simple measures discussed above are adequate for preoperative preparation.

CONDUCT OF OPERATION

Meticulous preparation of patients for surgery is no substitute for a well-performed operation. This is especially true in esophageal resection, because the procedure comprises many phases, each of which requires multiple discrete steps that are prone to failure. While the abdominal and neck phases are more straightforward, the thoracic dissection is complex as the surgeon has to balance the benefits and hazards of extensive radical surgery against a more limited resection which may compromise the possibility of cure. The difficulty of resection is increased when the tumor is infiltrative with obliteration of tissue planes. With the advent of multimodality treatment, although preoperative chemotherapy and radiotherapy may downstage cancer, tissue planes are also made less well-defined. Dissection may be more hazardous. Surgical complications are mostly related to technical faults, and in our experience accounted for 31% of 30-day mortality and 21% of hospital deaths.[13]

There are many variables for the different components of an esophagectomy. The choice of procedure, e.g., transhiatal versus transthoracic resection, the access route (through the right, left chest, minimal access surgery), the esophageal substitute used (stomach, colon, jejunum), the route of reconstruction (orthotopic, retrosternal, subcutaneous), the type of anastomosis (hand-sewn, stapled, number of layers, continuous or interrupted), and whether the operation should be staged, deserves careful consideration. A two-staged resection for instance is of value in patients with very high risk, and when intraoperative events (excessive bleeding and hypotension) make a one-staged reconstruction unsafe.[14,53] Postoperative complications may be closely related to intraoperative conduct and decisions.

Choice of procedure

One controversy concerning esophageal resection is the choice of surgical approach, in particular regarding whether a thoracotomy is necessary, or indeed desirable. Transhiatal esophagectomy without thoracotomy (THE) appears to result in less pulmonary complications and mortality compared with open thoracotomy resections (TTE).[2] There are added advantages of a shorter operating time, and placing the upper esophageal anastomosis in the cervical region where a longer resection margin is obtained. An anastomotic leakage is perhaps less lethal. Long-term survival is also comparable with that of TTE. Proponents of TTE criticize the THE for inadequate oncologic clearance, and the claimed advantage of a lower pulmonary complication rate is unproven. A review of THE in 1353 patients performed during the 1980s showed an overall mortality rate of 7%.[54] In experienced centers, the mortality rate is as low as 5%.[4] However, to date almost all comparative studies of the two approaches were retrospective,[55–58,93] making them less than adequate for proper and unbiased evaluation. A retrospective analysis in the authors' institute showed that pulmonary-related deaths occurred less frequently in THE than TTE for patients with high pulmonary risks for surgery.[59] Bolton et al.[56] also found that a lower pulmonary complication rate in THE resection, even though the patients had significantly worse American Society of Anesthesiologists (ASA) risk class in comparison with those undergoing TTE.

Randomized controlled trials comparing the two procedures are few in number, partly because both procedures are not practiced at the same institutions with equal skill and preference. Goldminc et al.[60] compared the clinical outcome of THE with TTE in a randomized trial of 67 patients with squamous cell cancer. There were no differences in morbidity rates (THE, 56% versus TTE, 46%), especially in the incidence of pulmonary complications (THE, 19% versus TTE, 20%). Mortality rates were also similar (THE, 6.2% versus TTE, 8.5%).[60] The lack of significant difference between the two techniques was also substantiated in our randomized trial comprising 39 patients. Intraoperative hypotension occurred more commonly in the THE group than the TTE group. This was likely the result of the operator's hand and forearm in the posterior mediastinum reducing venous return as well as compressing the heart. Although THE took significantly less time to perform, perioperative morbidity, mortality and long-term survival did not differ between the two groups. In this study however, only patients with lower-third tumors were included and both groups of patients were judged to have sufficient pulmonary reserve to undergo TTE before randomization.[61] The potential benefits of THE may therefore be lessened.

Significant complications from THE may result from the blind mobilization especially of the middle portion of the esophagus. Bleeding from the azygos vein or from esophageal branches of the aorta, tumor rupture and contamination, chylothorax, tracheobronchial injury, or recurrent nerve paresis may be associated with THE, and the surgeon should be prepared for urgent exploration.[4,57,59] In our experience, we reserve THE for patients with lower- or upper-third tumors where the dis-

section of the esophagus can be carried out under vision, and for patients with reduced pulmonary reserve, or in patients with obliterated pleural cavity. For patients with middle-third tumors, only early tumors may be resected safely via THE. A similar experience with worse outcome for middle-third tumor was also reported.[62] To avert complications, a specially designed mediastinoscope with operating channels, which allows microsurgical dissection of the esophagus under visual control, was reported to reduce significantly the incidence of recurrent laryngeal nerve injury and also pulmonary complications after THE.[63]

More recently, minimal access surgery applied to esophageal resection has been under investigation, with the aim of lowering in particular cardiopulmonary complications by reducing the trauma of conventional access. Different approaches have been utilized, including thoracoscopic esophageal mobilization,[64] video-assisted transmediastinal esophageal mobilization using a laparoscope inserted through the diaphragmatic hiatus,[65] laparoscopic gastric mobilization followed by thoracotomy,[66] and laparoscopic gastric and esophageal mobilization.[67] The most common is the thoracoscopic approach with open laparotomy for preparation of the esophageal substitute and a cervical anastomosis. In the authors' institute, thoracoscopic esophagectomy was introduced in 1994. Results in the first 22 patients showed that thoracoscopy took a median time of 110 min, and was successful in 82% of patients. Postoperatively, pneumonia affected 17% of the patients, but no mortality resulted. When compared with open thoracotomy resections performed in the same time period, no significant difference in morbidity and mortality rates were found. However, patients for thoracoscopy were selected with increased surgical risk (significantly worse ECOG score compared with those who underwent open thoracotomy resections).[68] Some patients would not have undergone surgical resection if only TTE and THE were available, as the risks were judged too high. A review of existing literature showed similar results.[64] The lack of clear advantages of minimal access techniques over conventional approaches may be related to the learning curve, patient selection, and the multifactorial nature in the genesis of cardiopulmonary complications. The benefit of smaller port sites compared with open thoracotomy may be offset by the reported lengthened time of single-lung anesthesia. The surgical trauma of mediastinal dissection is also independent of the incision size. Improvement in pain relief and perioperative care also lessen the deleterious effects of thoracotomy and laparotomy, while port site recurrence is another concern.[68]

In relation to the choice of approach and extent of resection used for esophageal resection, certain postoperative complications are closely related. Recurrent laryngeal nerve palsy is a known complication from esophagectomy, with its close proximity to the esophagus. Patients with vocal cord palsy are more prone to aspiration, and their cough effort is less effective because of inadequate glottic closure. The association of recurrent laryngeal nerve injury with THE has already been mentioned.

Extensive lymphadenectomy, especially three-field lymphadenectomy (lymph node dissection in the neck, mediastinum and upper abdomen), can result in up to 80% incidence of recurrent laryngeal nerve injury, and the cough reflex is significantly depressed.[69] Even without extensive mediastinal dissection, the recurrent laryngeal nerve is easily damaged in the cervical phase of the operation, and thus knowledge of the course of the nerve is important to avoid damage. The nerve runs a tortuous course and is somewhat hidden in a bed of connective tissue in close relationship with the esophagus, trachea, and thyroid gland. Dissection should be made as close as possible to the esophageal wall, and traction, compression to the tracheoesophageal groove, or blind stripping of the connective tissue should be avoided.[70]

Proponents of three-field lymphadenectomy also suggest ways to preserve pulmonary function which are related to surgical techniques. In experimental animals, preservation of the tracheopulmonary branches of the vagus nerve was shown to produce significantly less extravascular lung water after radical esophagectomy compared with their severance. Vagal preservation was therefore suggested. Preservation of the bronchial arteries also reduced tracheal ischemia.[30] Experimental data were produced to support the deleterious effect of overhydration after esophagectomy, though whether these measures can be translated into clinical benefit is difficult to prove.

Other components of surgery may be related to postoperative cardiopulmonary complications. Reconstruction using the posterior mediastinum after THE have been shown in a randomized trial to result in shorter intensive care stay, shorter time to normalize the cardiac index, less cardiopulmonary complications, and lower mortality compared with the retrosternal route.[71] Similar results were reported by others.[19]

Anastomotic leakage
Etiology

Anastomotic leakage between the esophagus and the conduit used for esophageal replacement is a dreaded complication. It remains a principal cause of surgical sepsis, and its associated morbidity and mortality are high. The incidence of this complication varies widely. A review of surgical series reported in the 1980s revealed an average leakage rate of 12%,[2] and even in some relatively recent reports, leak rates of up to 30% were still reported.[72]

Factors explaining why the esophageal anastomosis is so prone to failure were summarized by Urschel.[73] There are inherent factors of the esophagus: unlike the rest of the gastrointestinal tract, it has no serosa and its longitudinal muscle holds sutures poorly, and the anastomosis is carried out in poorly exposed, awkward positions. Local factors include vascular (both arterial and venous) insufficiency to the gastric fundus (the most commonly used esophageal substitute), tension at the anastomosis, gastric distention in the early postoperative period, and compression at the thoracic inlet compromising a cervical anastomosis. Systemic factors include severe malnutrition, hypoalbuminemia, perioperative hypoxia, or hypotension.

The esophageal conduit requires careful preparation and transposition to a distant site for anastomosis. Inexperienced preparation of the conduit may result in bruising, or kinking of the supplying vessels, resulting in ischemia. The degree of gastric fundal oxygenation measured by oximetry after stomach mobilization correlated with anastomosis healing.[74] Various innovative methods were proposed to improve vascular supply to the stomach tube. Some authors recommended using the splenic hilar vasculature following a splenectomy to preserve blood supply to the gastric fundus.[75] Additional grafting of the vessel arcades of the substitute organ using microvascular techniques was reported,[76] while preoperative embolization of the left gastric and splenic artery was advocated to "open up" vascular supply via the right gastroepiploic artery.[77]

Ischemia is in fact rarely a problem as the esophagus has a rich submucosal vascular network. The stomach also has an adequate blood supply if it is prepared with care. A corrosion cast study of the gastric conduit showed that the stomach blood flow can rely on the right gastroepiploic artery alone, with the best blood supply to a 4-cm gastric tube on the greater curvature.[78] The right gastric artery can be divided if preservation results in tension to the esophagogastric anastomosis.[79] The colon's blood supply is more variable, but preoperative arteriography may help in identifying reliable vasculature and lessen the risk of graft failure. Arterial anatomic features are favorable in at least 80% of patients with arteriographic examination, and anastomotic leakage rate and graft failure can be < 2%.[80]

Technical errors probably account for most cases of anastomotic leaks.[81,82] A careful analysis of the causes of anastomotic leaks in the authors' unit showed that 53% had an identifiable technical error and were therefore potentially avoidable.[13]

The advent of the stapling device has lowered the incidence of leakage, and was advocated as the preferred method of anastomosis.[83–85] The result using a circular stapler is perhaps more uniform and less operator-dependent. Most surgeons prefer to staple high thoracic anastomosis and suture cervical anastomosis. With experience, the hand-sewn method is as safe, if not more so, and certainly less expensive. In the author's unit, between 1964 and 1982, leak rates were nearly 25%, though this has improved to <5% and was recently 3%.[86,87] Moreover, with increasing experience with the hand-sewn method, the stapler is used less often and all of our anastomoses are now hand-sewn, regardless of the anatomic site.

A variety of techniques are favored for hand anastomosis, and the use of absorbable or nonabsorbable, one- or two-layered, continuous or interrupted sutures remain controversial.[81,82,88–90] Although the results of most of these techniques are comparable, other methods have been designed to lower leak rates. These include covering the anastomoses with omentum, pleura, or pericardial fat, and using fibrin glue to spray the anastomosis.[55,72,84,91] However, none of these is of proven value.

The site of the esophageal anastomosis was implicated as an important factor predisposing to leakage. Cervical anastomoses seem to have a higher tendency to leak compared with intrathoracic anastomoses. Less than 10% of thoracic anastomoses, and 10–25% of cervical anastomoses develop insufficiency.[58,73,92,93] Some surgeons advocate routine subtotal esophagectomy with cervical anastomosis because a longer resection margin can be achieved, a cervical leak is easier to manage, and is less lethal compared with a thoracic leak.[92] Mortality rates associated with cervical and thoracic leaks were estimated to be around 20% and 60%, respectively.[2,94,95] A higher leakage rate in the neck may be due to a longer route used and hence tension created, and compression of the conduit at the thoracic inlet. In this respect, the retrosternal route has higher leakage rates compared with the orthotopic route.[90] The higher leak rate in the neck is not universal, it has been reported by us and others that similar leakage rates occurred at the two sites.[96,97] In our experience, leakage rates are both at below 5% (including clinical and radiologic leaks), and the mortality associated with a leak is similar at around 40% for clinically obvious leaks. A similar length of resection margin could be obtained comparing the two sites because a near-total esophagectomy is accomplished in the chest. The anastomosis at the apex of the pleural cavity is situated at or above the level of the clavicle.[85,97] A cervical leak may not be truly confined to the neck, since mediastinal contamination is usual. Together with other factors that are associated with leakage which may be present in both groups (advanced disease, hypoalbuminemia, malnutrition), similar mortality rates could thus be explained.

The use of the distal stomach after esophagogastrectomy, when the proximal part of the stomach is resected, is reported to be more prone to leakage,[82,98] though we could not confirm this finding. Only when the stapler was used for the distal stomach was a higher leakage rate found. The fact that a gastrotomy is required to introduce the stapler, in addition to stapling the anastomosis either across or near another staple line, may contribute to anastomotic failure.[99]

Other inconsistent factors predisposing to leakage include radiotherapy, chemotherapy, diabetes, age of patient, cirrhosis, and cardiopulmonary diseases,[73] while malignant infiltration of the esophageal resection margin was implicated in some studies,[73,94] but not in others.[82,100]

Prevention

The choice of anastomotic technique is perhaps less important than its proper application. The principles of sound anastomosis still hold true, notably that the preparation of the esophageal substitute should be meticulous and rough handling avoided to prevent bruising, while the blood supply is carefully preserved. Tension should be minimized by preparing a sufficient length of conduit to reach the site of anastomosis. For the gastric tube, full kocherization of the duodenum allows the pylorus to reach the diaphragmatic hiatus, although in our experience this is rarely necessary except in the case of pharyngolaryngoesophagectomy. Compression at the thoracic inlet for cervical anastomosis, especially when the retrosternal route is used, may be alleviated by resecting part of the manubrium, first rib, and clavicle.[101,102]

The esophagus is prepared with equal care. The strength of the esophagus lies in its mucosa. Esophageal mucosa tends to retract proximally when divided. The division of the esophagus can be performed by first dividing a ring of muscular wall with cautery; the exposed mucosa is then divided carefully so that the mucosa lies level with the muscular layer. Placement of stay sutures which include the full thickness of the esophageal wall prevents inadvertent exclusion of the mucosa during anastomosis. In the authors' unit, a one-layer continuous suture with a monofilament suture is used.[103] For the posterior layer, full thickness bites of the esophagus and the esophageal substitute should be taken at least 5 mm from the edge. For the anterior layer, full thickness of the esophageal wall with less mucosa should be taken, and on the substitute only the seromuscular layer should be incorporated; this allows proper inversion of the mucosa. The esophagus and the conduit is only lightly apposed such that mucosa-to-mucosa apposition is encouraged. Knots are tied without excessive force to avoid tissue strangulation. For a stapled anastomosis, the purse-string is carefully placed and a complete "doughnut" ascertained after firing. The use of mechanical device is not a replacement for careful technique.[103,104]

A drainage procedure in the form of a pyloroplasty or pyloromyotomy of the vagotomized stomach, and the placement of a nasogastric tube, help decompression of the gastric conduit in the early postoperative period. This helps avoid distention and hence tension at the anastomosis, and also averts delayed gastric emptying.[81,105,106] When the colon is used for anastomosis, the placement of a "nasocolonic" tube may be difficult and is, in our experience, not necessary.

Avoiding excessive blood loss during surgery, and good postoperative pulmonary and cardiovascular support to avoid hypoxia and hypotension are also important. A low serum albumin reduces tissue oncotic pressure and predisposes to edema of the anastomosis. Although variably reported as a significant factor in anastomotic failure,[81,82] serum albumin concentration should be maintained by exogenous albumin infusion as the consequence of leakage more than justifies its cost.

Detection of leakage and management

Postoperative leaks were classified by Urschel into early fulminant, clinically apparent thoracic, clinically apparent cervical, and clinically silent leaks.[73] This serves as a good guide to management.

Early fulminant leaks within the first 48 h are usually due to necrosis and gangrene of the conduit. The patient may present with septicemia, and foul chest tube discharge may be evident. Timely intervention is mandatory. The conduit should be "taken down," appropriate débridement and drainage of the thoracic cavity and mediastinum established, a cervical esophagostomy performed and a feeding enterostomy done for nutritional support.[98,100] Maximum esophageal length should be preserved to ease future reconstruction.

Clinically apparent thoracic leaks usually take place within the first week, but we have experienced leaks up to 3 weeks after surgery. It should be suspected if there is excessive output from the chest drain, which may be turbid in color or bile-stained. Pleural collections on chest radiography or computed tomography (CT) scans may be evident. Confirmation can be made by giving the patient methylene blue dye orally and observing the appearance of the dye in the chest drainage. The location and magnitude of the leak can be visualized by a water-soluble contrast study. A carefully performed flexible endoscopic examination is also helpful to appreciate the site and size of leakage, and would not worsen the leak. The treatment of anastomotic leaks should be individualized. For small contained leaks, chest tube drainage with or without the addition of CT-guided drainage of pockets of collection may suffice (**Figures 12.1** and **12.2**), though in septic patients with a sizable leak, exploration is often warranted. Direct repair is seldom possible or effective, though in selected cases with adequate healthy surrounding tissue, this can be attempted. Buttress with pleura, pericardial fat or muscle may be useful;[107] otherwise, treatment along the lines of early fulminant leaks should be established. In selected cases, endoscopic placement of a sump nasogastric tube through the leak into the thoracic abscess cavity for irrigation and drainage has a place in non-operative management.[108]

For a cervical anastomosis, leakage is suspected when there is inflammation and pain of the neck wound. Turbid infected discharge is found when the skin stitches are removed and the wound laid open. Leaks truly confined to the neck are simply treated by laying the wound open with daily washing and frequent change of dressing. The patient is usually not septic. Leaks that communicate with the mediastinum may require formal exploration and placement of mediastinal drains.

In all leaks, treatment with broad-spectrum antibiotics is required and guided by culture and sensitivity results. Nutritional support is essential, and careful placement of a fine-bore feeding tube distal to the leak is often possible. With a thoracic stomach, endoscopic placement of a fine-bore tube using a guidewire in the duodenum is useful for enteral feeding. A nasogastric tube in the intrathor-

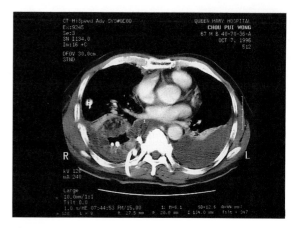

Figure 12.2 Computed tomography scan showing percutaneous drainage of mediastinal collection under radiologic guidance. This technique can be applied in selected patients.

acic stomach will help to decompress the stomach and avoid reflux of gastric contents through the anastomosis. A proton pump inhibitor helps lower the volume of gastric output. Parenteral nutrition is required if placement of feeding tube is not successful.

Subclinical leaks detected by contrast study only may be treated conservatively. Follow-up contrast study is done to monitor healing, and treatment is modified if clinical sepsis occurs or radiologic progression takes place. Drainage should also be considered in leaks close to the trachea or aorta, as fistulation has been reported.[107]

Prevention is preferable. The keys to avoid anastomotic leakage are optimization of the physiologic condition of the patient undergoing surgery, careful surgical technique, and perioperative care. Surgical experience will lead to lower leakage rates.[86,108a,109] At the authors' institute, the current anastomotic leak rate is 3%, half of which is subclinical. A high index of suspicion, timely diagnosis and intervention will lower mortality rate from this feared complication of esophageal surgery.

Anastomotic stricture

The development of anastomotic stricture must be considered a failure of surgical treatment since dysphagia from tumor stenosis is replaced by the same complaint from fibrotic stricture. The frequency of this complication is high, ranging from 5% to 45% in recent literature.[110] Previous anastomotic leak,

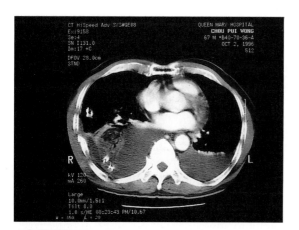

Figure 12.1 Computed tomography scan showing mediastinal collection and pleural effusion as a consequence of anastomotic leakage.

alkaline or acid reflux predispose to later stricture formation.[111] Prevention of leak in the first instance and avoidance of a low thoracic esophagogastrostomy to lessen gastroesophageal reflux are important. A one-layer anastomosis produces less stricture than a two-layered technique. In one study, the incidence of leak was 19% for both one- and two-layered anastomoses, but the stricture rates were 22% and 48%, respectively.[90]

In a retrospective study which was confirmed later by a prospective randomized trial, we have shown that the anastomotic technique (whether hand-sewn or stapled) had the most significant bearing on stricture, whereas the size of the esophagus was of secondary importance. A four-fold increase in stricture rate was found with the stapled technique (9% versus 39%). Although esophageal size was of secondary importance, the highest stricture rate occurred with a small esophagus using the stapler (44%).[87,89] The reasons why stricture was more common with the stapled method remain speculative, but the lack of accurate mucosa–mucosa apposition (with the edges separated by two thicknesses of bowel wall) may play a role, as the raw surface heals by second intention with granulation tissue formation. Tissue necrosis beyond the staple line, inflammation, and delayed epithelialization may then predispose to excessive fibrosis and stricture formation. In contrast, the hand-sewn method allows mucosa-to-mucosa apposition. When minimal tension is applied, a continuous single-layer suture offers coaptation with less risk of tissue strangulation than the stapled method or a two-layered hand-sewn technique. The median time to develop symptomatic stricture was 3 months, and no difference was found when the hand-sewn and stapled methods were compared. Although a nuisance, strictures can be easily and safely dealt with by endoscopic dilatation, with 80% of our patients requiring three or less dilatations.

The hand-sewn method was shown in colorectal cancer to be associated with a higher incidence of anastomotic recurrence and cancer-specific deaths,[112] though we could not confirm this in our study.[87] We have shown that anastomotic recurrence after esophageal resection was a function of resection margin and was uncommon if an adequate margin was obtained.[6,113,114]

For all the reasons mentioned, we recommend the one-layered hand-sewn technique for esophageal anastomosis as it has proved to be a safe, efficacious, and cost-effective method.

Gangrene of esophageal substitute and non-anastomotic leakage

Insufficient blood supply to the esophageal substitute produces ischemic necrosis of the conduit. An early analysis between 1964–1982 in the authors' unit showed an incidence of gangrene of 3.9%,[115] though this has dropped to 1% in recent years.[13] Gangrene was seen almost exclusively when the substitute was brought up to the neck for anastomosis; the relative risk was highest when the colon was used, less for the jejunum, and least for the stomach. These observations reflect the more precarious blood supply to the colon and long jejunal loops, and that a longer route (anastomosis in the neck) used for the conduit.[116,117] The importance of care in preparation of the conduits has been emphasized. In our experience, a redundant stomach can rotate on itself, compressing its blood supply and resulting in fundal gangrene. While prolonged postoperative hypotension from bleeding can be responsible for ischaemia,[13] such complications are avoidable.

Gangrene of the conduit carries with it a high mortality rate of over 70–90%.[115,117] Patients may present with fever and a shock state early after surgery (usually within the first 2 days), while chest drainage may become foul and bile-stained. Consequently, urgent re-exploration is warranted, with treatment following the same lines as discussed under early fulminant leaks. Staged reconstruction is considered later.

Chylothorax

The incidence of chylothorax after esophageal resection ranges from 0.6% to 3.9% and carries with it up to 50% mortality rate.[118–120] The thoracic duct may be damaged at operation because it is relatively collapsed in the fasting state. Increased incidence of chylothorax is reported after transhiatal resection,[119] though in centers experienced with this approach such complication is < 1%.[4] Routine ligation of the thoracic duct is recommended to prevent this complication.[119,121,122] With elective ligation of the thoracic duct, the incidence of chylous fistula was 2.1% compared with 9% without ligation.[121] The preferred site of ligation is the lower thoracic cavity where the duct runs next to the azygos vein and on the aorta. In the event that the duct could not be identified, mass ligation of the tissue between the aorta and azygos vein may be performed.[123]

After esophagectomy, the presentation of chylothorax should be suspected if there is increased drainage from the chest tube. In transhiatal resection, persistent pleural effusion may be found which requires repeated aspiration. The diagnosis may not be obvious since the fluid appears straw-colored or blood-stained in the postoperative fasting state. There may only be signs of low-grade pyrexia. When the pleura was not violated during surgery, unusual presentation of a mediastinal lymph collection has also been reported.[124] The diagnosis may be confirmed by administration of cream by mouth or by the nasogastric tube, which will turn the effluent milky in appearance. Lymphagiography provides useful information concerning the size and site of leak, and may help to distinguish complete transection or partial laceration of the duct.[125,126]

In a healthy adult, the thoracic duct transports up to 4 l of chyle per day. However, in a leak after esophagectomy, its output depends on the size of the leak and dietary intake. The effect of a chyle leak may be asymptomatic at first, apart from the increased drainage volume. Continuous leak leads to loss of protein (in particular albumin), fat, vitamins, and electrolytes. Thus, hyponatremia, acidosis, and hypocalcemia are common and both cell-mediated and humoral immunity are depressed. The patient may be prone to opportunistic infection, so that barrier nursing, sterile procedures, and regular microbiologic surveillance are important.

Management of chylothorax involves drainage of the effusion, correction of electrolyte disturbance, and nutritional support. Dietary oral fat, except medium-chain triglycerides (which bypass the chylous system) is withheld. This, combined with somatostatin analogs, reduces the volume of chylous output, permitting continued diet. Total parenteral nutrition may be required. Depending on the etiology and the damage, conservative treatment may be successful in almost 80% of cases,[127] though chemical pleurodesis has also been reported as effective.[128] Some authors are not in favor of conservative treatment and recommend early re-exploration and ligation of the thoracic duct.[129] and we too, favor early re-exploration.[13,122] Guidelines for surgery may include: chyle leak for >1 l per day for more than 5 days,

persistent leak of more than 2 weeks despite conservative treatment, and nutritional or metabolic complications.[118]

Re-exploration should aim at ligation of the thoracic duct and, if it is difficult to locate, mass ligation of periaortic tissue at the esophageal hiatus should be attempted. Administration of cream, with or without methylene blue, may help to identify the site of leak. Thoracoscopic ligation is reported to produce less morbidity,[130] while fibrin glue, if used under thoracoscopic guidance, can be used to seal leaks and results in minimal morbidity.[131]

Gastric outlet obstruction

Poor gastric emptying after esophagectomy is not only related to long term gastrointestinal symptoms of dysphagia, regurgitation, early satiety and vomiting, but is also related to immediate postoperative events. Delayed gastric emptying is thus associated with a higher incidence of anastomotic leakage, presumably due to gastric distention and tension on the anastomosis.[81] Patients are also more prone to aspiration because of retained gastric fluid.

The need for a drainage procedure for the gastric conduit has been controversial.[132–137] In a prospective randomized trial involving 200 patients undergoing Lewis–Tanner esophagectomy, we showed that in the absence of a pyloroplasty, 13% of patients developed gastric outlet obstruction compared with none in the pyloroplasty group. Long-term studies showed that gastric emptying was faster in the drainage group measured by scintigraphy. Long-term symptoms were worse for the no-drainage group, even at 6 months after surgery.[105] We consider that a drainage procedure is essential to avoid gastric outlet obstrution. No morbidity was experienced at the pyloroplasty site.

Pyloromyotomy is an alternative technique to pyloroplasty in effecting gastric drainage. It has the potential advantages over a pyloroplasty of avoiding disruption of the gastrointestinal mucosa, and so has less risk of leakage. Moreover, by avoiding a suture line at right-angles to the longitudinal axis of the stomach it does not shorten the conduit, resulting in tension at the esophagogastrostomy. In another randomized trial we have demonstrated that both pyloroplasty and pyloromyotomy were equally safe. No leakage occurred at the pyloro-duodenotomy site and the leakage rates at the esophagogastrostomy were both low at 2%. In our experience, a pyloroplasty did not create tension at the esophagogastric anastomosis. The stomach can reach the apex of the thoracic cavity and the neck, an anastomosis can be carried out without tension. Only in reconstruction after pharyngolaryngoesophagectomy (PLE) for hypopharyngeal cancer, when the anastomosis is very much higher in the neck, may a pyloromyotomy be more appropriate.[106] We routinely perform a pyloroplasty after esophagectomy, and a pyloromyotomy after PLE.

Emptying of the intrathoracic stomach depends not only on the presence of a drainage procedure, but also on body position, composition of the meal, and size of the esophageal substitute. Bemelman *et al.*[134] suggested that the rate of gastric emptying was related to the size of the stomach tube rather than the presence of a pyloroplasty. The performance of a drainage procedure may also lead to duodenogastric reflux and chronic active gastritis, and even gastric ulceration.[135] Biliary reflux could be demonstrated after esophagectomy with gastric bile acid aspiration or scintigraphic techniques,[133,135–138a] but there was poor relationship between gastric pathology and symptoms of biliary reflux.[137a,138] An intact pylorus was also no bar to reflux,[137a,138] although in our experience, we have not found bile reflux to be an important clinical problem.

Re-exploration after esophagectomy

Re-exploration after the primary operation is indicative of failure of the primary operation. Our detailed study of the reasons for re-exploration showed that most complications were potentially avoidable, such as a change or modification of the operative procedure. An apparent technical error was identified in 53% of patients who developed anastomotic leakage, and in 40% of patients who developed ischemia of the esophageal conduit. Bleeding was a problem, with inadequate hemostasis at the time of operation, and gastric outlet obstruction alleviated if a routine drainage procedure had been performed. Overall, in two-thirds of patients the complications requiring re-exploration could be ascribed to potentially avoidable technical faults.[13,122] If these errors were recognized and corrected, surgical outcome could be much improved.

Although other surgical complications are less frequently observed, one complication deserves special mention. During esophagectomy, the eso-

phageal hiatus is often enlarged and should be wide enough to prevent compression of the esophageal substitute if it is brought up through the orthotopic route. However, the hiatus should not be too wide to allow herniation of bowel into the chest, and should be closed if the conduit is brought up via another route, e.g., a retrosternal tunnel. A post-esophagectomy patient presenting with intestinal obstruction should have this complication considered. A "pleural effusion" may in fact be fluid filled bowel in the thoracic cavity (**Figures 12.3–12.5**).

ANESTHESIA FOR ESOPHAGEAL SURGERY

Postoperative patient care starts during the operation itself. Of particular importance is anesthesia

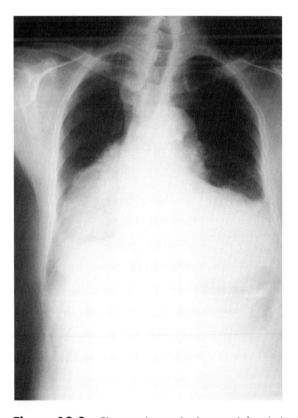

Figure 12.3 Chest radiograph showing left sided "pleural effusion" (which was in fact a fluid-filled bowel in the thoracic cavity) and distended intrathoracic stomach on the right side, as a result of herniation of the bowel through the diaphragmatic hiatus.

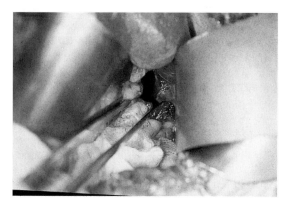

Figure 12.4 Intraoperative photograph showing the hiatus through which bowel has herniated into the chest.

which, if good, contributes significantly to outcome. The availability of an experienced anesthesiologist to place a double-lumen endobronchial tube reduces trauma to the airway. One-lung ventilation allows adequate exposure for the surgeon and makes the thoracic phase of esophageal resec-

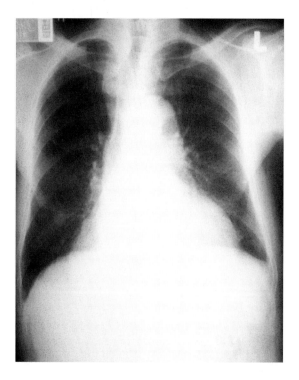

Figure 12.5 Postoperative radiograph showing resolution of the "pleural effusion" and decompression of the stomach.

tion easier and thus less prone to error. However, significant arteriovenous shunting occurs during one-lung ventilation. Episodic hypoxemia (SpO_2 <90%) and severe desaturation (SpO_2 <80%) was found in 50% and 41%, respectively, for patients under one-lung ventilation. Distention of the right lung using oxygen to maintain a continuous positive airway pressure (CPAP) of 5–10 cmH_2O will help to minimize hypoxemia.[139]

If intubation with a double-lumen endobronchial tube is difficult for technical reasons or due to unfavorable airway anatomy, multiple attempts should not be performed to avoid extra trauma. High-frequency jet ventilation using a smaller tidal volume with a single-lumen endotracheal tube should be used. A controlled trial showed that high-frequency ventilation resulted in less hypoxemia during thoracotomy compared with one-lung ventilation,[139] without significantly compromising surgical exposure. Fluid infusion should be adequate to avoid dehydration and hypotension, but not so excessive as to produce fluid overload. Plasma oncotic pressure should be maintained by infusion of albumin concentrate.

After esophagectomy and general anesthesia, the limited preoperative respiratory reserve is further compromised by deterioration in pulmonary mechanics, sputum retention, and immobilization in the immediate postoperative period. Pain aggravates pulmonary complications because it discourages the patient to take deep inspiration, cough effectively, and cooperate with the chest physiotherapist. Pain also causes sympathetic discharge which increases myocardial oxygen consumption (through hypertension and tachycardia) and predisposes to arrhythmia and deep venous thrombosis. Good pain relief enables better pulmonary function, chest expansion, effective cough effort and cooperation with chest physiotherapist.

The best quality of pain relief is achieved with epidural morphine. In a study comparing epidural morphine, epidural fentanyl, or intramuscular morphine for pain relief after esophagectomy, it was shown that epidural morphine was superior to the other two regimens assessed by the total dose of opioid administered, a visual analog scale, and pain score.[140] Since morphine is administered in close proximity to its site of action in the spinal cord, good quality analgesia can be achieved regionally at one-quarter the dose of intravenous morphine.

This is particularly suitable for post-esophagectomy patients, because better analgesia can be achieved with less sedation and other systemic side effects. The epidural catheter at T8 to L3 level is adequate to cover both the thoracotomy and abdominal incisions, since epidural morphine diffuses extensively in cerebrospinal fluid to block higher dermatome levels. Morphine is given early at induction, allowing time for its migration upwards to block the thoracic dermatomes. Subsequent infusion can be started in the recovery room or in the intensive care unit (ICU) and continued for 48 h or longer. One further advantage of an epidural morphine over epidural local anesthetic agent is circulatory stability, as the latter produces sympathetic blockade and may require fluid loading to avert hypotension.

The impact of pain control on outcome after esophagectomy was investigated in a study comparing patients with epidural analgesia or patient-controlled intravenous analgesia with conventional intramuscular opioid for pain relief. Cardiopulmonary complications, the need for postoperative tracheostomy, hospital stay, and mortality were significantly less for the former group. Surgical complications were not significantly different.[141] The benefits of epidural analgesia on outcome after esophagectomy was similarly demonstrated by another study, with respiratory complications decreasing from 30% to 13% after the introduction of epidural analgesia.[142]

The traditional practice of routine ventilatory support after esophagectomy has become obsolete. Patients who had routine overnight ventilation were shown in one study to require prolonged postoperative ventilation and reventilation more often, ICU stay was longer, and hospital mortality was significantly higher compared with patients with early extubation.[143] Preliminary data from a prospective randomized trial comparing early extubation (within 6 h after procedure) with prolonged ventilation (for at least 24 h) showed that early extubation benefited patients who underwent transhiatal resection, the complication rates being 20% and 38%, respectively. No significant difference was found for transthoracic resections.[144] Routine extubation in the operating or recovery room after esophagectomy is practiced in 74% of patients at the authors' institute. The decision for elective ventilation depends on first, preoperative factors, including patients with severe chronic obstructive pulmonary disease and grossly abnormal blood gases, and second, intraoperative factors, including those in whom there has been a technical problem, when the operation is prolonged, and when blood loss is excessive. Preoperative finding of suboptimal lung function is not an absolute indication for postoperative ventilation if the operation is smooth and uneventful. Preoperative indices have not proved to be reliable predictors for successful weaning.[145]

POSTOPERATIVE CARE

It is during the postoperative period that complications have a most visible causal relationship with mortality. The development, early detection, prevention, and management of these complications depend on the vigilance of the surgical and nursing staff, whether this is in an ICU or a specialized ward environment.

Complications that occur in the first 24 h are usually related to bleeding from inadequate hemostasis during surgery, hypotension from insufficient volume replacement, and occasionally respiratory depression in patients with morphine given intravenously or via an epidural catheter. Arrhythmia, usually in the form of atrial fibrillation and supraventricular tachycardia, may occur in the first few days after surgery. Sputum retention, atelectasis, and hypoxia from shunting are common.

If sufficient care has been taken during surgery for hemostasis, bleeding should be avoidable. If bleeding occurs, hypotension may jeopardize the viability of the esophageal substitute. At best, it may lead to anastomotic leakage; at worst gangrene of the loop may result. Hemorrhage may be occult initially, the chest tube drainage may not be excessive, and blood may collect within the pleural cavity. When a right thoracotomy is used for resection, occasionally blood may flow into the left chest when the left-side pleura was breached at operation. Unexpected tachycardia, and a fall in hematocrit should prompt the surgeon to look for sites of bleeding even before the drop in blood pressure. Needle aspiration of the chest and urgent chest radiography may help to locate the bleeding. Unexpected laceration of the spleen during the abdominal phase of the operation may present soon after surgery is finished.

Respiratory complications from sputum retention, atelectasis, and bacterial infection are most common during the first week after surgery, and are still the major causes of death. The preoperative and intraoperative pulmonary care should be carried into the postoperative phase, with chest physiotherapy, incentive spirometry, good pain relief, and avoidance of fluid overload essential. Though unproven, fluid restriction in the early postoperative period and albumin infusion are recommended. In elderly patients where the stress hormone response is blunted, fluid restriction assumes more importance.[16] The urine output in most patients after esophagectomy in the first 48 h will be reduced. This is a normal response to major surgery and we are conservative in administering fluid challenge in order to avoid excessive fluid. In the presence of stable blood pressure, normal preoperative renal function, and if the patient does not appear underperfused, administration of a renal dose of dopamine sometimes helps to improve urine output. Renal failure due to "overdehydration" is very unlikely.

In patients who require ventilator care, early tracheostomy has been shown to reduce duration of ventilation, and ICU and hospital stay compared with translaryngeal intubation.[146] Sputum retention due to poor cough effort may be aided by sputum aspiration by a flexible fiberoptic bronchoscope. A tracheostomy is considered early in selected patients if sputum clearance is suboptimal. A mini-tracheostomy inserted percutaneously is also a good alternative, and has the advantages of being comfortable, minimal air leak, minimal scarring, and preservation of glottic function for expulsive cough, phonation, eating, and drinking. A shorter hospital stay was shown after esophagectomy.[147]

Early ambulation aids pulmonary mechanics recovery, and drains are removed as soon as practicable. In this regard, we have also in recent years employed a small 18-Fr suction drain after thoracotomy in place of the conventional larger Argyle drains. These smaller drains are equally efficacious and allow earlier and easier ambulation after surgery.[148]

Cardiac arrhythmia in the form of atrial fibrillation and supraventricular tachycardia is common, and some authors consider prophylactic digitalization. In our experience, arrhythmia is commonly related to sputum retention and respiratory complications. Although treatment with amiodarone is usually more effective than digitalis, identification and treatment of pulmonary problems and surgical sepsis, when present, are more important.

SUMMARY

Much has improved in the management of esophageal cancer in recent years. While better long-term survival has been difficult to achieve, perioperative mortality has been reduced. Surgical experience, changes in operative techniques and perioperative care with time, have been shown repeatedly to correlate with postoperative outcome.[2,108a,109] In the authors' experience, hospital mortality rates have fallen from 16% (1982–1986), to 13% (1987–1991), and to 6% (1992–1996). Indeed, in the last few years, the mortality rate has been 2%.

It cannot be overemphasized that progress in preoperative assessment, perioperative care and surgical technique has been derived from the experience and vigilance of physicians, anesthesiologists, surgeons, and nurses alike. Moreover, with further refinement, it is hoped that mortality can be eliminated after esophagectomy.

REFERENCES

1. Earlam R & Cunha-Melo JR Oesophageal squamous cell carcinoma: I A critical review of surgery. *Br J Surg* 1980; **67**: 381–90.
2. Muller JM, Erasmi H, Stelzner M, Zieren U & Pichlmaier H. Surgical therapy of oesophageal carcinoma. *Br J Surg* 1990; **77**: 845–57.
3. O'Rourke I, Tatt N, Bull C, Gebski V, Holland M & Johnson DC. Oesophagael cancer: outcome of modern surgical managment. *Aust N Z J Surg* 1995; **65**: 11–16.
4. Orringer MB, Marshall B & Stirling MC. Transhiatal esophagectomy for benign and malignant disease. *J Thorac Cardiovasc Surg* 1993; **105**: 265–76.
5. DeMeester TR, Zaninotto G & Johansson KE. Selective therapeutic approach to cancer of the lower esophagus and cardia. *J Thorac Cardiovasc Surg* 1988; **95**: 42–54.
6. Law SY, Fok M, Cheng SW & Wong J. A comparison of outcome after resection for squamous cell carcinomas and adenocarcinomas of the esophagus and cardia. *Surg Gynecol Obstet* 1992; **175**: 107–12.
7. Zhang DW, Cheng GY, Huang GJ *et al.* Operable squamous esophageal cancer: current results from the East. *World J Surg* 1994; **18**: 347–54.

8. Watson A. Operable esophageal cancer: current results from the west. *World J Surg* 1994; **18**: 361–6.

9. Bumm R. Staging and risk-analysis in esophageal carcinoma. *Dis Esoph* 1996; **9**: 20–9.

10. Liedman BL, Bennegard K, Olbe LC & Lundell LR. Predictors of postoperative morbidity and mortality after surgery for gastro-oesophageal carcinomas. *Eur J Surg* 1995; **161**: 173–80.

11. Griffin S, Desai J, Charlton M, Townsend E & Fountain SW Factors influencing mortality and morbidity following oesophageal resection. *Eur J Cardiothorac Surg* 1989; **3**: 419–23.

12. Ferguson MK, Martin TR, Reeder LB, Olak J & Mick R. Determinants of pulmonary complications following esophagectomoy. In: Peracchia A, Rosati R, Bonavina L, Fumagalli U, Bona, S & Chella B. (eds) *Recent Advances in Diseases of the Esophagus*. Bologna: Monduzzi Editore 1996: 527–32.

13. Law SY, Fok M & Wong J. Risk analysis in resection of squamous cell carcinoma of the esophagus. *World J Surg* 1994; **18**: 339–46.

14. Tsutsui S, Moriguchi S, Morita M *et al.* Multivariate analysis of postoperative complications after esophageal resection. *Ann Thorac Surg* 1992; **53**: 1052–6.

15. Fan ST, Lau WF, Yip WC *et al.* Prediction of postoperative pulmonary complications in oesophagogastric cancer surgery. *Br J Surg* 1987; **74**: 408–10.

16. Nishi M, Hiramatsu Y, Hioki K *et al.* Risk factors in relation to postoperative complications in patients undergoing esophagectomy or gastrectomy for cancer. *Ann Surg* 1988; **207**: 148–54.

17. Peracchia A, Bardini R, Ruol A *et al.* Carcinoma of the esophagus in the elderly (70 years of age or older). Indications and results of surgery. *Dis Esoph* 1988; **1**: 147-52.

18. Poon R, Law S, Chu KM, Branicki FJ & Wong J. Esophagectomy for carcinoma of the esophagus in the elderly: results of current surgical management. *Ann Surg* 1997; **227**: 357–64.

19. Nishi M, Hiramatsu Y, Hioki K, Htano T & Yamamoto M. Pulmonary complications after subtotal oesophagectomy. *Br J Surg* 1988; **75**: 527–30.

20. Nagawa H, Kobori O & Muto T. Prediction of pulmonary complications after transthoracic oesophagectomy. *Can J Surg* 1994; **81**: 860–2.

21. Hennessy TPJ. Respiratory complications in oesophageal surgery. In: Peracchia A, Rosati R, Bonavina L, Fumagalli U, Bona S & Chella B. (eds) *Recent Advances in Diseases of the Esophagus*. Bologna: Monduzzi Editore 1996: 533–5.

22. Daly JM, Redmond HP & Gallagher H. Perioperative nutrition in cancer patients. *J Parenter Enteral Nutr* 1992; **16**: 100S–105S.

23. DeWys WE, Begg C, Lavin PT *et al.* Prognostic effect of weight loss prior to chemotherapy in cancer patients. *Am J Med* 1980; **69**: 491–7.

24. Windsor JA & Hill GL. Risk factors for post-operative pneumonia: the importance of protein depletion. *Ann Surg* 1988; **208** 209–14.

25. Belghiti J & Fekete F. Surgical implications of malnutrition and immunodeficiency in patients with carcinoma of the oesophagus. *Br J Surg* 1983; **70**, 339–341.

26. Fekete F & Belghiti J. Nutrition factors and oesophageal resection. In: Jamieson, GG. (ed.) *Surgery of the Oesophagus*. Edinburgh: Churchill Livingstone 1988: 110–24.

27. Brandmair W, Lehr L & Siewert JR. Nutritional status in esophageal cancer: assessment and significance for preoperative risk assessment. *Langenbecks Arch Chir* 1989; **374**: 25–31.

28. Saito T, Shimoda K, Kinoshita T *et al.* Prediction of operative mortality based on impairment of host defense systems in patients with esophageal cancer. *J Surg Oncol* 1993; **52**: 1–8.

29. Fan ST, Lau WY, Wong KK & Chan YPM. Preoperative parenteral nutrition in patients with oesophageal cancer: a prospective, randomised, clinical trial. *Clin Nutr* 1989; **8**: 23–7.

30. Kakegawa T, Fujita H & Yamana H. Illustrations of surgery for carcinoma in the thoracic esophagus. In: Sato T & Lizuka T. (eds) *Color Atlas of Surgical Anatomy for Esophageal Cancer*. Tokyo: Springer-Verlag 1992: 91–116.

31. Pettigrew RA & Hill GL. Indicators of surgical risk and clinical judgement. *Br J Surg* 1986; **73**: 47–51.

32. Fekete F, Belghiti J, Cherqui D, Langonnet F & Gayet B. Results of esophagogastrectomy for carcinoma in cirrhotic patients: a series of 23 consecutive patients. *Ann Surg* 1987; **206**: 74–8.

33. Belghiti J, Cherqui D, Langonnet F & Fekete F. Esophagogastrectomy for carcinoma in cirrhotic patients. *Hepatogastroenterology* 1990; **37**: 388–91.

34. Ruol A, Rossi M, Baldan N *et al.* Esophageal and cardial cancers concomitant with liver cirrhosis: prevalence and treatment results in 273 consecutive cases. In: Peracchia A, Bonavina

L, Fumagalli U, Bona S & Chella B. (eds) *Recent advances in diseases of the esophagus.* Bologna: Monduzzi Editore 1996: 183–8.

35. Horvath OP & Lukacs L. Palliative resection and bypass surgery. *Dis Esoph* 1996; **9**: 117–22.

36. Moghissi K. Surgical resection for stage I cancer of the oesophagus and cardia. *Br J Surg* 1992; **79**: 935–7.

37. Bonavina L. Early oesophageal cancer: results of a European multicentre survey. *Br J Surg* 1995; **82**: 98–101.

38. Windsor JA & Hill GL Weight loss with physiologic impairment – a basic indicator of surgical risk. *Ann Surg* 1988; **207**: 290–6.

39. Muehrcke DD, Kaplan D & Donnelly RJ. Oesophagogastrectomy in patients over 70. *Thorax* 1989; **44**: 141–5.

40. Lund O, Kimose HH, Aagaard MT, Hasenkam JM & Erlandsen M. Risk stratification and long-term results after surgical treatment of carcinomas of the thoracic esophagus and cardia – A 25-year retrospective study. *J Thorac Cardiovasc Surg* 1990; **99**: 200–9.

41. Imdahl A, Munzar T, Schulte-Monting J, Ruckauer KD, Kirchner R & Farthmann EH. Perioperative risk factors in esophageal cancer: a prospective study of independent variables. *Zentralbl-Chir* 1993; **118**: 190–6.

42. Hall JC, Tarala R, Harris J, Tapper J & Christiansen K. Incentive spirometry versus routine chest physiotherapy for prevention of pulmonary complications after abdominal surgery. *Lancet* 1991; **337**: 953–6.

43. Daly JM, Massar E, Giacco G *et al.* Parenteral nutrition in esophageal cancer patients. *Ann Surg* 1982; **196**: 203–8.

44. Muller JM, Dienst C & Brenner U. Preoperative parenteral feeding in patients with gastrointestinal carcinoma. *Lancet* 1982; **1**: 68.

45. Moghissi K, Hornshaw J, Teasdale PR & Dawes EA. Parenteral nutrition in carcinoma of the oesophagus treated by surgery: nitrogen balance and clinical studies. *Br J Surg* 1977; **64**: 125.

46. Lim STK, Choa RG, Lam KH, Wong J & Ong GB. Total parenteral nutrition versus gastrostomy in the preoperative preparation of patients with carcinoma of the oesophagus. *Br J Surg* 1981; **68**: 69–72.

47. Buzby GP. Perioperative total parenteral nutrition in surgical patients. *N Engl J Med* 1991; **325**: 525–32.

48. Page CP. The surgeon and gut maintenance. *Am J Surg* 1989; **158**: 485–94.

49. Baigrie RJ, Devitt PG & Watkin S. Enteral versus parenteral nutrition after oesophagogastric surgery: a prospective randomized comparison. *Aust N Z J Surg* 1996; **66**: 668–70.

50. Gerndt SJ & Orringer MB. Tube jejunostomy as an adjunct to esophagogastrectomy. *Surgery* 1994; **115**: 164–9.

51. Swails WS, Baineau TJ, Ellis FH, Kenler AS & Forse RA. The role of enteral jejunostomy feeding after esophagectomy: a prospective, randomized study. *Dis Esoph* 1995; **8**: 193–9.

52. Christie PM & Hill GL. Effect of intravenous nutrition and function in acute attacks of inflammatory bowel disease. *Gastroenterology* 1990; **99**: 730–6.

53. Sugimachi K, Kitamura M, Maekawa S, Matsufuji H, Kai H & Okudaira Y. Two-stage operation for poor risk patients with carcinoma of the esophagus. *J Surg Oncol.* 1987; **36**: 105–9.

54. Katariya K, Harvey JC, Pina E & Beattie EJ. Complications of transhiatal esophagectomy. *J Surg Oncol* 1994; **57**: 157–63.

55. Mathisen DJ, Grillo HC, Wilkins E, Jr, Moncure AC & Hilgenberg AD. Transthoracic esophagectomy: a safe approach to carcinoma of the esophagus. *Ann Thorac Surg* 1988; **45**: 137–43.

56. Bolton J, Sardi A, Bowen J & Ellis J. Transhiatal and transthoracic esophagectomy: a comparative study. *J Surg Oncol* 1992; **51**: 249–53.

57. Tilanus HW, Hop WC, Langenhorst BL & van-Lanschot JJ. Esophagectomy with or without thoracotomy. Is there any difference? *J. Thorac Cardiovasc Surg* 1993; **105**: 898–903.

58. Hankins JR, Attar S, Coughlin TRJ *et al.* Carcinoma of the esophagus: a comparison of the results of transhiatal versus transthoracic resection. *Ann Thorac Surg* 1989; **47**, 700-705.

59. Fok M, Law S, Stipa F, Cheng S & Wong J A comparison of transhiatal and transthoracic resection for oesophageal carcinoma. *Endoscopy.* 1993; **25**: 660–3.

60. Goldminc M, Maddern G, Le Prise E, Meunier B, Campion JP & Launois B. Oesophagectomy by a transhiatal approach or thoracotomy: a prospective randomized trial. *Br J Surg* 1993; **80**: 367–70.

61. Chu KM, Law SYK, Fok M & Wong J. A prospective randomized comparison of transthoracic and transhiatal resection for lower-third esophageal carcinoma. *Am J Surg* 1997; **174**: 320–4.

62. Hurley JP & Keeling P. Transhiatal oesophagectomy – its role for tumours of the middle

third of the intrathoracic oesophagus. *Ir Med J* 1990; **83**: 23–5.

63. Bumm R, Holscher AH, Feussner H, Tachibana M, Bartels H & Siewert, J. Endodissection of the thoracic esophagus. Technique and clinical results in transhiatal esophagectomy. *Ann Surg* 1993; **1**: 97–104.

64. Fumagalli U. Resective surgery for cancer of the thoracic esophagus. Results of a Consensus Conference held at the VIth World Congress of the International Society for Diseases of the Esophagus. *Dis Esoph* 1996; **9**: 30–8.

65. Sadanaga N, Kuwano H, Watanabe M *et al.* Laparoscopy-assisted surgery: a new technique for transhiatal esophageal dissection. *Am J Surg* 1994; **168**: 355–7.

66. Perniceni T, Boudet M, Le Guillou J, Laurent P & Gayet B. Laparoscopic gastrolysis and esogastric resection for esophageal cancer. A prospective study in 27 patients. *O. E. S. O. Fifth World Polydisciplinary Congress. The Esophagogastric Junction. Paris. V30* (Abstract), 1996.

67. DePaula A, Hashiba K, Ferreira E, DePaula R & Grecco E. Laparoscopic transhiatal esophagectomy with esophagogastroplasty. *Surg Laparosc Endosc* 1995; **5**: 1–5.

68. Law S, Fok M, Chu KM & Wong J. Thoracoscopic esophagectomy for esophageal cancer. *Surgery* 1997; **122**: 8–14.

69. Nishihira T, Mori S & Hirayama K. Extensive lymph node dissection for thoracic esophageal carcinoma. *Dis Esoph* 1992; **5**: 79–90.

70. Liebermann-Meffert D and Siewert JR. Surgical aspects regarding the distribution of the recurrent laryngeal nerves (RLN) in esophagogastric anastomosis. In: *Recent Advances in Diseases of the Esophagus.* Bologna: Monduzzi Editore 1996: 199–202.

71. Bartels H, Thorban S & Siewert JR. Anterior versus posterior reconstruction after transhiatal oesophagectomy: a randomized controlled trial. *Br J Surg* 1993; **80**: 1141–4.

72. Hsu HK, Hsu WH & Huang MH. Prospective study of using fibrin glue to prevent leak from esophagogastric anastomosis. *J Surg Assoc Republic of China* 1992; **25**: 1248–52.

73. Urschel JD. Esophagogastrostomy anastomotic leaks complicating esophagectomy: A review. *Am J Surg* 1995; **169**: 634–40.

74. Salo JA, Perhoniemi VJ & Heikkinen LO. Pulse oximetry for the assessment of gastric tube circulation in esophageal replacements. *Am J Surg* 1992; **163** 446–7.

75. Ueo H, Abe R, Takeuchi H, Arinaga S & Akiyoshi T A reliable operative precedure for preparing a sufficiently nourished gastric tube for esophageal reconstruction. *Am J Surg* 1993; **165**: 273–6.

76. Hirabayashi S, Miyata M, Shoji M & Shibusawa H. Reconstruction of the thoracic esophagus, with extended jejunum used as a substitute, with the aid of microvascular anastomosis. *Surgery* 1993; **113**: 515–19.

77. Akiyama S, Ito, S, Sekiguchi H. *et al.* Preoperative embolization of gastric arteries for esophageal cancer. *Surgery*, 1996; **120**: 542–6.

78. Liebermann-Meffert DMI, Meier R & Siewert JR. Vascular anatomy of the gastric tube used for esophageal reconstruction. *Ann Thorac Surg* 1992; **54**: 1110–15.

79. Siewert JR, Stein HJ, Liebermann-Meffert D & Bartels H. Esophageal reconstruction: the gastric tube as esophageal substitute. *Dis Esoph* 1995; **8**: 11–19.

80. Peters JH, Kronson JW, Katz M & DeMeester TR. Arterial anatomic considerations in colon interposition for esophageal replacement. *Arch Surg.* 1995; **130**: 858–63.

81. Dewar L, Gelfand G, Finley RJ, Evans K, Inculet R & Nelems B. Factors affecting cervical anastomotic leak and stricture formation following esophagogastrectomy and gastric tube interposition. *Am J Surg* 1992; **163**: 484–9.

82. Peracchia A, Bardini R, Ruol A, Asolati M & Scibetta D. Esophagovisceral anastomotic leak. A prospective statistical study of predisposing factors. *J Thorac Cardiovasc Surg* 1988 **95**: 685–91.

83. Hopkins RA, Alexander JC & Postlethwait RW. Stapled esophagogastric anastomosis. *Am J Surg* 1984; **147**: 283–7.

84. Fekete F, Breil PH, Ronsse H, Tossen JC & Langonnet F. EEA stapler and omental graft in esophagogastrectomy: experience with 30 intrathoracic anastomoses for cancer. *Ann Surg* 1981; **193**: 825–30.

85. Wong J. Stapled esophagogastric anastomosis in the apex of the right chest after subtotal esophagectomy for carcinoma. *Surg Gynecol Obstet* 1987; **164**: 568–72.

86. Lorentz T, Fok M & Wong J. Anastomotic leakage after resection and bypass for esophageal cancer: lessons learned from the past. *World J Surg* 1989; **13**: 472–7.

87. Law S, Fok M, Chu KM & Wong J. Comparison of hand-sewn and stapled esophagogastric

anastomosis after esophageal resection for cancer: A prospective randomized controlled trial. *Ann. Surg* 1997; **226**: 169–73.

88. Bardini R, Bonavina L, Asolati M, Ruol A, Castoro C & Tiso E. Single-layered cervical esophageal anastomoses: a prospective study of two suturing techniques. *Ann Thorac Surg* 1994; **58**: 1087–90.

89. Fok M, Ah Chong AK, Cheng SW & Wong J Comparison of a single layer continuous hand-sewn method and circular stapling in 580 oesophageal anastomoses. *Br J Surg* 1991; **78**: 342–5.

90. Zieren HU, Muller JM & Pichlmaier H. Prospective randomized study of one- or two-layer anastomosis following oesophageal resection and cervical oesophagogastrostomy. *Br J Surg* 1993; **80**: 608–11.

91. Goldsmith HS, Kiely AA & Randall HT. Protection of intrathoracic esophageal anastomoses by omentum. *Surgery* 1968; **63**: 464–8.

92. Chasseray VM, Kiroff GK, Buard JL & Launois B. Cervical or thoracic anastomisis for esophagectomy for carcinoma. *Surg Gynecol Obstet* 1989; **169**: 55–62.

93. Shahian DM, Neptune WB, Ellis FHJ & Watkins EJ. Transthoracic versus extrathoracic esophagectomy: mortality, morbidity, and long term survival. *Ann Thorac Surg* 1986; **41**: 237–46.

94. Patil P, Patel S, Mistry R, Deshpande R & Desai P. Cancer of the esophagus: esophagogastric anastomotic leak – a retrospective study of predisposing factors. *J Surg Oncol.* 1992; **49**: 163–7.

95. Giuli R & Gignoux M. Treatment of carcinoma of the esophagus: retrospective study of 2400 patients. *Ann Surg* 1980; **192**:44–52.

96. Goldfaden D, Orringer MB, Appelman HD & Kalish R. Adenocarcinoma of the distal esophagus and gastric cardia: comparison of results of transhiatal esophagectomy and thoracoabdominal esophagogastrectomy. *J Thorac Cardiovasc Surg* 1986; **91**: 242–7.

97. Lam TC, Fok M, Cheng SW & Wong J. Anastomotic complications after esophagectomy for cancer. A comparison of neck and chest anastomoses. *J Thorac Cardiovasc Surg* 1992; **104**: 395–400.

98. Hermreck A & Crawford D. The esophageal anastomotic leak. *Am J Surg* 1976; **132**: 794.

99. Lam TCF, Fok M, Cheng SWK & Wong J. Anastomotic leakage following oesophageal reconstruction using whole stomach and distal stomach. *Gullet* 1991; **1**: 114–18.

100. Wilson SE, Stone R, Scully M, Ozeran L & Benfield JR. Modern management of anastomotic leak after esophagogastrectomy. *Am J Surg* 1982; **144**: 95–101.

101. Orringer MB & Sloan H. Substernal bypass of the excluded thoracic esophagus for palliation of esophageal carcinoma. *J Thorac Cardiovasc Surg* 1975; **70**: 836–51.

102. DeMeester TR, Johansson KE, Franze I *et al.* Indications, surgical technique, and long-term functional results of colon interposition or bypass. *Ann Surg* 1998; **208**: 460–73.

103. Wong J & Fok M. The esophageal anastomosis in excision of the esophagus. In: Nyhus L, Baker R & Fischer J. (eds) *Mastery of Surgery.* 3rd edn. Boston: Little, Brown and Company 1996: 793–801.

104. Wong J, Cheung HC, Lui R, Fan YW, Smith A & Siu KF. Esophagogastric anastomosis performed with a stapler: the occurence of leakage and stricture. *Surgery* 1987; **101**: 408–15.

105. Fok M, Cheng SW & Wong J. Pyloroplasty versus no drainage in gastric replacement of the esophagus. *Am J Surg* 1991; **162**: 447–52.

106. Law S, Cheung MC, Fok M, Chu KM & Wong J. Pyloroplasty and pyloromytomy in gastric replacement of the esophagus after esophagectomy: a prospective randomized controlled trial. *J. Am Coll Surg* 1997; **184**: 630–6.

107. Orringer MB. Complications of esophageal resection and reconstruction. In: Waldhausen JA & Orringer MB (eds) *Complications in Cardiothoracic Surgery.* St. Louis: Mosby Year Book 1991: 354–69.

108. Jorgensen JO & Hunt DR. Endoscopic drainage of esophageal suture line leaks. *Am J Surg* 1993; **165**: 362–4.

108a. Swisher SG, Hunt KK, Holmes C, Zinner MJ, & McFadden DW. Changes in the surgical management of esophageal cancer from 1970 to 1993. *Am. J Surg* 1995; **169**: 609–14.

109. Matthews HR, Powell DJ & McConkey CC. Effect of surgical experience on the results of resection for oesophageal carcinoma. *Br J Surg* 1986; **73**: 621.

110. Bardini R, Asolati M, Ruol A, Bonavina L, Baseggio S & Peracchia, A. Anastomosis. *World J Surg* 1994; **18**: 373–8.

111. Wang LS, Huang MH, Huang BS & Chien KY. Gastric substitution for resectable carcinoma of the esophagus: an analysis of 368 cases. *Ann Thorac Surg* 1992; **53**: 289–94.

112. Akyol AM, McGregor JR, Galloway DJ, Murray G & George WD. Recurrence of colorectal

cancer after sutured and stapled large bowel anastomosis. *Br J Surg* 1991; **78**: 1297–300.

113. Tam PC, Siu KF, Cheung HC, Ma L & Wong J. Local recurrences after subtotal esophagectomy for squamous cell carcinoma. *Ann Surg* 1987; **205**: 189–94.

114. Law SY, Fok M & Wong J. Pattern of recurrence after oesophageal resection for cancer. Clinical implications. *Br J Surg* 1996; **83**: 107–111.

115. Moorehead RJ & Wong J. Gangrene in esophageal substitutes after resection and bypass procedures for carcinoma of the esophagus. *Hepatogastroenterology* 1990; **37**: 364–7.

116. Ngan SYK & Wong J. Lengths of different routes for esophageal replacement. *J Thorac Cardiovasc Surg* 1986; **91**: 790–2.

117. Hanaoka T, Nakata Y, Hamakubo S *et al.* Necrosis in esophageal reconstruction organs after esophageal cancer resection. In: Peracchia A, Rosati R, Bonavina L, Fumagalli U, Bona S & Chella B. (eds) *Recent Advances in Diseases of the Esophagus*. Bologna: Monduzzi Editore 1996: 267–71.

118. Merrigan BA, Winter DC & O'Sullivan GC. Chylothorax. *Br J Surg* 1997; **84**: 15–20.

119. Bolger C, Walsh T, Keeling P & Hennessy T. Chylothorax after oesophagectomy. *Br J Surg* 1991; **78**: 587–8.

120. Lam KH, Lim STK, Wong J & Ong GB. Chylothorax following resection of the oesophagus. *Br J Surg* 1979; **66**: 105–9.

121. Dougenis D, Walker W, Cameron EW & Walbaum ER. Management of chylothorax complicating extensive oesophageal surgery. *Surg Gynecol Obstet* 1992; **174**: 501–6.

122. Tam PC, Fok M & Wong J. Reexploration for complications after esophagectomy for cancer. *J Thorac Cardiovasc Surg* 1989; **98**: 1122–7.

123. Patterson GA, Todd T, Delarue N, Ilves R, Pearson F & Cooper JD. Supradiaphragmatic ligation of the thoracic duct in intractable chylous fistula. *Ann Thorac Surg* 1981; **32**: 44–9.

124. Lautin JL, Baran S, Dumitrescu O, Sakurai H, Halpern N & Lautin EM. Loculated mediastinal chylothorax resulting from esophagogastrectomy: a case report. *J Thorac Imaging* 1993; **8**: 313–15.

125. Sachs PB, Zelch M, Rice T, Geisinger M, Risius B & Lammert GK. Diagnosis and localization of laceration of the thoracic duct: usefulness of lymphangiography and CT. *Am J Roentgenol* 1991; **157**: 703–5.

126. Ngan H, Fok M & Wong J. The role of lymphography in chylothorax following thoracic surgery. *Br J Radiol* 1988; **61**: 1032–6.

127. Marts BC, Naunheim K, Fiore A & Pennington D. Conservative versus surgical management of chylothorax. *Am J Surg* 1992; **164**: 532–4.

128. Nakano A, Kato M, Watanabe T *et al.* OK-432 chemical pleurodesis for the treatment of persistent chylothorax. *Hepatogastroenterology* 1994; **41**: 568–70.

129. Orringer MB, Bluett M & Deeb GM. Aggressive treatment of chylothorax complicating transhiatal oesophagectomy without thoracotomy. *Surgery* 1988; **104**: 720–6.

130. Kent RP & Pinson RW. Thoracoscopic ligation of the thoracic duct. *Surg Endosc* 1993; **7**: 52–3.

131. Inderbitzi RG, Krebs T, Stirneman T & Althaus U. Treatment of postoperative chylothorax by fibrin glue application under thoracoscopic view with the use of local anaesthetic. *J Thorac Cardiovasc Surg* 1994; **104**: 209–10.

132. Finley RJ, Lamy A, Clifton J, Evans KG, Fradet G & Nelems B. Gastrointestinal function following esophagectomy for malignancy. *Am J Surg* 1995; **169**: 471–5.

133. Bonavina L, Anselmino M, Ruol A, Bardini R, Borsato N & Peracchia, A. Functional evaluation of the intrathoracic stomach as an oesophageal substitute. *Br J Surg* 1992; **79**: 529–32.

134. Bemelman WA, Taat CW, Slors JFM, van Lanschot JJB & Obertop H. Delayed postoperative emptying after esophageal resection is dependent on the size of the gastric substitute. *J Am Coll Surg* 1995; **180**: 461–4.

135. Hinder RA. The effect of posture on the emptying of the intrathoracic vagotomized stomach. *Br J Surg* 1976; **63**: 581–4.

136. Gupta S, Chattopadhyay TK, Gopinath PG Kapoor VK & Sharma LK. Emptying of the intrathoracic stomach with and without pyloroplasty. *Am J Gastroenterol* 1989; **84**: 921–3.

137. Chattopadhyay TK, Gupta S, Padhy AK & Kapoor VK. Is pyloroplasty necessary following intrathoracic transposition of stomach? Results of a prospective clinical study. *Aust NZ J Surg* 1991; **61**: 366–69.

137a. Chattopadhyay TK, Shad SK & Kumar A. Intragastric bile acid and symptoms in patients with an intrathoracic stomach after oesophagectomy. *Br J Surg* 1993; **80**: 371–3.

138. Mannell A, Hinder RA & San-Garde BA. The thoracic stomach: a study of gastric emptying, bile reflux and mucosal change. *Br J Surg* 1984 **71**: 438–41.

138a.   Holscher A, Voit H, Buttermann G & Siewert J. Function of the intrathoracic stomach as esophageal substitute. *World J Surg* 1988; **12**: 835–44.

139.   Tsui SL, Chan CS, Chan ASH, Wong SJ, Lam CS & Jones RDM. A comparison of two-lung high frequency positive pressure ventilation and one-lung ventilation plus 5cm H_2O non-ventilated lung CPAP, in patients undergoing anaesthesia for oesophagectomy. *Anaesth Intens Care* 1991; **19**: 205–12.

140.   Tsui SL, Chan CS, Chan ASH, Wong SJ, Lam CS & Jones RDM. Postoperative analgesia for oesophageal surgery: a comparison of three analgesic regimens. *Anaesth Intens Care* 1991; **19**: 329–37.

141.   Tsui S, Law S, Fok M *et al.* Postoperative analgesia reduces morbidity and mortality after esophagectomy. *Am J Surg* 1997; **173**: 472–8.

142.   Watson A & Allen PR. Influence of thoracic epidural analgesia on outcome after resection for esophageal cancer. *Surgery* 1994; **115**: 429–32.

143.   Caldwell MTP, Murphy PG, Page R, Walsh TN & Hennessy TPJ. Timing of extubation after esophagectomy. *Br J Surg* 1993; **80**: 1537–9.

144.   Bartels H, Stein H & Siewert JR. Early extubation versus prolonged ventilation after esophagectomy: a randomized prospective study. In: Peracchia A, Rosati R, Bonavina L, Fumagalli U, Bona S & Chella B. (eds) *Recent Advances in Diseases of the Esophagus.* Bologna: Monduzzi Editore: 537–39.

145.   Yang K & Tobin M. A prospective study of indices predicting the outcome of trials of weaning from mechanical ventilation. *N Engl J Med* 1991; **324**: 1445–50.

146.   Rodriguez JL, Steinberg SM, Luchetti FA, Gibbons KJ, Taheri PA & Flint LM. Early tracheostomy for primary airway management in the surgical critical care setting. *Br J Surg* 1990; **77**: 1406–10.

147.   Van Raemdonck D, Coosemans W, De Leyn P, Deneffe G & Lerut T. Experience with minitracheostomy following oesophageal resection. In: Peracchia A, Rosati R, Bonavina L, Fumagalli U, Bona S & Chella B. (eds) *Recent Advances in Diseases of the Esophagus.* Bologna: Monduzzi Editore 1996: 542–5.

148.   Lau H, Law S & Wong J. Prospective evaluation of vacuum plerual drainage after thoracotomy in patients with carcinoma of the esophagus. *Arch Surg* 1997; **132**: 749–52.

PART

4

Palliation

13
RADIATION

LAWRENCE R. COIA
ROBERT IVKER

ESOPHAGEAL CANCER

INTRODUCTION

The need for palliation of symptoms from esophageal cancer is a not uncommon problem faced by physicians. Significant detriments to quality of life are often caused by these malignancies in their advanced stage, and unfortunately most patients present with advanced malignancies. Pain, weight loss, difficulty with swallowing, or bleeding lead patients and their physicians to seek rapid methods of relief.

Despite the need for rapid palliation, the physician must take time to establish reasonable goals for palliation and choose treatment judiciously. Whereas in the past surgical resection or bypass were two of only few options for palliation, there are presently a variety of options available. Among highly effective means for palliating esophageal cancer is chemotherapy combined with radiation. This along with other options are further described in this chapter.

Patients with carcinoma of the esophagus often present at an advanced stage when palliation is the only reasonably achievable goal. However, even patients with potentially curable cancers (1983 AJC Stage I or II), significant swallowing problems often exist. The technical and clinical emergencies faced in the palliation of esophageal cancer are similar, whether the cancer is early or advanced. Furthermore, since cancer of the esophagus afflicts the older and more debilitated population, patient tolerance to treatment is also a particularly important consideration.

CLINICAL PRESENTATION

The modal decade of life at presentation with cancer of the esophagus is between 60 and 70 years, with a median age of 66 years.[1] The overall incidence rate in the United States is approximately 5 per 100 000, with a mortality rate which approaches that of the incidence rate. The mortality rate increases with age. In Japan, for example, the mortality rate for patients over 80 years of age is 78 per 100 000 in men and 24 per 100 000 in women.[2] Clinically, patients frequently present with symptoms of weight loss and dysphagia. Although a period of weight loss of 6 months or more prior to diagnosis is not uncommon, the amount lost before treatment is important. For example, a weight loss >10% was associated with a median survival of only 6 months, while a median survival of 15 months was reported for weight loss of <10%.[3] When the esophageal lumen circumference progressively decreases to below one-third of its normal size, dysphagia for first solids, then liquids, is usually described. A typical distribution of symptom status at presentation for radiation treatment is shown in **Table 13.1**.[4] Less than 5% of patients are completely obstructed and cannot swallow anything at presentation, while 5% are without dysphagia on presentation. Radial growth into the trachea or bronchus may result in hemoptysis or a fistula formation. Involvement of the recurrent laryngeal nerve may lead to hoarseness and therefore examination of the larynx is essential in evaluation. Symptoms of pleural effusion, sympathetic nerve involvement, phrenic nerve involvement, or percardial involvement are much less common. With

Table 13.1 Swallowing status before and at maximal improvement after radiation treatment

	SWALLOWING STATUS	
SWALLOWING SCORE	NO. OF PATIENTS BEFORE TREATMENT (%)	NO. OF PATIENTS AT MAXIMAL IMPROVEMENT (%)
1 Asymptomatic	5 (4)	85 (71)
2 Eats solids with some dysphagia	48 (40)	16 (13)
3 Eats soft or puréed foods only	50 (42)	3 (2.5)
4 Drinks liquids only	8 (7)	2 (1.6)
5 No swallowing at all	5 (4)	0 (0)
x Unknown	4 (3.5)	14 (11.7)

Reproduced from Coia et al.[4]

complete obstruction of the esophagus patients may also have problems with difficulty in swallowing saliva, which can result in aspiration of saliva and potential development of pulmonary complications. Debatably, a pharyngostomy may be useful in such patients to prevent problems with aspiration, though such a procedure is also associated with morbidity and is not easily handled by the patient.

GOALS OF PALLIATION

The median survival of patients with esophageal cancer is 12–18 months,[5–7] though patients with extraesophageal extension of cancer or distant metastases have a median survival of only 5–8 months.[8] Therefore, treatment goals of palliation need to include rapid, lasting improvements of symptoms and the treatment must not be a burden to the patient in terms of time, commitment, or morbidity. The use of radiation alone, chemoradiation, and endocavitary radiation will be discussed below, highlighting – when possible – their palliative benefits.

RADIATION ALONE

External beam radiation alone has been shown to be an effective palliative modality for advanced esophageal cancer, resulting in rates of palliation of dysphagia of 52% to 76% and duration of dysphagia palliation of 5–10 months (**Table 13.2**) Wara et al.[12] reported significant relief of dysphagia in two-thirds of patients with a mean dysphagia-free interval of 6 months and median survival of 7 months. A dose response for palliation has been noted,[13,14] with patients treated to doses of 45–50 Gy (or higher) having a greater rate of palliation than when lower doses were used. Langer et al. used >50 Gy in 80% and >60 Gy in 60% of patients treated with radiation at Massachusetts General Hospital, and found that 60% had dysphagia relief with a median duration of 4.5 months.[10] The actuarial survival rate was 11% at 2 years, with a median of 8.8 months. Complications including

Table 13.2 Radiation therapy for palliation of esophageal cancer

REFERENCE	NO. OF PATIENTS	XRT DOSE FX	PALLIATION (%)	DURATION OF PALLIATION
Wara et al.[12]	169	50–60 Gy	66	Mean 6 months
Langer et al.[10]	44	56–60 Gy	60	Median 4.5 months
Petrovich et al.[11]	133	55 Gy	52	34% > 6 months
Caspers et al.[13]	127		76	
	52	< 50 Gy/5 wk		Median 5 months
	75	≥ 50 Gy/5 wk		Median 10 months
Stoller and Brumwell[9]	53	20–55 Gy	55	–

Reproduced from Ahmad et al.[19]

severe esophagitis, stenosis, and fistula formation were seen in 30% of patients. Overall, approximately 30–50% of patients may develop a non-malignant stricture following radiation alone.[9,14] Additional therapy such as repeated esophageal dilatation may be required to maintain swallowing function. Caspers et al.[13] found a median duration of palliation of 5 months with doses of < 50 Gy compared with 10 months for doses of ≥ 50 Gy. In general, half the patients with stricture have benign stricture, and half stricture secondary to tumor recurrence.[15]

Treatment with external beam radiation for palliation is often considered a preferable alternative to surgical resection for palliation of patients with advanced cancer since it is not invasive, it is less morbid, and it is more readily applicable. Stoller et al. compared the palliation of symptoms achieved by radiation therapy with that attained by surgery,[9] and found no significant difference between the two regimes (at 50–60%). Moreover, these authors noted that although 45% of irradiated patients required subsequent minor intervention to maintain swallowing, 20% of surgically treated patients also needed such therapy.

CHEMORADIATION

Chemoradiation results in better survival than treatment with radiation alone, and provides palliation of dysphagia in the majority of patients.[16–18] Chemoradiation is a preferable alternative to radiation alone or surgery alone for dysphagia relief in patients with advanced esophageal cancer, where the only goal is palliation. The studies in which chemoradiation alone have been used provide valuable information about the palliative efficacy of a non-surgical approach. Such studies have usually combined radiation therapy with doses of ≥ 50 Gy along with infusional 5-fluorouracil (5-FU) in either mitomycin C or cisplatin. For example, Coia et al. reviewed the results of combined chemotherapy and radiation in relieving dysphagia caused by esophageal cancer in over 100 patients treated at Fox Chase Cancer Center.[4,17] All patients received combined chemotherapy with infusional 5-FU at $1 \, g/m^2$ body surface area per day for 24-h infusion for 4 days during weeks one and five, along with a single bolus of mitomycin C at $10 \, mg/m^2$ for day two concurrent with external beam radiation therapy to 50–60 Gy. Initial

improvement in dysphagia occurred in 88% of patients, with a median time to improvement of less than 2 weeks. There was no difference in percent improvement or time to improvement in patients treated with 50 or 60 Gy. Furthermore, there was no difference in percent improvement or time to improvement for patients with adenocarcinoma compared with squamous cell cancer. However, patients with distal lesions, whether adenocarcinoma or squamous cell carcinoma, improved somewhat earlier and to a greater extent than patients with proximal esophageal cancers. [4] Long-term follow-up of patients treated indicate that, among 25 patients who remained free of disease for more than one year, approximately 12% had some degree of dysphagia to soft solid foods due to benign strictures which were generally effectively treated by dilatation. Of the patients who were treated with palliative intent, i.e., those who presented with stage III and IV cancer, the median survival was only 8 months. However, palliation was quite good as 77% of the patients were rendered free of dysphagia following treatment, and 60% remained free of dysphagia until death, with a median relief duration of 5 months. The morbidity of chemoradiation, as given in this study, was mild to moderate with symptoms of esophagitis, nausea, and vomiting and myeloid suppression usually of grade II–III, while < 10% of patients had severe acute toxicity of grade IV.

In a landmark study reported by Herskovic et al.[16] which randomized patients to chemoradiation (cisplatin, 5-FU and 60 Gy) versus radiation alone (50 Gy), a significant improvement in survival was reported with 2-year actuarial survival rate of 38% compared with only 10% in the radiation-alone arm. An update of this study by Al-Saraf et al.[18] has indicated survival at 5 years to be 27% for patients treated with chemoradiation versus 0% for radiation alone. Dysphagia improvement with radiation alone was 66% compared with 58% for those treated with chemoradiation, though this difference was not significant statistically. Acute effects from this aggressive chemoradiation regimen resulted in a 44% rate of severe side effects, and a 20% rate of life-threatening effects, compared with 25% and 3%, respectively, for radiation alone. In contrast, there was only one fatal acute complication caused by bone marrow suppression and renal failure in the chemoradiation arm. Thus, chemoradiation results in better survival and equivalent palliation of dysphagia compared with radiation alone, but this improved survival must be weighed against greater morbidity associated with chemoradiation. Given their dismal outcome, it is reasonable to treat patients with esophageal cancer aggressively as long as they can be adequately monitored and supported through the period of acute toxicity. Late toxicity has not been reported to be higher with chemoradiation than with radiation alone for patients treated with esophageal cancer.[18] For patients with disseminated disease, treatment must be individualized depending on the patient's overall performance status and medical condition. Radiation alone remains a viable option for those patients too ill to tolerate chemotherapy.

ENDOCAVITARY RADIATION

A variety of endoscopic and endocavitary approaches in the palliation of esophageal cancer are available, including dilatation, stent placement, laser therapy, the use of bi-cap tumor probe, and photodynamic therapy. Details of the features of endoscopic modality used in esophageal cancer are beyond the scope of this chapter, but have been expertly reviewed by Ahmad *et al.*[19] Endocavitary radiation is another technique for localized treatment which may aid in local tumor control in patients in whom improved palliation or improved survival are the goal. Selected studies of high-dose rate (HDR) brachytherapy and low-dose rate brachytherapy in cancer of the esophagus are highlighted in **Table 13.3**. Petrovich *et al.*[20] compared results of patients treated with external beam radiation alone to a mean dose of 55 Gy with those from patients who received a combination of external beam to a mean dose of 50 Gy plus mean brachytherapy of 40 Gy low-dose rate to a 0.5 cm depth from the surface of the applicator. In their study, a palliative effect was felt to be good if there was complete disappearance of dysphagia

Table 13.3 Selected studies of HDR brachytherapy in cancer of the esophagus

	STUDY 1	STUDY 2	STUDY 3	STUDY 4
No. of patients	148	161	32	32
Pathology	Squamous	Squamous	Squamous	NS
Extent of disease	LD 66	LD 101	T1–2 26	Stage III–IV
	ED 82	ED 60	T3 6	
Chemotherapy	–	–	DDP 70 mg/m^2 q 2–3 wk (5 pts)	Mit-C 10 mg/m^2 d2,29 5-FU 1000 mg/m^2/d × 4d
Radiation therapy (Gy)/wks	60 Gy/6 wk	50–60 Gy/5.5–6.0 wk	60–64 Gy/NS	55.8 Gy/6 wk
HDR dose/fraction	6 Gy	4–10 Gy	5 Gy	7 Gy
No. of fractions	2	1–3	2	2
Dose prescription point (mm)	10	10	10	10
Interfx interval	3–4 d	1 wk	1 wk	2 wk
Applicator diameter (mm)	10	10	10	NS
Complication				
Stricture	4%	} 3%	–	–
Ulcer	28%		12%	–
Fistula	10%	–	–	–
Local control	LD 2 yr 64% ED 2 yr 45%	5 yr 31%	Primary 36% Nodal 89%	NS
Survival	Median 13 mo LD 5 yr 18%* ED 2 yr 7%*	LD 5 yr 43% stage I* 21% stage II ED 5 yr 0%	5 yr Stage I 44% II 20% III 9%	1 yr 48% 2 yr 24% Median actuarial 15 mo

*Actuarial.
ED, extensive disease; LD, limited disease; NS, not stated.

and return to normal weight and diet for more than 6 months, while a moderate effect was improvement of dysphagia with mildly impaired swallowing of solid foods for more than 3 months. Using these criteria, after external beam radiation alone 34% of patients had good palliation, and 18% had moderate palliation of symptoms. For the group receiving combined external beam and intracavitary radiation, 48% had a good result and 28% a moderate result. Although these results suggest the possible improvement of palliation with the use of high-dose rate brachytherapy in conjunction with external beam compared with external beam alone, a prospective randomized study comparing external beam radiation alone to external beam plus brachytherapy boost has not been carried out. Hishikawa et al.[21] found a significant improvement in 2-year local control with external beam radiation median dose 50 Gy and 12 Gy of HDR brachytherapy (6 Gy given in two fractions) compared with external beam radiation alone to a dose of 50 Gy. Conversely, Chatani and colleagues[22] found that local control was higher with external beam radiation alone (79%) compared with external beam plus HDR brachytherapy (56%).

Relatively few studies have examined the use of concurrent chemotherapy and brachytherapy. Dinshaw et al.[23] reported the results for a randomized trial designed to assess the efficacy of intraluminal radiation with or without concurrent 5-FU infusion following 50 Gy of radiation therapy in 6 weeks. There was no significant difference in 2-year survival whether intraluminal radiation was given alone or with 5-FU. Overall, improvement of dysphagia was excellent, as three-fourths of the patients had relief of dysphagia. A recent study by Gaspar et al.[24] combined the successful regimen reported by Herskovic et al. of 50 Gy along with infusional 5-FU and cisplatin followed by HDR brachytherapy of 5 Gy in three fractions delivered starting 3 weeks following completion of chemoradiation. The first of these three fractions was given concurrently with infusional 5-FU and cisplatin. Unfortunately, there was a high rate of morbidity with the combination of intracavitary radiation along with concurrent chemotherapy, resulting in significant esophagitis and fistula formation, causing early closure of the study. Clearly, further investigations to optimize the use of intracavitary radiation with or without chemotherapy are required before it should be considered as part of the standard management of esophageal cancer.

MANAGEMENT OF THE TRACHEOESOPHAGEAL FISTULA

Approximately 5–15% of patients with esophageal cancer will develop fistula formation between the esophagus and bronchial tree.[25–27] This is a devastating clinical condition which results in continuous contamination of the bronchial tree by saliva and food, and resultant cough and aspiration pneumonia. The median survival for patients with tracheoesophageal fistula who are untreated is only 6 weeks; usually, the patient succumbs to sepsis.[26] The survival of patients who are treated is only somewhat better at 2–5 months. Retrospective studies would suggest that although tracheoesophageal fistula may be treated by stent placement alone, esophageal bypass or radiation therapy appear to result in better survival. It had been maintained that radiation therapy should not be used in the treatment of tracheoesophageal fistula because it might enlarge the fistula with tumor shrinkage. However, more recent experience provides evidence to the contrary. Gschossmann et al.[27] reported the results of radiation therapy for tracheoesophageal fistula secondary to esophageal cancer in a limited number of patients treated at the Mayo Clinic. Patients received 30 to 66 Gy at 1.8 to 3.0 Gy per fraction. The median survival was 4.8 months, and although radiation therapy did not worsen the tracheoesophageal fistula, all patients eventually died of esophageal cancer.

Overall, one must bear in mind that the development of tracheoesophageal fistula is a dismal prognostic indicator for patients with esophageal cancer. Although a wide variety of treatment options exists, only radiation therapy and bypass surgery appear to prolong survival. For patients too ill even to undergo radiation treatment, intubation remains a practical option.

FUTURE DIRECTIONS

Few studies examining the most efficient and cost-effective manner for palliating esophageal cancer exist. Nonetheless, such studies are needed since palliation is generally a more realistic goal than cure in the management of esophageal cancer. In designing future studies, a careful assessment of the risks and benefits is necessary, whether patients are treated palliatively or with curative intent. Improvements in treatment planning, the use of appropriate patient positioning, altered fractionation, brachytherapy, and optimization of chemotherapy scheduled with radiation, all offer the possibility of improving tumor control while remaining within the tolerance of surrounding normal tissues.

SUMMARY

The challenge for the physician managing esophageal cancer is to select the appropriate palliative therapy for a given patient, taking into account the stage of disease, coexisting medical problems, and performance status, as well as patient desires. An algorithm for the treatment of patients with symptomatic advanced esophageal cancer has been proposed by Ahmad et al.[19] (**Table 13.4**). For patients with reasonably good performance status and in whom adequate support of care is available, chemoradiation is the treatment of choice. When chemotherapy cannot be included as part of the treatment regimen, radiation alone offers excellent palliation, though the chance of long-term survival is slim. Placement of a feeding gastrostomy or jejunostomy tube often is useful in the patient who is to be treated with a regimen which will likely induce a high degree of esophagitis, and in the patient in whom significant obstructive symptoms are present. Additionally, endoscopic

procedures may be used to augment the results obtained with chemoradiation and radiation alone such as dilatation, laser treatment, tumor probe or stent placement. For patients who cannot tolerate either radiation treatment or chemoradiation and who have failed first line treatment, endoscopic palliation may offer prompt, although short-term, relief of symptoms.

GASTRIC CANCER

NEED FOR LOCOREGIONAL CONTROL IN GASTRIC CANCER

Although the incidence of gastric cancer in the United States has declined, most gastric cancers are diagnosed at an advanced stage.[28] Presenting symptoms are often non-specific and include pain, bleeding, obstruction, and weight loss.[29] The rationale and eventual need for radiation therapy in the treatment of advanced, i.e., recurrent or unresectable gastric cancer is to diminish the problems attendant with the high risk of local progression, such as bleeding, pain, and obstruction. Studies analyzing the likelihood of local failure following "curative" resection (i.e., surgery in which all macroscopic tumor has been resected with no evidence of metastatic cancer) of gastric tumors have consistently indicated that over 50% will have some component of local failure, which often results in pain or bleeding.[30] The likelihood increases in patients with either nodal involvement or disease that extends through the gastric wall.

Table 13.4 Treatment of patients with dysphagia secondary to advanced esophageal cancer

TEF present?

    Yes $\longrightarrow$ assess performance status
               Rx options: radiation/chemotherapy
                            stent
                            surgical bypass
    No $\longrightarrow$ assess performance status

ECOG 0,1,2:total obstruction?	ECOG 3:total obstruction?

Yes → laser or dilate, then proceed as for "no"	Yes → assess tumor characteristics
	Rx options:
	    laser
	    dilate
	    tumor probe
	    stent

No → chemoradiation	No → radiation/chemotherapy

Reproduced from Ahmad et al.[19]
TEF, tracheo-esophageal fistula

Gunderson et al.[31] reported the results of second-look laparotomies in patients at the University of Minnesota who had undergone resection of their primary gastric tumor. Among patients who had been found to have pathologically positive lymph nodes at the time of their original surgery, 87% were discovered to have regional recurrence at the time of second surgery.

In a study conducted at Massachusetts General Hospital, Landry et al.[32] found that most recurrences occurred in the gastric bed or the gastric stump. These findings match those reported by Waggensteen, who found close to 80% of recurrences in the gastric bed, 34% in the anastomosis, and 68% in the regional lymph nodes. Patients with unresectable gastric cancer without evidence of metastatic disease can be expected to survive 5 to 6 months without any treatment.[33]

No form of adjuvant treatment has yet been convincingly demonstrated to be of benefit following surgical resection of stage I–III disease versus observation following surgical resection of gastric cancer. The use of adjuvant chemoradiation is presently being investigated in several randomized trials. Many centers use postoperative moderate dose radiation (45 Gy) along with 5-FU in patients with serosal involvement, nodal involvement, positive margins, or gross residual disease.

RELIEF OF SYMPTOMS WITH EXTERNAL RADIATION THERAPY

Though few studies have been undertaken solely to determine the efficacy of radiation in the palliation of gastric cancer, it is clear that there is an established role for radiation therapy in this setting. One such study was reported in 1982 by Mantell et al.[34] In it, they reported on the results of attempted palliation of carcinoma of the gastric cardia with external beam therapy. Of the 17 patients enrolled, all but one received at least 3000 cGy in daily fractions of 300 cGy. Before therapy, 15 of the 17 had described varying degrees of dysphagia; after completion of radiation therapy, four of the 17 reported that their swallowing had become normal, while, overall, 13 "experienced a useful improvement" in swallowing. It should be noted that in current practice, patients would most likely be treated with lower daily fractions to a higher total dose. Nonetheless, the outcome of these patients with regard to functional improvement is noteworthy.

The results of the study are all the more noteworthy when the age and extent of symptoms is considered. Eleven of the 17 were 65 or older, with eight at least 70 years old (the oldest was 85). Of the five patients who originally reported either total obstruction or dysphagia for fluids, all were able to at least swallow liquids after completion of radiation.

Because these symptoms of obstruction are common only when disease is located in the gastric cardia, other studies must be reviewed to evaluate the efficacy of palliation in the gastric body.

A study published by Tsukiyama et al.[35] described palliation in terms of post-treatment radiologic findings. Ultrasound and barium studies were used to evaluate the response to treatment. Of the 75 patients who received radiation (10 of whom received no chemotherapy), complete response (CR) was noted in 6%, while partial response (PR) was reported in another 61% of patients. (CR was defined as complete disappearance of tumor, PR as >50% reduction in tumor size.) While the authors did not indicate the rate of relief of symptoms, they stated that "in some patients, improvement in subjective symptoms was also taken into consideration."

Falkson et al.[36] treated patients with split-course external radiation therapy, with or without chemotherapy, and palliation was reported to be only 36%. However, as with most studies, palliative response to treatment was measured in terms of radiologic response rather than measurement of symptom relief. It is likely that reduction in tumor size correlates with relief of pain and reduction in bleeding as it does in cancers of other sites.

SURVIVAL WITH RADIATION THERAPY IN THE PALLIATIVE SETTING

There are conflicting results with regard to the survival benefit of radiation therapy in the treatment of locally advanced/unresectable gastric carcinoma. Moertel et al.[37] found an improvement in 5-year survival rate from 5% in patients who received surgery alone, to 20% with the addition of adjuvant radiation therapy (37.5 Gy) and 5-FU for three days.

The Gastrointestinal Tumor Study Group (GITSG) randomized patients to receive either chemotherapy alone (5-FU and methyl CCNU) or chemotherapy combined with 5000 cGy.[38] All patients had either locally advanced unresectable tumor or gross residual disease after an attempted curative resection. While there were severe treatment-related toxicities associated with the chemoradiation arm, the 5-year survival rate was 18% for patients receiving chemoradiation, compared with 7% for those in the chemotherapy only arm. In a 1985 ECOG study,[39] patients with locally unresected or gross residual disease after surgery were randomized to receive either 600 mg/m^2 weekly of 5-FU until the progression of disease, or radiation therapy, 4000 cGy plus 600 mg/m^2 of 5-FU on the first three days of radiation therapy. (Maintenance 5-FU was then given once weekly until there was evidence of progression of disease.) This study failed to confirm an advantage for chemoradiation.

TECHNICAL CONSIDERATIONS

The aggressiveness with which radiation oncologists have treated gastric cancer has been tempered by the radiation tolerance of normal tissue adjacent to the stomach. Also, the mobility of both the stomach and small bowel make accuracy and reproducibility of radiation treatments quite challenging.

Initially, areas at risk (gastric bed, regional nodes) are treated using parallel opposed anterior and posterior fields using standard fractionation (180–200 cGy per fraction) to 4500 cGy. Subsequently, radiation may be given to a smaller area using lateral or oblique fields, taking into account the limited tolerance to radiation of the liver, small bowel, and kidneys.

INTRAOPERATIVE RADIATION

Because of the location of the stomach and its close proximity to organs with lower tolerances for radiation, intraoperative radiation may hold advantages over external beam radiation since surrounding structures can be removed from the radiation beam.

Abe and colleagues[40,41] randomized patients to receive either surgery alone or intraoperative radiation therapy. Although criticized for their failure to stratify the patients by prognostic factors, i.e., weight loss and extent of disease, the results nonetheless were intriguing. They found that patients with stage III and IV cancer who received the intraoperative radiotherapy showed significant advantages in survival. Of the patients with stage IV cancers, nearly 20% were alive at 5 years, compared with none of those treated with surgery alone. However, this form of treatment remains largely investigational.

MORBIDITY OF RADIATION THERAPY

Actue problems such as nausea, vomiting, abdominal cramping, and diarrhea are not uncommon with gastric radiation,[42] and concurrent administration of 5-FU may exacerbate these symptoms. At doses over 5000 cGy, the likelihood of gastric bleeding and ulceration increases. As mentioned earlier, tolerance of kidneys, liver, and spinal cord must also be considered.

SUMMARY

The number of patients with advanced gastric cancer has declined, but for those patients with gastric cancer the prognosis remains relatively poor. External beam radiation can palliate bleeding, dysphagia and pain – symptoms which commonly occur with gastric or gastroesophageal junction cancers. Despite the often weak and debilitated condition of these patients, radiation can be relatively well tolerated with appropriate treatment techniques.

REFERENCES

1. Blow WJ. Esophageal cancer trends and risk factors. *Semin Oncol* 1994; **21**: 403–10.
2. Yang Z. Long term survival of radiotherapy for esophageal cancer. *Int J Radiat Oncol Biol Phys* 1983; **9**: 1769–73.
3. Roth JA, Pass HI, Flanigan MM *et al.* Randomized clinical trial of pre-operative and post-operative adjuvant chemotherapy with cisplatin, indesine and bleomycin for cancer of the esophagus. *J Thorac Cardiovas Surg* 1988; **96**: 242–8.
4. Coia LR, Soffen EM, Schultheiss TE, Martin EE & Hanks GE. Swallowing function in patients with esophageal cancer treated with concurrent radiation and chemotherapy. *Cancer* 1993; **71**: 281–6.
5. Blot WJ & Fraumeni JF, Jr. Trends in esophageal cancer mortality among US blacks and whites. *Am J Public Health* 1987; **77**: 296–8.
6. MacDonald WC & MacDonald JB. Adenocarcinoma of the esophagus and/or gastric cardia. *Cancer* 1987; **60**: 1094–8.

7. Coia LR. The esophagus In: Cox J (ed) *Moss' Radiation Oncology: Rationale, Techniques, Results.* 2nd edn. St. Louis: Mosby-Year Book, 1994: 409.

8. Ajani J. Contributions of chemotherapy in the treatment of carcinoma of the esophagus: results and commentary. *Semin Oncol* 1994; **21**: 474–82.

9. Stoller JL & Brumwell MI. Palliation after operation and after radiotherapy for cancer of the esophagus. *Can J Surg* 1984; **27**: 491–5.

10. Langer M, Choi NC, Orlow E *et al.* Radiation therapy alone or in combination with surgery in the treatment of carcinoma of the esophagus. *Cancer* 1986; **58**: 1208–13.

11. Petrovich Z, Langholz B, Formenti S *et al.* Management of carcinoma of the esophagus: the role of radiotherapy. *Am J Clin Oncol* 1991; **14**: 80–6.

12. Wara WM, Mauch PM, Thomas AN *et al.* Palliation for carcinoma of the esophagus. *Radiology* 1976; **121**: 717–20.

13. Caspers RJL, Welvaart K, Verkes RJ *et al.* The effect of radiotherapy on dysphagia and survival in patients with esophageal cancer. *Radiother Oncol* 1988; **12**: 15–23.

14. Albertsson M, Ewers S-B, Widmark H *et al.* Evaluation of the palliative effect of radiotherapy for esophageal carcinoma. *Acta Oncol* 1989; **28**: 267–70.

15. O'Rourke IC, Tiver K, Bull C *et al.* Swallowing performance after radiation therapy for carcinoma of the esophagus. *Cancer* 1988; **61**: 2022–6.

16. Herskovic A, Martz K, Al-Sarraf M *et al.* Combined chemotherapy and radiotherapy compared with radiotherapy alone in patients with cancer of the esophagus. *N Engl J Med* 1992; **326**: 1593–8.

17. Coia LR, Engstrom PF, Paul AR *et al.* Long-term results of infusional 5-FU, mitomycin-C, and radiation as primary management of esophageal carcinoma. *Int J Radiat Oncol Biol Phys* 1991; **20**: 29–36.

18. Al-Sarraf M, Martz K, Herskovic A *et al.* Progress report of combined chemoradiotherapy versus radiotherapy alone in patients with esophageal cancer: an intergroup study. *J Clinic Oncol* 1997; **15**: 277–84.

19. Ahmad N *et al.* Palliative treatment of esophageal cancer. *Semin Radiat Oncol* 1994; **4**: 202–14.

20. Petrovich Z, Langholz B, Formenti S *et al.* Management of carcinoma of the esophagus: the role of radiotherapy. *Am J Clinic Oncol* 1991; **14**: 80–6.

21. Hishikawa Y, Kurisu K, Tanigushi M *et al.* High-dose-rate intraluminal brachytherapy for esophageal cancer. *Int J Radiat Oncol Biol Phys* 1991; **21**: 1133–5.

22. Chatani M, Matayoshi Y & Masaki N. Radiation therapy for the esophageal carcinoma: external irradiation vs. high-dose-rate intraluminal irradiation. *Strahlewther Onkol* 1992; **168**: 328–32.

23. Dinshaw KA, Sharma V, Pendse AM *et al.* The role of intraluminal radiotherapy and concurrent 5-FU infusion in the management of carcinoma of the esophagus: a pilot study. *J Surg Oncol* 1991; **47**: 155–60.

24. Gaspar L, Barnett R, Kocha WI *et al.* High-dose-rate esophageal brachytherapy: Initial experience. *Endocuriether Hypertherm Oncol* 1992; **8**: 5–10.

25. Boyce HW, Jr. Palliation of advanced esophageal cancer. *Semin Oncol* 1984; **11**: 186–95.

26. Burt M, Diehl W, Martini N *et al.* Malignant esophagorespiratory fistula: management options and survival. *Ann Thorac Surg* 1991; **52**: 1222–9.

27. Gschossmann JM, Bonner JA, Foote RL *et al.* Malignant tracheoesophageal fistula in patients with esophageal cancer. *Cancer* 1993; **72**: 1513–21.

28. Silverberg E, Boring CC & Squires TS. *Cancer Statistics* 1990; **40**: 9–26.

29. Moertel CG. The stomach. In: Holland JF, Frei E III (eds) *Cancer Medicine.* Philadelphia: Lea and Febiger, 1982: 1760–74.

30. Wisbeck WM, Becher EM & Russell AH. Adenocarcinoma of the stomach: autopsy observations with therapeutic implications for the radiation oncologist. *Radiother Oncol* 1986; **7**: 13–18.

31. Gunderson L & Sosin H. Adenocarcinoma of the stomach: areas of failure in a re-operative series clinicopathologic correlation and implications for adjuvant therapy. *Int J Radiat Oncol Biol Phys* 1982; **8**: 1–11.

32. Landry J, Tepper Wood W, Moulton E, Koerner F & Sullinger J. Patterns of failure following curative resection of gastric carcinoma. *Int J Radiat Oncol Biol Phys* 1990; **19**: 1357–62.

33. Childs D, Moertel C, Holbrook M, Reitemeyeir R & Colby M. Treatment of unresectable adenocarcinomas of the stomach with a combination of 5-FU and radiation. *Am J Roentgenol Radium Ther Nucl Med* 1968; **102**: 541–4.

34. Mantell BS. Radiotherapy for dysphagia due to gastric carcinoma. *Br J Surg* 1982; **69**: 69–70.

35. Tsukiyama I, Akine Y, Kajiura Y, Ogina T, Yamashita K & Egawa S. Radiation therapy for advanced gastric cancer. *Int J Radiat Oncol Biol Phys* 1988; **15**: 123.

36. Falkson G. A controlled clinical trial of fluorouracil plus imidazole carboxamide dimethyl triazeno plus vincristine plus bis-chloroethyl nitrosurea plus radiotherapy in stomach cancer. *Med Pediatr Oncol* 1976; **2**: 111–17.

37. Moertel C, Childs D, O'Fallon J, Holbrook M, Schutt A & Reitemeir R. Combined 5-FU and radiation therapy as a surgical adjuvant for poor prognosis gastric carcinoma. *J Clin Oncol* 1984; **2**: 1249–54.

38. Gastrointestinal Tumor Study Group. A comparison of combination chemotherapy and combined modality therapy for locally advanced gastric carcinoma. *Cancer* 1982; **49**: 1771–7.

39. Klaassen D, MacIntyre J, Cotton G, Engstrom & Moertel C. Treatment of locally unresectable cancer of the stomach and pancreas: a randomized comparison of 5-FU alone with radiation plus concurrent and maintenance 5-FU – an Eastern Cooperative Oncology Study Group. *J Clin Oncol* 1985; **3**: 373–8.

40. Abe M. Intraoperative radiation therapy for gastric cancer. In: Delbower RR & Abe M (eds) *Intraoperative Radiation Therapy*. Boca Raton, Florida: CRC 1991: 166–74.

41. Takahashi T & Abe M. Intraoperative radiotherapy for carcinoma of the stomach. *Eur J Surg Oncol* 1986; **12**: 247–52.

42. Minsky B. The role of radiation therapy in gastric cancer. *Semin Oncol* 1996; **23**: 390–6.

14
OTHER MODALITIES

STEPHEN ATTWOOD

INTRODUCTION

Surgical resection offers the patient with cancer of the esophagus the greatest chance of cure. However, in Western societies, the majority of patients are not curable and there are a host of alternative treatments, some very recently developed, which are now available to treat the symptoms and maintain the quality of life of patients with cancer of the esophagus. While the application of these new technologies is covered in some detail below, the most important factors in clinical practice relate directly to the patient (**Table 14.1**), and not the technology. Thus, the general principles of palliation and the specific symptoms which require palliation are discussed in some detail.

This chapter deals with a variety of technologies including dilatation, rigid intubation, expanding metallic stents, lasers, photodynamic therapy, argon beam plasma coagulation, and injection of toxins which can be used to treat patients with either advanced cancer of the esophagus or recurrence after previous resection, chemotherapy, or radiotherapy. There is an almost bewildering array of combinations in which these treatments can be given, and some guidance is given on the more rational combinations.

The clinical indications for using palliative treatments for cancer of the esophagus are because the disease is too advanced, usually because of metastases, less commonly because of involvement of adjacent vital organs, or because the patient is unfit for – or does not want – resection (**Table 14.2**).

GENERAL ISSUES

Treatment of patients with carcinoma of the esophagus rarely achieves cure. Indeed, overall, < 15% of the patients survive for 5 years.[1,2] In some areas this figure may be even less, such as the 3-year survival rate of 8.5% which was found during a population study in the North-West region of the UK.[3] Thus, care of patients with this cancer is palliative in a major portion of cases no matter what kind of treatment is applied. Surgery, radiotherapy, and combinations of chemotherapy with these two modalities have been discussed in previous chapters, but these treatments are applied to only a minority of the total number.

Surgery is the modality which offers the greatest hope of cure, but most resections are palliative in their effect. Surgical series quote resection rates varying from 45% to 85%.[4,5] These may be biased by referral pattern, and a true picture of operability rate is difficult to get as patients with inoperable disease may not be referred to the surgical unit. In the literature, the treatment options offered to patients with cancer of the esophagus seem to vary depending on the author and their specialty. Indeed, published series often are based on the availability of a new technology, and decisions are based on whether the patient suits the modality rather than the treatment best suiting the patient.

Few studies have actually examined what happens to the totality of patients with this disease. In our recent study, we found 1400 patients with carcinoma of the esophagus and stomach who

Table 14.1 Symptoms of esophageal carcinoma that require palliation

Dysphagia
Hiccup
Regurgitation of food and saliva
Nausea and vomiting
Bleeding
Pain
    Local (thoracic)
    Metastatic
Cachexia
Respiratory complications
    Pneumonia – due to aspiraton
    Cough
    Copious productive cough (fistulation)
    Hoarseness

Table 14.2 Conditions that categorize a patient into a palliative approach

Spread of tumor outside the esophagus and regional lymph nodes
    adjacent essential structures (aorta, bronchus, trachea)
    distal metastases (liver, lung, bone, brain)
Insufficient respiratory or cardiac function for major surgery
General debility or immobility
Patient's preference

presented in one year in a region of England with a population of 4.2 million, giving an incidence rate 33 per 100 000 for esophageal and gastric cancer. These data were derived from detailed population study and were not based on a single institution. They revealed that 27% of the tumors involved the esophagus alone, 31% crossed the esophagogastric junction, and 42% were only in the stomach. The true resection rate in this region for cancers of the esophagus and the esophagogastric junction were 21% and 39%, respectively. Many of these patients were not referred to a surgical practice and palliative treatment was administered as the only clinical objective. An esophageal stent or tube was used in 45% who had an esophageal carcinoma, supplemented with radiotherapy, chemotherapy, laser, or photodynamic therapy in < 25%. The data suggest that there is a nihilistic attitude to the treatment of cancer of the esophagus in this area.

MULTIDISCIPLINARY APPROACH

It is clear from the range of potential treatments that, for the best decision to be taken, the involvement of a multidisciplinary team is helpful. However, the committee approach is probably not the best way of deciding treatment for individual patients. A team leader with pre-discussed protocols and channels of communication with other specialist therapists is in the best position to make such a decision. This infers that individual patients meet with an individual clinician, and the decision for care of all new patients is discussed at regular team meetings.

This upper gastrointestinal cancer team needs a leader, and in many circumstances the surgeon is well placed to be that leader. The surgeon is often the clinician who makes the diagnosis at endoscopy, and is the person who performs the staging investigations. The surgeon delivers the mode of therapy with the greatest chance of cure (i.e., resection) and often possesses the skills to palliate with lasers, endoprostheses, and other modalities if resection is not appropriate.

In the care of patients with carcinoma of the esophagus it is most important to ensure that the most appropriate therapy is offered to the patient based on its inherent value in the patient's individual case. In practice, this will require teams of clinicians who communicate effectively so that the therapies of their own discipline are placed in the overall perspective of available treatments. While the results of all forms of therapy for carcinoma of the esophagus are disappointing, this means that many patients may need to undergo a number of therapies during their illness. The order in which they are applied will depend on the symptoms and the general condition of the patient. For instance, it is common to combine radiotherapy with other modalities including laser and intubation. In some circumstances, radiotherapy is advisable before a stent is placed in order to avoid the complication of a stent falling into the stomach after the tumor responds to the radiation treatment. In other circumstances, an esophagobronchial fistula may need to be stented prior to radiotherapy as the respiratory complications of fistula require immediate treatment.

The multidisciplinary team may include a surgeon, a physician gastroenterologist, an interventional radiologist, a physician oncologist, a radiotherapist, and the medical services of hospice support teams. In addition to these medical staff, paramedical and nursing staff such as dietitians, physiotherapists and specialist palliative care nurses (McMillan nurses in the UK) play a major role in the support and care of patients with progressive cancers of the esophagus. As well as communicating with each other, the hospital-based team needs to keep the general practitioner informed of their activities, as it is in the community that the patients may end up needing most of their care. The geographic location of the patient – in hospital, hospice or home – depends on the symptoms and the treatment modalities being used and how often therapeutic changes are required. Social support is critical, and the carers of such patients need a considerable amount of education into the problems they will face and how to seek assistance. In a previous era, patients expected to be cared for in institutions, but increasingly they express a wish to be treated at home, such that the services are moved to the community rather than the patient moved to the services.

Despite the depressing statistics in terms of cure of esophageal carcinoma it is most important that patients feel that their symptoms can be treated. An explanation that there is a wide variety of treatments available should encourage a patient to report his or her symptoms. A nihilistic attitude is rarely of any benefit to the patient. Conversely, while miraculous resolution of tumors has been described,[6] it is more reassuring for the patient with advanced cancer to be encouraged to seek effective symptomatic therapy than wish for the rare cure. Indeed, in the words of Murray Brennan when a patient, faced with a surgical decision of inoperability, asks the surgeon "Is there nothing more that you can do?" the right answer is "This treatment may not cure you, but I will always care for you."

THE SYMPTOMS OF PROGRESSION OF ESOPHAGEAL CARCINOMA

Dysphagia

This is the most common symptom and is usually the first to affect patients with cancer of the esophagus. Before dysphagia becomes significant, the tumor usually occupies > 50% of the circumference of the esophagus, or is a polypoid exophytic growth occupying > 50% of the available lumen. At this size, the tumors are usually at an advanced stage of invasion and hence the overall prognosis is poor. Dysphagia may or may not be painful, and is usually progressive for solids and liquids. Odynophagia may occur and bolus obstruction may happen occasionally. The management of dysphagia is usually the primary aim of any therapy of cancer of the esophagus. Surgery, radiotherapy, lasers, stents, and injections of toxic materials are all aimed at restoring swallowing and maintaining oral nutrition.

Conditions which aggravate dysphagia include drugs which dry the mouth and reduce saliva secretion, pharyngoesophageal candidiasis (common in the malnourished patients), anxiety with esophageal spasm, drowsiness, and disinterest.

Hiccup

This is a pathologic respiratory reflex characterized by spasm of the diaphragm and causing sudden inspiration with associated closure of the vocal cords. In cancer of the esophagus the hiccup may be secondary to a swallowed bolus becoming lodged in the obstructed or partially obstructed esophagus. It may also be due to direct irritation of the diaphragm or crurae by the tumor mass. Thirdly, it is said to be psychogenic in some patients. There are many treatments for hiccup in other forms of malignant disease, but for cancer of the esophagus the relief of esophageal obstruction (by stenting or endoscopic tissue ablation) or, if an obstruction is not present by drug therapy (chlorpromazine), are almost always effective.[7]

Regurgitation of food and saliva

This occurs either secondary to the obstructive nature of the tumor or is due to the placement of a rigid stent across the esophagogastric junction, allowing uninhibited gastroesophageal reflux. It is common for physicians to prescribe an acid suppressant such as a proton pump inhibitor or an H_2-receptor antagonist to prevent heartburn from refluxed gastric juice.

Nausea and vomiting

These symptoms are not common in patients with primary carcinoma of the esophagus. However, they do occur as a side effect of other treatment such as radiotherapy and chemotherapy, and may also be secondary to drugs used for analgesia. The actions and indications of drugs used to treat nausea and vomiting are summarized in **Table 14.3.**

Vomiting may also occur in patients after esophagectomy where stasis may occur in the intrathoracic stomach. Poor gastric emptying in this circumstance may be due to the stomach being placed too low in the chest, the result of vagotomy, too wide a conduit, or it may be due to an outflow obstruction such as pyloric stenosis. Pyloromyotomy, pyloroplasty, and postoperative balloon dilatation are all methods of dealing with this gastric stasis. Medications such as cisapride or the prokinetic side effect of the antibiotic erythromycin may be used to stimulate gastric activity.

Bleeding

This is a relatively rare problem in cancer of the esophagus. It may occur secondary to surface abrasion of the tumor by a swallowed bolus, or may occur *de novo*. While lasers or argon beam plasma coagulation may arrest local bleeding by thermal injury, the tamponade and protection provided by covered stents is probably the best relief from bleeding tumors.

Pain
Local (thoracic) pain

This occurs due to tumor invasion of the chest wall, nerve invasion in the chest, abdomen or neck and occasionally intercostal pain from thoracotomy. This is best treated with opioid analgesia, or if one or two intercostal segments are involved a nerve block may help.

Metastatic pain

Bony pain may occur anywhere in the skeleton, but the most common is probably in the vertebral column. Bony pain is resistant to analgesia in some patients, but may respond to the combination of narcotic analgesia with non-steroidal analgesia (we use combinations of long-acting morphine (MST) and naprosyn or ibuprofen). In others, radiotherapy is useful to alleviate resistant bony pain. It is wise to ensure that a bone scan confirms metastatic disease in the bones to be irradiated. Painful soft tissue metastases respond poorly to radiation, especially in the neck because soft tissue metastases here can invade the brachial plexus. Not only do these not respond well to radiotherapy, but radiation of the brachial plexus may also produce uncomfortable secondary effects in the affected arm.

Abdominal pain may be due to the progression of soft tissue disease – involved lymph nodes or diffuse invasion of the retroperitoneum and irritation of the sympathetic plexuses. Pain may also occur from the rapid growth of liver metastases. MST is the mainstay of pain relief and needs careful dose adjustment to achieve the desired effect. Some patients may suffer nausea or be unable to take analgesia by mouth, and in these cases a dermal patch (fentanyl) is very useful. Subcutaneous portable infusion pumps for morphine or diamorphine are also effective alternatives. Liver metastases, when painful, may respond to opioids or steroids, but rarely, celiac plexus block and embolization are used. Nursing and medical staff responsible for pain control medication need to be well

Table 14.3 The role of specific antiemetics for esophageal cancer

DRUG GROUP	EXAMPLES	MECHANISMS AND MAIN INDICATION
Anticholinergics	Hyoscine; atropine	Reduction of salivary secretion in the presence of esophageal fistula
Phenothiazines	Prochlorperazine; chlorpromazine; methotrimeprazine	D_2 receptor activity at chemoreceptor trigger zone with additional sedative effects
Butryophenones	Haloperidol; droperidol	Suppresses cytotoxicity-induced emesis
Antihistamines	Cyclizine; promethazine	For short-term narcotic-related emesis
Gastrokinetic	Domperidone; metoclopramide	Suppresses cytotoxicity-induced emesis
5-HT3 receptor antagonists	Odansetron	Suppresses cytotoxicity-induced emesis
Miscellaneous	Erythromycin; cisapride	Useful for postesophagectomy stasis in the intrathoracic stomach

trained in palliative care and it is desirable to have specialist palliative care nursing staff involved.

Cachexia

Combinations of dehydration and malnutrition occur if dysphagic patients are not relieved of their symptoms. In addition to this input deficiency, there are numerous other mechanisms of cancer cachexia, and a detailed discussion of them is beyond the scope of this book. An excellent description of the causes and metabolic effects of cancer cachexia is given in the *Oxford Textbook of Palliative Medicine*. Current information implicates endogenously produced cytokines, particularly tumor necrosis factor and interleukin-1 as principal mediators of cancer cachexia. While some therapies may have measurable and favorable influences on some metabolic parameters, no treatment directed towards the amelioration of cachexia has been dramatically successful. Importantly, parenteral nutrition has been shown to be of no benefit and is not indicated for the correction of malnutrition in isolation in patients with esophageal cancer.

It is desirable that patients can maintain themselves on a self-administered diet rather than become dependent on tube feeding, as neither nasogastric feeds nor gastrostomy provide a quality of life or dignity. Thus, it is most important to avoid these methods and attempt to maintain a transesophageal route for normal swallowing until such time as the patient reaches the terminal phase of the illness. At the terminal stages, the use of tube feeds – whether enteral or intravenous – is unlikely to help the patient's quality of life and thus are best avoided.

Respiratory complications

These include pneumonia (due to aspiration) cough, copious productive cough (fistulation), and hoarseness. This collection of pulmonary and airway symptoms relates to the problems of regurgitation and aspiration due to either an obstructed esophagus or sometimes to reflux through a tube stent which allows uncontrolled regurgitation of gastric contents. Alternatively, direct invasion of the tumor may cause erosion into the neighboring organs, the right main stem bronchus usually being responsible for bronchoesophageal fistulas, while recurrent laryngeal nerve invasion is usually the cause of the development of hoarseness. Fistulas

are best corrected by covered stent insertion (see below). Recurrent nerve involvement is not reversible, but occasionally it may be worthwhile injecting the cords with Teflon.

ASSESSMENT OF SYMPTOMS

Previously, it was common practice to care for patients with advanced carcinoma of the esophagus in a hospital or hospice institution. This is still common in some areas, but in our practice the patient preference is to remain out of the hospital environment and treatment in the community is maintained. The effect of this is to remove the opportunity for hospital-based staff to observe patients' symptoms. What is now needed is monitoring of patients' progress in their homes and visits by the community physician, palliative nursing staff, and other support. These carers need to understand the range of symptoms, the possible causes, and the range of treatments available if they are going to help maintain a comfortable life for the patient with advanced carcinoma of the esophagus.

In order to improve objective assessment it is useful to measure the "quality of life" using a questionnaire such as a Rotterdam Symptoms Checklist, a Dysphagia Score, and Activities of Daily Living Score. In practice, these are mostly used for the prospective comparative evaluation of treatment protocols for patients with advanced esophageal cancer.[8–11] These are a most useful objective comparison between groups. However, quality of life questionnaires have yet to become accepted for day-to-day management of single patients, and are also too cumbersome for the longitudinal documentation of a patient's symptoms and for therapeutic decision-making in individual patients.[12]

The issue of quality of life has been addressed earlier in this book, and the reader is referred to Chapter 3 for a detailed discussion.

METHODS OF PALLIATION

Non-resectional surgery

Surgical resection as a means of palliation has been fully discussed in previous chapters. Non-resectional surgery has been regarded as too invasive for palliation, as the discomfort, risks and residual symptoms are too great for satisfactory routine treatment. Non-surgical means of palliation are becoming increasingly popular in carcinoma of the esophagus because of improved efficacy, greater patient tolerance, and much improved procedure-related morbidity and mortality.[13]

However, at the same time, reports of improved survival by surgical palliation including bypass procedures means that non-surgical improvements need to be tested against current surgical techniques and not historic controls, if at all possible. For instance, results of bypass using the substernal stomach have improved from >21% hospital mortality rate[14] to 11%.[15] Mannell et al.[15] reported an operative mortality rate of only 4% and 7% postoperative mortality in 126 patients undergoing bypass surgery, where the whole stomach was used and brought substernally to the neck without thoracotomy and without attempt at resection of the primary tumor. Symptomatic results were very good, but the mean survival was only 5 months. In this study, survival was extended by combination with radiotherapy by about 3 months, but the majority of patients had died by 8 months. Even in this series of good results the morbidity was high, with a 25% rate of neck wound sepsis and a pulmonary sepsis rate of 18%. Re-operations were required for obstruction of feeding jejunostomy (two), delayed gastric emptying (two), drainage of subphrenic abscess (two), and adhesive small bowel obstruction.

Colon bypass has even more problematic results, with anastomotic leak rates of up to 44% and mortality rates as high as 45%.[16,17] Problems with these surgical approaches supports the view held by many physicians that palliation without open surgical intervention is preferable.

In a large retrospective review of 732 patients with advanced carcinoma, who were not considered suitable for curative resection, Segalin et al.[18] recorded that intubation was used in 254 patients, lasers in 50, palliative resection was the option in 156, and palliative bypass in 49. No procedure, other than staging, was performed in 223 cases. The mortality rate in this series was 10% for resection, 20% for bypass, 10% for intubation with rigid stents, and 0% for laser. The modern technologies of endoscopy and interventional radiology must be assessed against this background.

Dilatation and rigid intubation

The simplest way to relieve dysphagia due to esophageal stricture is to dilate the esophagus. However, when the stricture is due to the presence of tumor, the benefits of dilatation are either short-lived or limited in quality. One of the best results of simple dilatation is the report by Lundell et al.[19] who used dilatation in 41 patients with two perforations, and averaged three dilatations at monthly intervals. The problems are the need for repeated treatments and the associated morbidity. The risks in terms of perforation are usually higher than the 5% achieved by Lundell et al., and most authors believe that the results are too short-lived to relieve dysphagia adequately.

Once a tumor has been dilated, it is relatively simple to place a tube across the stricture, and both Celestin and Atkinson designed effective tubes for such inoperable tumors. The Celestin tube is designed for perioperative placement using a traction technique, but its popularity has fallen because improved diagnostic methods for staging such as laparoscopy, computed tomography (CT) scanning, and endoscopic ultrasonography usually predict the diagnosis of inoperability before exploration. The Atkinson tube is a rigid plastic tube which is placed by a pulsion technique at endoscopy after dilatation to an appropriate diameter.[20] It was the most popular method of stenting before the introduction of expandable stent devices.

EXPANDING METALLIC STENTS

The technique of placement of a tube across the tumor in the esophagus has been available for 30 years. However, the approach has recently become much more popular due to improvements in the design of the stents, which allow a much safer placement and more effective palliation of dysphagia. The expandable metallic stents are easier to insert, require less pre-dilatation, are therefore associated with less risk of perforation, and provide a better palliation due to their wider lumen.[21–23] A prospective randomized comparison of metallic expanding stents versus rigid plastic tubes has been carried out by Knyrim et al.[24] and De Palma et al.[25] These both showed a significant reduction in complications (0% versus 21%) and mortality (0% versus 16%) with the expanding metallic stents, with similar improvements in dysphagia scores. Migration was less, perforation was less, and management of the expandable stents after insertion was more simple.

The advantages of stents include ease of insertion, a low complication rate, and low re-intervention rates. The newer stents have a very low insertion profile and less pre-insertion esophageal dilatation is required. The perforation rate previously associated with stent insertion was predominantly due to the splitting of the tumor by dilators prior to inserting large rubber tubes. Stents bring about a dramatic relief of dysphagia. The newer expandable stents have a large internal luminal diameter (16–25 mm compared with 7–11 mm for rigid tubes; **Table 14.4**, **Figure 14.1**) which allows normal diet in most patients. They are also inserted using a minimally invasive technique and this allows a short hospital stay. In our unit, we keep patients in hospital overnight to check their swallow with barium the following day. This not only allows fine adjustments to be made to the stent if necessary, but also allows the patient to receive support and meet other members of the team. A stent could be placed as an outpatient procedure, but very rapid discharge has some disadvantages in terms of allowing full communication with the patient, and the need for repeated trips to the hospital.

It has been a perception that the cost of expandable stents is a limiting factor. However, the high initial cost of the stent itself (£600–800; $1000–1500) is easily offset by the short hospital stay (one or two nights), the reduction in readmissions, and the low frequency of complications.

Indications for expanding metallic stents

The indications for an expandable metallic stent in the esophagus (**Table 14.5**) include relief of dysphagia in primary esophageal carcinoma,[25–27] relief of dysphagia in anastomotic recurrence, and relief of dysphagia in recurrence or failed response to radiotherapy or chemotherapy.[28] They are also particularly helpful in relieving the distressing symptoms of tracheoesophageal fistula,[29,30] and the even more rare oesophagopericardial fistulas.[31] Moreover, they have been used for the tamponade of bleeding tumors, but this is a circumstance that is rare and not easy to solve.

Expandable stents are also indicated for rescue of iatrogenic perforation such as after laser or dilatation injury.[32,33] Most laser-associated perforations have actually been in relation to the pre-laser dilatation. In these cases, an alternative policy is to institute a conservative course of action,[34] as long as the perforation is recognized and laser or other thermal injury has not been used to aggravate the injury. However, since the patients will still require palliation of their dysphagia once they have recovered from their perforation, it may be preferable to place a covered expanding metallic stent which occludes the site of perforation and which allows earlier discharge of patients and does not require their readmission for further palliative procedures.

The quality of life of patients who have received a stent has been assessed by Cwikiel et al.[11] who identified a good-quality swallow which was close to normal in 81% of patients, compared with 56% and 49% for radio- and chemotherapy respectively

---

Table 14.4 Commonly used esophageal stents

NAME	MATERIAL	INTRODUCER	INSERTION TECHNIQUE	LENGTH	LUMEN
Atkinson	Plastic tube, reinforced	Nottingham pulsion	Endoscopy + radiography	7–15 cm	9–12 mm
Celestin	Plastic tube, reinforced with nylon	Traction introducer	Laparotomy	to 30 cm	7–11 mm
Schneider	Polyurethane-covered expanding metallic	Telestep device	Radiography ± endoscopy	10–1 cm	20–25 mm
Gianturco	Polythene-covered expanding metallic	Introducer sheath + tapered dilator	Radiography ± endoscopy	10,12 + 14 cm	16–20 mm
Ultraflex	Knitted alloy of titanium and nickel	Introducer sheath, self-expanding after gelatin dissolves	Radiography ± endoscopy	7,10 + 15 cm	18 mm

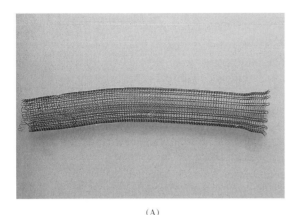

(A)

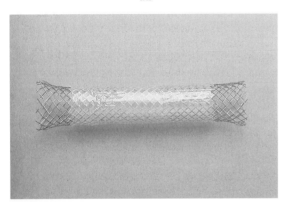

(B)

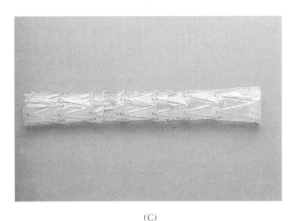

(C)

Figure 14.1 Detail of esophageal expandable metallic stents, illustrating: A. Nitinol; B. Wallstent; and C. Gianturco stents.

in a retrospective study. Few studies have clearly addressed the global quality of life after stenting with expandable metallic stents, and none has been instigated as a prospective randomized comparison with surgery.[8–10] Non-randomized compar-

isons are of limited value, as referral bias and patient characteristics hinder a true evaluation, and most comparative studies have included rigid, as well as expandable, stents.

Tracheoesophageal fistulas have not been successfully palliated by rigid rubber or plastic stents in the past due to a failure to obtain an adequate seal across the fistula. Persistent aspiration of gastric or esophageal fluids into the trachea or bronchus results in a productive cough, and aspiration pneumonia, and in some patients rigid esophageal tubes may compress the airway, causing stridor and dyspnea. Airway stenting has been tried with some success,[35] using a bifurcated foam-covered stent in the trachea, or by using a combination of a dynamic airway stent along with an esophageal tube (**Figure 14.2**).[36] While there is logic to this double stenting technique, the majority of centers now use covered expandable metallic stents in the esophagus alone, with very good results. Indeed, the covered Gianturco stent or Wallstent give excellent results with both relief of symptoms of fistula and radiologic sealing being reported.[30,37–41]

As well as sealing the fistula in 90% of reported cases, the esophageal expanding stent provides relief of the dysphagia, and airway stenting is rarely necessary. The main indication currently for using airway stenting routinely is when the fistula is due to a tumor of the bronchus or trachea, rather than arising from the esophagus.[42] The main problem after stenting tracheo- or bronchoesophageal

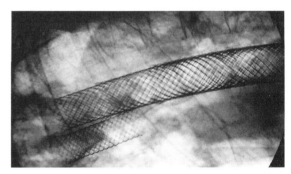

Figure 14.2 Radiograph of a double stent for tracheoesophageal fistula. A small expanding metallic stent has been placed in the trachea and a large expanding metallic stent in the esophagus. (Illustration kindly supplied by R. Mason, Guy's Hospital, London.)

Table 14.5 Indications for expanding metallic stents

Relief of dysphagia in primary esophageal carcinoma
Relief of dysphagia in anastomotic recurrence
Relief of dysphagia in recurrence or failed response to radiotherapy or chemotherapy
Occlusion of tracheoesophageal fistula
Occlusion of esophagopericardial fistulae[31]
Tamponade of bleeding tumors
Rescue of iatrogenic perforation such as after laser or dilatation injury

fistulas has been hemorrhage in the airway, or progression of a previously established pneumonia. The other scenario where an airway stent alone is useful is postoperative fistula between the bronchus and the thoracic stomach. The stomach tube will not hold a stent, and if conservative management does not allow healing, then an airway stent may be helpful to reduce the emptying of gastric juice into the bronchus.

Methods of stent insertion

Preparation

Oropharyngeal analgesia with lignocaine is used. Sedation (midazolam and pethidine) and routine monitoring is needed, including pulse oxymetry along with routine administration of oxygen and intravenous access. The teeth or gums are protected with a mouthguard.

Endoscopy

This is not routinely necessary for placement of stents. It is of help to prevent high stents from impinging on the cricopharyngeus. Stents can be placed in the mid and lower esophagus under endoscopic guidance, but the tumor must be negotiable by the scope for this to be done safely. It is therefore recommended that, for routine use, radiology with fluoroscopy should be the primary imaging modality for stent insertion and endoscopy used as a complementary tool.

Radiology

Prior to stent insertion a barium swallow is performed to assess the position and length of the tumor, and to identify if there is any bronchoesophageal fistula. A steerable catheter (e.g., 6.5 Fr biliary manipulation catheter) is then passed over a guidewire into the mouth, down to the lesion. Contrast is injected through the catheter to find the upper limit of the tumor, and the level

marked with a metallic marker on the skin.[43] The catheter is then passed through the tumor into the stomach. It is useful to use a hydrophilic guidewire to aid this passage. Contrast can then be injected below the lesion and the lower limit of the lesion identified. The skin at the level of the tumor's lower limit is then marked. The fine hydrophilic guidewire is then removed and replaced with a stiff guidewire before removing the catheter. Balloon dilatation to 10–15 mm should then be achieved, depending on the stent being used. Each stent requires a different balloon dilatation technique; the Strecker stent needs full dilatation to 15 mm, but the Gianturco or Wallstent need only 10 mm dilatation before allowing them to expand under their own recoil pressure. The stent insertion device can be measured according to the distance between the skin markers and then passed safely and positioned radiographically. **Figure 14.3** shows the detail of insertion of the Ultraflex Nitinol stent; **Figure 14.4** shows the insertion sheath and unloading of the Gianturco stent.

Post stent care is minimal, except for occasional analgesia if the expanding stent causes pain. Oral fluids are usually allowed the same day as the stent is placed. The next day a barium swallow is performed to check that the stent is in good position, well-dilated, and sealing any fistula. If so, then diet may be started.

Problems with stents

Despite the dramatically improved results with expandable metallic stents over their rigid predecessors, there is still an impressive collection of complications (**Table 14.6**) that can occur after their insertion.[44] Most of these are rare and many may be related to poor training of the staff who insert them. These stents are not difficult to place, but expert tuition is helpful to prevent the operator from learning by his or her mistakes. Poor stent expansion is uncommon with Cook Gianturco

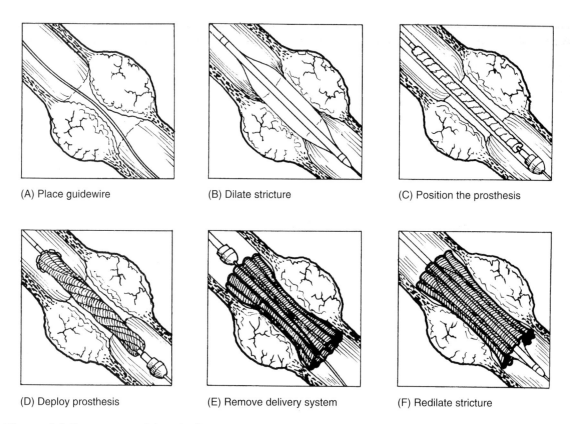

(A) Place guidewire

(B) Dilate stricture

(C) Position the prosthesis

(D) Deploy prosthesis

(E) Remove delivery system

(F) Redilate stricture

Figure 14.3 Diagram of the Ultraflex Nitinol stent insertion and release using sheath-mounted stents. A. A guidewire is placed across the carcinoma. B. The tumor is dilated with a balloon dilator 12 mm in diameter. C. A metallic stent introducer is placed across the tumor extending to more than 2 cm above and below the limits of the lesion by checking with fluoroscopy. D. The prosthesis is deployed and as the gelatin dissolves the prosthesis self-expands. E. Once the expansion is sufficient the delivery system is removed under fluoroscopic control. F. The stent is redilated with a 12 mm diameter balloon.

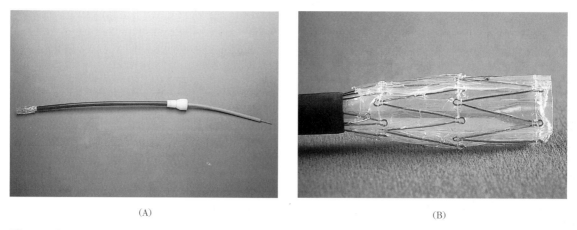

(A)

(B)

Figure 14.4 A. Broad view of the insertion sheath of a Gianturco covered stent. B. Detail of the stent being unloaded from the sheath.

Table 14-6 Complications of expandable metallic stents used in the treatment of esophageal carcinoma

Poor stent expansion	Ingrowth through the metallic latticework
Migration	Overgrowth above or below the ends of the stent
Reflux symptoms	Fracture of Nitinol stents
Food impaction	Stent torsion
Retrosternal pain	Erosion of the right main stem bronchus
Neck pain	Delayed bleeding
Odynophagia	Mediastinal fistula
Psychogenic dysphagia	

and Schneider Wallstent,[45] but is more common with the Ultraflex Nitinol stent.[46] If this is identified on the barium swallow performed on the first postoperative day, then it can be corrected by endoscopic or radiologic balloon distention.[47]

Complications that relate to the stents themselves are very infrequent. Migration may still occur, despite elaborate anchorage devices. Retrieving a poorly positioned or migrated stent can be difficult because of the effectiveness of the anchorage devices. Methods of retrieval vary,[48,49] depending on the stent used. With the Ultraflex stent it is relatively simple to catch a strand of the wire, and traction on this allows the whole stent to unravel due to the stent being constructed with a simple knitted fabric.[50] With simple wall stents a flexible endoscope may be placed within them to reposition them, but the barbs on the Gianturco and other similar stents makes retrieval almost impossible.[51-53] In circumstances where a stent has migrated into the stomach it may be wise to leave it there, as it is most unlikely to obstruct gastric outflow. If migration is only partially through the tumor, a second stent should be placed above the first to anchor the lower stent and relieve any proximal obstruction.[54]

Stents placed high in the esophagus with the funnel in the post cricoid region have in the past proved troublesome, with a sensation of globus and problems with aspiration of regurgitated food. With modifications, the new expandable stents are much more acceptable to patients when placed in these positions than were the rubber Atkinson or Celestin tubes.[55,56]

Reflux symptoms occur in only 10% of patients after stenting. As this frequency is low, it is suggested not to use routine acid suppression or prokinetics, but to reserve them for treating patients who suffer reflux symptoms.[52,57] The aim of treatment in patients with symptomatic reflux or regurgitation through the stent should be to reduce the volume of gastric contents by aiding gastric emptying (domperidone or cisapride), and reducing the acid content with either an H_2-receptor antagonist or proton pump inhibitor (ranitidine, omeprazole, or lanzoprazole). In some patients, gastric emptying may be particularly poor because of the invasion by the tumor of the vagus nerves. In these patients it is much more important to improve gastric emptying than to suppress acid, as their acid production may already be low.

Retrosternal pain may occur after stent insertion and in my experience in approximately 20% of cases there will be a need for symptomatic treatment within the first 24–48 h. This is usually managed simply with orally administered narcotics, but the patients may benefit from being kept in hospital overnight after the stent has been placed.

Long-term problems with stents relate usually to recurrent dysphagia.[58] The reasons include poor stent expansion, ingrowth through the metallic latticework of uncovered stents, and overgrowth above or below the ends of the stent. In comparative studies there is a range in frequency of recurrent dysphagia from 10% with Wallstents to 36% with the Ultraflex Nitinol stent.[59] The incidence correlates with survival time.[44] For ingrowth, the best options of treatment are laser or argon beam coagulation (**Figure 14.5**), while for overgrowth, intubation with a second stent is both safe and relatively easy.[60] If this is not feasible, it may be worthwhile using laser or gas plasma coagulation of the overgrowth.

Rare complications which have been reported include fracture of Nitinol stents,[61] stent torsion, odynophagia, psychogenic dysphagia, erosion of the right main stem bronchus,[62] delayed bleeding, and mediastinal fistula.[52]

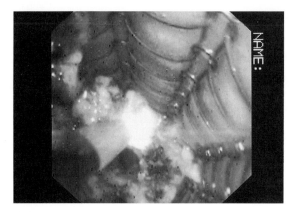

Figure 14.5 Argon beam plasma coagulator being used to remove tumor which has grown in through the open latticework of an uncovered expanding metallic stent that has been in the esophagus for the previous 4 months.

Despite optimistic reports about stent insertion, the complications are likely to continue. The true rate of complications is often higher than the summation of literature reports and it is important to take heed of reports such as Wu et al.[41] who, in a series of 32 patients, documented a migration in four patients (12%), food impaction in two (6%), tumor ingrowth through disrupted membrane (one), overgrowth (one), hemorrhage (one) and late pressure necrosis with sepsis (one), which gave a 30% problematic stent rate. The rate of complications can probably be reduced realistically to 10% with training to achieve good placement and appropriate after-treatments for tumor extension.[63,64]

Which expandable stent is best?

The stent which is the cheapest, associated with the lowest complication rate overall, and provides the best functional result in the hands of the operator concerned is the best stent to use. This will vary depending on local costs, local training, and facilities. May et al.[65] compared the problems of three types of stent (Schneider Wallstent, Ultraflex Nitinol, and Cook covered Gianturco-Z) (see **Table 14.5**). We favour the Gianturco covered stent, but there are certainly patients, such as those with very high tumors, who might benefit from the knitted stents.

COMBINATIONS OF STENTS AND RADIOTHERAPY

In theory, the addition of radiotherapy to palliation by intubation should have some survival advantage, but this has not been demonstrated in practice. The only study to show a difference in favor of combined radiotherapy and intubation was not randomized and clearly biased the more favorable patients into the combined treatment arm.[66] Indeed, if the data are reanalyzed after removing the deaths within 30 days there is no difference in survival. The only effect seems to be a very long hospitalization for those treated with radiotherapy (46 days versus 23 days). In a small study, Reed et al.[67] compared three treatment groups: (i) intubation with an Atkinson tube; (ii) radiotherapy combined with a tube; and (iii) laser combined with radiotherapy, and identified no inter-group differences in survival. Schmid et al.[68] also compared intubation with and without radiotherapy and found no difference statistically, although the group treated with intubation alone showed a trend towards longer survival (15 versus 9 weeks).

LASERS

Lasers were introduced for palliation of cancer of the esophagus during the 1980s as a significant advance over the rigid intubation methods available at that time. Endoscopic application of lasers became feasible and carcinoma of the esophagus was regarded as one of the primary targets for their application. Numerous papers have reported their use,[69–74] but the initial enthusiasm has declined because of the introduction of improved intubating techniques, as well as problems of the time, expertise, and cost of laser application. The neodimium-ytrium aluminium garnet laser (Nd-YAG) is the preferred type for esophageal tumors because it has a more useful tissue penetration and vaporization power than the pulsed dye lasers of KTP or argon.

Principles of laser application

The principle behind laser application is that tumor can be ablated to achieve a reasonable caliber of patency. The technique is usually performed under sedation and with topical pharyngeal anesthesia. The safest method of laser ablation is to pass a guidewire through the tumor under fluoroscopic control and pre-dilate the tumor to the size of the endoscope – usually 11 mm. The endoscope is passed through the tumor and the ablation commenced from below; progressive tissue ablation is then executed during gradual withdrawal of the endoscope. The initial reaction of the malignant tissue is a white, circular burn, though with continued application of laser energy there is vaporization of the tissue. Some charring and smoke is produced and this can either be aspirated through the endoscope (convenient if a dual-channel endoscope), or by passing a nasogastric tube alongside the scope to vent the insufflated gas and smoke.

The most popular laser technique in Britain is the non-contact Nd-YAG laser using a coaxial gas flow and delivering 2000–10 000 J per treatment session. The use of non-contact or contact probes has been debated[75] because, in theory, the contact lasers may have had a lower perforation rate, but the two techniques have been shown to be equivalent. This lack of benefit may be related to the mechanism of perforation during laser treatment. The incidence of perforation is related to the pre-dilatation necessary,[34] as well as to the transgression of the beams through the full thickness of the esophageal wall. As most of the perforations occurred after pre-dilatation, these are usually recognized and as long as they are managed conservatively survival is good. Using a management strategy of stenting only if a contrast swallow 3 days later showed persistent leak, Tyrrell et al.[34] showed that only three of 20 patients with perforation after dilatation died. In contrast, the two perforations attributable to the laser therapy resulted in death in both cases. The overall death rate from laser therapy was low (1.4%); however, the cost of managing perforations after laser therapy is expensive both in terms of money and in terms of the proportion of active life remaining to the patient with cancer of the esophagus.

The procedure is time-consuming, especially in long tumors, and most of the comparative studies observed the best results with short strictures. Repeat applications are necessary. A delay of up to 1 week between initial treatment and relief of dysphagia is typical. Some patients suffer substernal pain, and many have a fever and leukocystosis.

Problems with lasers

The use of a laser through an endoscope is not a universal skill, and the expertise needed is not readily available. In addition, the set-up costs for laser treatment are expensive, as the instruments cost £50 000–100 000 ($75 000–150 000) and the safety measures associated with their installation and use are expensive. The instruments are potentially dangerous to staff and patients if the laser beams are not effectively controlled. Perforations are kept to a minimum in centers with expertise, but still range between 6% and 13% in reported series.[76,77] One of the largest series is that of Mason et al.,[76] who have reported laser treatment of more than 350 patients with cancer of the esophagus and a 6% perforation rate. With such a large experience it is likely that this is the best result possible and centers with less experience might suffer considerably higher perforation rates.

Combined laser and standard radiotherapy

Radiotherapy has been used in combination with lasers in order to reduce the frequency of repeat laser treatment sessions. However, the addition of radiotherapy adds little in practice as the patient must attend for radiotherapy and the days spent in hospital are no less. Also, esophageal tumors that respond well to radiotherapy often heal with fibrosis, and a significant number require further dilatation to relieve dysphagia.[78]

Combined laser and afterloading radiotherapy

The concept of intraluminal radiotherapy with some form of tissue ablation is appealing because, with radiation alone, dysphagia takes some weeks to improve while with luminal tissue ablation the lack of injury to deeper tumor allows rapid recurrence. By combining the two treatments, a number of authors have shown significant improvements.[79–82] However, the combination of this equipment is expensive and not widely available, and this treatment is currently limited to a few specialist centers. Brachytherapy alone and radiotherapy alone have been discussed in Chapter 13.

Stents versus lasers

During the 1980s, laser treatment became the mainstay of palliation for dysphagia in many units.[72,83] Lasers were perceived to give a better quality of palliation than the rigid rubber or plastic stents, had a lower complication rate,[76] and enabled near-normal swallowing for malignant dysphagia. However, laser therapy has to be repeated, usually every 6 weeks, and in some patients the dysphagia free interval becomes progressively shorter as the disease progresses. While the complication rate is lower than rigid stents, there is still a perforation rate[26,32] which is significantly greater than the complication rate for the new expandable metallic stents.

Prospective comparison of endoscopic laser therapy with the placement of self-expandable metallic prostheses has been performed in a number of institutions, although few have been properly randomized. The series from Guys Hospital London[84] randomized 60 patients to three treatment arms: (i) laser; (ii) covered expandable stents; and (iii) uncovered expandable stents, and showed a substantially improved quality of swallow with the stents.

Even comparisons of laser with rigid stents showed a similar quality of swallow improvement for mid-esophageal tumors and, for those tumors crossing the cardia, intubation was better.[85] In this study, the perforation rate of lasers at 13% was considerably more than the 2% with expandable stents. Similarly, Alderson et al.,[86] in a non-randomized comparison in 40 patients, showed comparable quality of swallow of laser recanalization with rigid stents except for short tumors, where lasers produced a better result. Carter et al.[87] in a very similar study, again in 40 patients, showed some advantage for quality of swallow in patients treated with lasers. In neither trial was there any difference in the survival of patients in the differing treatment arms. However, for both of these trials the new pliable metallic stents would probably negate the quality of swallow advantage that lasers had in short tumors.

For palliation of post-cricoid tumors or bulky growths, lasers have been regarded as better than intubation as the pressure of the stent in the neck can cause discomfort in breathing, pain, and pressure on the larynx with cough.[88] For most other indications, expanding metallic stents are the preferred method of palliating dysphagia or fistula.

Cost-effectiveness

Comparisons of costs are very difficult from the published literature because of variations in the pattern of practice and costs in different geographic locations. In addition, the constantly changing practice makes meaningful comparisons out of

date. Sculpher et al.[89] from the Health Economics Research Group in Brunel University, Middlesex, UK, identified that the costs of laser palliation were between £153 and £710 more than intubation. However, their stent assumptions were based on statistics reporting rigid stents and not expandable metallic stents. The latter are certainly more expensive to insert than rigid stents, but this cost is offset by the cost of treating the complications of rigid stent insertion.

ARGON BEAM PLASMA COAGULATION

This is a recently developed technology for safely ablating surface tissue. It is not a laser, but an electrified stream of argon gas which is readily applied through a gastroscope and effective in the destruction of upper gastrointestinal lesions. The argon plasma is a stream of ionized argon gas which carries monopolar diathermy current in a controlled manner from the end of the applicator to the tissue. A particularly useful feature of the current is its controlled application to the surface. Once the surface has been coagulated and dried, current needs to find an easier electrical path, and passes through the tissue adjacent to the initial coagulated area. The longer the energy is applied, the wider the area of tissue ablation with minimal deep extension. It is therefore very suitable for endoscopic application in the esophagus, reducing the risk of perforation. The high gas flow (2 l/min) into the esophagus requires regular aspiration to prevent dangerous gastric distention, but otherwise no special precautions are needed over normal diathermy.

The technique of argon beam plasma coagulation is easy to learn and the instrument is relatively cheap, being only a small additional cost over a standard diathermy machine. Compared with the costs of a laser it is cheap, and does not require the eye protection and room safety features that lasers necessitate.

While the application of argon beam plasma coagulation in the upper gastrointestinal tract has been limited, it shows promise as a tool of palliation.[90] In our own unit we have found it particularly useful in clearing ingrowth of tumor through stents and for tumor overgrowth at the ends of stents (see **Figure 14.5**).

Combined stenting and tissue ablation

Tissue ablation can be helpful before and after stenting. Laser recanalization has been used to allow the passage of a stent safely through the esophageal tumor. Barr *et al.*[91] compared laser only with laser plus intubation and found a very high rate of complications in patients who were recanalized with laser and then intubated with a rigid stent. It is clear that complication rates from the insertion of expandable stents now is significantly less than this, and there is only a rare indication for using lasers prior to stent placement. Indeed, to place an expandable stent or pass a laser probe, a wire must be placed across the tumor; once this is achieved, an expandable stent can usually be placed without the need for tissue ablation.

Lasers and argon beam ablation are very useful for releasing blockage of an esophageal stent by tumor. The new expandable stents have two problems which relate to tumor growth: (i) growth over the upper or lower ends of the stent; or (ii) growth inward through the latticework of the metal. Covered stents avoid this latter complication, but have the disadvantage of slippage and migration. Tumor growth above, below, or into expandable metallic stents is relatively easy to deal with by laser or argon beam ablation,[6,60,92–94] and these deal with stent blockage in the majority of patients, avoiding the need for the placement of a second tube. By the time stents become blocked (which occurs in only 15–20% of patients), the survival of the patients is very limited and a median of only one treatment is needed to maintain tube patency for the remainder of the patient's life.

PHOTODYNAMIC THERAPY

Photodynamic therapy (PDT) is an application of light, usually from an argon pumped dye laser source, but where the tissue destruction relies on the principle of activation of a chemical in the affected tissues. The photosensitizing chemical may be acridine orange, hematoporphyrin derivative (HpD; protoporphyrin I), or purified dihematoporphyrin ether (protoporphyrin II), or aminolevulinic acid (ALA).[95,96] The protoporphyrin is administered some time before the light is applied. HpD is given 48 h before irradiation by intravenous infusion and at a dose of 2.5–5.0 mg/ kg. ALA is more easily administered as it can be given orally. The dose is important in balancing the side effects against the efficacy. Photosensitization of the skin is a temporary, but limiting, factor and patients may suffer nausea, malaise and fever. The restriction from natural sunlight may be quite upsetting to patients who may have only a very limited life span and sunburn has been reported in >25% of cases.[97] The orally administered ALA seems to be very much less skin toxic, but most of the published series to date have used the injected protoporphyrins.

The selectivity of PDT for neoplasms appears to be related to the uptake of the photosensitizing drug. This apparent selectivity may occur because of the increased permeability of tumor vasculature that allows the relatively large photosensitizing molecules to leak into the intercellular space. This effect is compounded by a decreased lymphatic drainage within the tumor, which decreases drug removal. The drugs also localize to intracellular (hydrophobic) membranes, especially the cytoplasmic, mitochondrial, and nuclear membranes. Cytotoxicity depends on a reaction of the light, the drug, and oxygen. The drug becomes energized by a light photon and transfers its energy to surrounding oxygen, producing active forms such as singlet oxygen free radical or peroxide.

The light is very easily applied, but requires some pre-dilatation in obstructive tumors in order to allow the beam to access the full length of the lesion. This pre-dilatation accounts for the low but documented rate of perforation at 1%, which is significantly better than the 6–13% perforation rate for laser therapy.[97,98] However, the application is much easier than Nd-YAG laser, and has possibly wider application if laser skills are not available. Exposure times vary from 5 to 40 min, and some centers use two applications over 2 days while others single treatments. To achieve an adequate intensity (of red light at 630 nm wavelength), a laser is used but the power output is much less than thermal injury Nd-YAG lasers. Red light at 630 nm wavelength is used because it has the deepest penetration.

A major drawback of PDT using hematoporphyrin derivative is the altered quality of life, because the patient must avoid direct sunlight for one month. Another complication is the frequent esophageal stenoses requiring dilatation in 30% of patients. While this is perhaps unavoidable and common to any procedure which produces circumferential injury to the esophagus, it is a major limitation for a technique which is being considered as palliation for dysphagia. Another important limitation is that the depth of tissue destruction is < 1 cm, and only T1 and T2 tumors are ideal candidates for PDT. The most impressive results from this therapy come from Sibille et al.[95] in France, where 123 patients unfit for resectional surgery with early tumors were treated with PDT and 5-year disease-specific survival rates of 75% were achieved. However, this was not as good as surgical resection for similar staged tumors, and the authors recommended PDT only where resection is not a safe option.[99]

Photodynamic therapy in palliation of advanced lesions produces few, if any, long-term cures, but so-called complete responses with good palliation have been achieved. The results in the early series[100–102] suggested that frequent complete responses might be feasible, but these results have not been achieved in subsequent larger prospective studies.[103–105] This may be due to differences in disease (all three earlier Japanese studies treated squamous carcinoma exclusively) or differences in methodology. Patrice et al.[106] in France also reported a high complete response rate, but their study group contained patients with rectal cancer, gastric cancer, and esophageal cancer; moreover, the esophageal cancer cure rates when examined were less optimistic.

The most comprehensive prospective study to date is by Lightdale et al.[98] from New York who compared, in a randomized study, 110 patients treated with PDT and 108 patients treated with Nd-YAG laser. At 1 month after treatment, the PDT group showed greater tumor response (32% compared with 20% reduction) but few patients had a complete response (8% versus 2%). Tumors in the mid-esophagus were equally well palliated by laser or PDT, but those at the upper and lower ends of the esophagus and those with a very long middle stricture showed the greatest advantage with PDT, which was not surprising given that these are difficult to palliate well with laser.

There are, however, few studies comparing PDT with expanding metallic stents and it would appear that, except for the centers with a special interest in PDT, expanding metallic stents are now preferred due to their low complication rate and rapid palliation without side effects. Photodynamic therapy

has also been used to treat tumor overgrowth in patients with esophageal cancer and metal stents.[107]

Photodynamic therapy is thus best suited to early lesions. Indeed, it has been used for high-grade dysplasia and while not coming under the heading of palliation, PDT treatment is now being used increasingly in order to prevent the development of carcinoma in patients with Barrett's esophagus.[108] PDT has not yet established its role in either advanced or early esophageal carcinoma, and further investigation of this method is required to improve its application and side effects.

LOCAL ALCOHOL AND POLIDOCANOL INJECTION

While alcohol as a tissue toxin has been used in open surgery for many years, endoscopic injection of tumors has only been popularized in the past decade. It is a simple endoscopic technique that requires no special equipment and is extremely cheap.[109,110] The results of treatment have been reported as equivalent to the palliation of dysphagia that is achieved with lasers. Despite being cheap, simple and more widely available, polidocanol injection has not become a commonly used technique. It is not without complication and perforation, necrosis, and bleeding are potential problems. However, the technique deserves further study.

Other forms of injection of chemical material into a tumor allows a number of other modalities greater versatility. For instance, preloading a tumor with photosensitizer locally may reduce the side effects of systemically administered porphyrin derivatives or ALA. Another potential future option will be chemotherapy injection into the tumor with microcapsules for delayed release of the cytotoxic agent. By administering the therapy directly and allowing the microcapsules to drain through the lymphatics prior to release of chemotherapy, the systemic side effects of very high doses can theoretically be minimized. Microcapsule radiotherapy injection is also a potential future development.

PALLIATIVE CHEMOTHERAPY WITH OR WITHOUT RADIOTHERAPY

Palliative chemotherapy is not recommended routinely for esophageal cancer because of disappointing response rates and associated toxicity in patients who are often elderly and of poor performance status. The stimulus for continued investigation comes with the increasing number of young and active patients presenting with advanced or metastatic carcinoma, and there is a rising demand for any form of therapy that will extend their life. Intubation with a good quality stent allows a patient to maintain a community-based life and a normal diet. It does not, however have any impact on the rate at which the tumor grows, and despite improvement in the nutrition of the patient it will have little effect in lengthening the life of the patient.

Chemotherapy is often regarded as the only hope in extending useful life and the literature is constantly being updated with new regimens which seem to offer some hope. Most current chemotherapy regimens use combinations of cisplatinum, 5-fluorouracil (5-FU), mitomycin C and paclitaxel.[111] Ajani et al.[112] showed some benefit after the new agent paclitaxel was introduced, but results have not been as promising as in gynecology or other areas of oncology. Trials of radical chemotherapy with immunologic rescue or immunologic manipulation have not yet shown results which would justify their routine use. Javed et al.[113] administered paclitaxel, cisplatinum and 5-FU in relatively high doses, and followed this by white cell rescue with granulocyte colony-stimulating factor (G-CSF), documenting excellent response in epidermoid and adenocarcinoma of the esophagus. However, this aggressive treatment is tolerable by only a small proportion of patients with cancer of the esophagus. In a Phase II clinical trial, Wadler et al.[114] used 5-FU, recombinant interferon alpha-2b, and cisplatinum for patients with metastatic or regionally advanced carcinoma of the esophagus. Both of these two combined regimens are probably too aggressive in terms of side effects to be regarded as palliative,[115] and they are being developed with the ambition of significant life extension.

The recent literature shows that both adenocarcinoma and squamous carcinoma are equally chemosensitive, and in trials associated with subsequent resection[116] where the measurement of response to chemotherapy could be assessed objectively at surgery, there was clearly a good response in patients with either lesion. In unusual tumors such as small cell (oat cell) carcinoma, responses may be dramatic[117] but where complete necrosis of the tumor occurs there can be the risk of perforation of the esophagus, as reported by Clark et al.[118]

As with much of the literature on palliation in esophageal carcinoma, proper randomized prospective trials are rare. Schmid et al.[68] published a well-controlled randomized trial (albeit with small numbers; 120 in total) and showed no advantage of adding chemotherapy or radiotherapy after intubation.

Where improvements are documented they are measured in terms of months, rather than years, so that no chemotherapy treatment to date has been shown to improve 5-year survival statistics. However, improvements in 1- and 2-year survival rates may be clinically relevant when treating younger patients whose family and life commitments may benefit from such short-term life extension. The benefit of any such life extension must be balanced with the side effects of the treatment, so that extended life is useful to the patient. Despite the many reports published, further work is required before there is convincing evidence of an overall benefit. At present, palliative chemotherapy remains experimental and should be considered only in the context of a clinical trial.

SUMMARY

Expanding metallic stents are now the preferred option in palliating the dysphagia of unresectable carcinoma of the esophagus. They are not without complication and are relatively expensive to insert, but produce the best quality of palliation with the least intervention and fewer complications compared with lasers. The injection of toxins produces a good palliation, but leads to the same problems as lasers in requiring repeated therapy. Newer methods of tissue ablation using photodynamic therapy and argon beam plasma coagulators are still experimental, and should be deployed in centers with research facilities to analyze the results. Chemo- and radiotherapy may be used to supplement these methods, but should be considered only where the merits of short-term life extension are worthwhile in the context of the patient's quality of life and cost-effectiveness. Patients with advanced cancer of the esophagus need a multidisciplinary approach to the palliation of a wide variety of potential symptoms.

REFERENCES

1. Watson A. Carcinoma of the esophagus. In: Misiewicz JJ, Pounder, RE & Venables CW (eds) *Diseases of the Gut and Pancreas.* Oxford, UK: Blackwell 1994: 159–72.

2. Giuli R & Sancho-Garnier H. Diagnostic, therapeutic and prognostic features of cancers of the oesophagus : results of the international prospective study by the OESO group (190 patients). *Surgery* 1986; **99**; 614–22.

3. Byrne J, Parry J, Attwood SEA & Woodman C. The epidemiology of adenocarcinoma at the oesophago-gastric junction in the North West of England. In: Guili R, Galmiche J-P, Jamieson GG & Scarpignato C (eds) *The Esophago-Gastric Junction.* Paris: OESO 1998: 1140–4.

4. McKeown KC. Trends of oesophageal resection for carcinoma. *Ann R Coll Surg Engl* 1972; **51**: 213–38.

5. Ellis FH Jr. Treatment of carcinoma of the oesophagus or cardia. *Mayo Clin Proc* 1989; **64**: 945–50.

6. Cwikiel W, Tranberg KG & Willen R. Disappearance of esophageal carcinoma after stenting combined with endoscopic laser therapy. *Cardiovasc Intervent Radiol* 1995; **18**: 247–50.

7. Doyle D, Hanks GW & Macdonald N. Pathophysiology of cancer cachexia. In: Alexander RH & Norton JA (eds) *Oxford Textbook of Paliative Medicine.* Oxford: Oxford University Press 1993: 316–29.

8. Loizou LA, Rampton D, Atkinson M, Robertson C & Bown SG. A prospective assessment of quality of life after endoscopic intubation and laser therapy for malignant dysphagia. *Cancer* 1992; **70**: 386–91.

9. O'Hanlon DM, Harkin M, Karat D, Sergeant T, Hayes N & Griffin SM. Quality of life assessment in patients with oesophageal carcinoma. *Br J Surg* 1995; **82**: 1682–5.

10. Watson A. A study of the quality and duration of survival following resection, endoscopic intubation and surgical intubation in oesophageal carcinoma. *Br J Surg* 1982; **69**: 585–8.

11. Cwikiel M, Cwikiel W & Albertsson M. Palliation of dysphagia in patients with malignant esophageal strictures. Comparison of results of radiotherapy, chemotherapy and esophageal stent treatment. *Acta Oncol* 1996; **35**: 75–9.

12. Reed CE. Comparison of different treatments for unresectable esophageal cancer. *World J Surg* 1995; **19**: 828–35.

13. Griffin SM & Robertson CS. Non-surgical treatment of cancer of the oesophagus. *Br J Surg* 1993; **80**: 412–13.

14. Conlan AA, Nicolaou N, Hammond CA, de Nobrega C & Mistry BD. Retrosternal gastric bypass for inoperable esophageal cancer: a report of 71 patients. *Ann Thorac Surg* 1983; **36**: 396–400.

15. Mannell A, Becker PJ & Nissenbaum M. Bypass surgery for unresectable esophageal cancer: early and late results in 124 cases. *Br J Surg* 1988; **75**: 283–6.

16. Postlethwait RW, Sealy WC, Dillon ML & Young WG. Colon interposition for esophageal substitution. *Ann Thorac Surg* 1971; **12**: 89–94.

17. Stephens HB. Colon bypass of the esophagus. *Am J Surg* 1971; **122**: 217–221.

18. Segalin A, Little AG, Ruol A *et al.* Surgical and endoscopic palliation of esophageal carcinoma. *Ann Thorac Surg* 1989; **48**: 267–71.

19. Lundell L, Leth R, Lind T, Lonroth H, Sjovall M & Olbe L. Palliative endoscopic dilatation in carcinoma of the esophagus and esophagogastric junction. *Acta Chir Scand* 1989; **155**: 179–84.

20. Ogilvie AL, Dronfield MW, Ferguson R & Atkinson M. Palliative intubation of oesophagogastric neoplasms at fibreoptic endoscopy. *Gut* 1982; **23**: 1060–7.

21. Lishman AH, Dellipiani AW & Devlin HB. The insertion of oesophagogastric tubes in malignant oesophageal strictures. *Br J Surg* 1980; **80**: 257–9.

22. Cusumano A, Ruol A, Segalin A *et al.* (1992) Push-through intubation: effective palliation in 409 patients with cancer of the esophagus and cardia. *Ann Thorac Surg* 1992; **53**: 1010–14.

23. Liakakos TK, Ohri SK, Townsend ER & Fountain SW. Palliative intubation for dysphagia in patients with carcinoma of the esophagus. *Ann Thorac Surg* 1992; **53**: 460–3.

24. Knyrim K , Wagner HJ, Bethge N, Keymling M & Vakil N. A controlled trial of an expansile metal stent for palliation of esophageal obstruction due to inoperable cancer. *N Engl J Med* 1993; **329**: 1302–7.

25. De Palma GD, di Matteo E, Romano G, Fimmano A, Rondinone G & Catanzano C. Plastic prosthesis versus expandable metal stents for palliation of inoperable esophageal thoracic carcinoma: a controlled prospective study. *Gastrointest Endosc* 1996; **43**: 478–82.

26. Ellul JPM, Watkinson A, Khan RJK, Adam A & Mason RC. Self expanding metal stents for the palliation of dysphagia due to inoperable oesophageal carcinoma. *Br J Surg* 1995; **82**: 1678– 81.

27. Hill J, Nicholson DA & Bancewicz J. Endoscopic intubation of oesophagogastric malignancy. *Eur J Gastroenterol Hepatol* 1995; **7**: 815–6.

28. Bethge N, Sommer A, von Kleist D & Vakil N. A prospective trial of self-expanding metal stents in the palliation of malignant esophageal obstruction after failure of primary curative therapy. *Gastrointest Endosc* 1996; **44**: 283–6.

29. Hause DW, Kagan AR, Fleischman E & Harvey JC. Tracheo-esophageal fistula complicating carcinoma of the esophagus. *Am Surg* 1992; **58**: 441–2.

30. Cook TA & Dehn TCB. Use of expandable metal stents in the treatment of oesophageal carcinoma and tracheo-oesophageal fistula. *Br J Surg* 1996; **83**: 1417–8.

31. Tukkie R, Hulst RW, Sprangers F & Bartelsman JF. An esophagopericardial fistula successfully treated with an expandable covered metal mesh stent. *Gastrointest Endosc* 1996; **43**: 165–7.

32. Watkinson A, Ellul J, Entwisle K, Farrugia M, Mason R & Adam A. Plastic-covered metallic endoprostheses in the management of esophageal perforation in patients with oesophageal carcinoma. *Clin Radiol* 1995; **50**: 304–9.

33. Nicholson AA, Royston CM, Wedgewood K, Milkins R & Taylor AD. Palliation of malignant oesophageal perforation and proximal oesophageal malignant dysphagia with covered metal stents. *Clin Radiol* 1995; **50**: 11–14.

34. Tyrrell MR, Trotter GA, Adam A & Mason RC. Incidence and management of laser-associated oesophageal perforation. *Br J Surg* 1995; **82**: 1257–8.

35. Albes JM, Schafers HJ, Gebel M & Ross UH. Tracheal stenting for malignant tracheoesophageal fistula. *Ann Thorac Surg* 1994; **57**: 1263–6.

36. Freitag L, Tekolf E, Steveling H, Donovan TJ & Stamatis G. Management of malignant esophagotracheal fistulas with airway stenting and double stenting. *Chest* 1996; **110**: 1155–60.

37. Mohammed S & Moss J. Palliation of malignant tracheo-oesophageal fistula using covered metal stents. *Clin Radiol* 1996; **51**: 42–6.

38. Wong K & Goldstraw P. Role of covered esophageal stents in malignant esophagorespiratory fistula. *Ann Thorac Surg* 1995; **60**: 199–200.

39. Do YS, Song IIY, Lee BH *et al*. Esophago-respiratory fistula associated with esophageal cancer: treatment with a Gianturco stent tube. *Radiology* 1993; **187**: 673–7.

40. Ell C, May A & Hahn EG. Gianturco-Z stents in the palliative treatment of malignant esophageal obstruction and esophagotracheal fistulas. *Endoscopy* 1995; **27**: 495–500.

41. Wu WC, Katon RM, Saxon RR *et al*. Silicone-covered self-expanding metallic stents for the palliation of malignant esophageal obstruction and esophagorespiratory fistulas: experience in 32 patients and a review of the literature. *Gastrointest Endosc* 1994; **40**: 22–33.

42. Weigert N, Neuhaus H, Rosch T, Hoffmann W, Dittler HJ & Classen M. Treatment of esophago-respiratory fistulas with silicone-coated self-expanding metal stents. *Gastrointest Endosc* 1995; **41**: 490–6.

43. Raijman I, Kortan P, Haber GB & Marcon NE. Contrast injection to identify tumor margins during esophageal stent placement. *Gastrointest Endosc* 1994; **40**: 222–4.

44. Acunas B, Rozanes I, Akpinar S, Tunaci A, Tunaci M & Acunas G. Palliation of malignant esophageal strictures with self-expanding nitinol stents: drawbacks and complications. *Radiology* 1996; **199**: 648–52.

45. Messmann H, Vogt W, Gmeinwieser J, Scholmerich J & Holstege A. Delayed spontaneous opening of a self-expanding metal stent bridging a malignant esophageal stenosis. *Hepatogastroenterology* 1994; **41**: 571–2.

46. Winkelbauer FW, Schofl R, Niederle B, Wildling R, Thurnher S & Lammer J. Palliative treatment of obstructing esophageal cancer with nitinol stents: value, safety, and long-term results. *Am J Roentgenol* 1996; **166**: 79–84.

47. Hoepffner N, Foerster E & Domschke W. A new balloon system for complete dilation of self-expanding mesh stents in malignant esophageal stenosis. *Endoscopy* 1996; **28**: 472–3.

48. Tampieri I, Triossi O, Melandri G, Michieletti G & Casetti T. Distal migration of an esophageal prosthesis: a new technique for endoscopic retrieval. *Endoscopy* 1994; **26**: 268.

49. Rosen C & Goldberg RI. Repositioning of a migrated esophageal stent using a retroflexed endoscope (letter) *Gastrointest Endosc* 1995; **42**: 278–9.

50. Axelrad AM, Fleischer DE & Gomes M. Nitinol coil esophageal prosthesis: advantages of removable self-expanding metallic stents. *Gastrointest Endosc* 1996; **43**: 155–60.

51. Feins RH, Johnstone DW, Baronos ES & O'Neil SM. Palliation of inoperable esophageal carcinoma with the Wallstent endoprosthesis. *Ann Thorac Surg* 1996; **62**: 1603–7.

52. Song HY, Do YS, Han YM *et al*. Covered, expandable esophageal metallic stent tubes:

experiences in 119 patients. *Radiology* 1994; **193**: 689–95.

53. Moores DW & Ilves R. Treatment of esophageal obstruction with covered, self-expanding esophageal Wallstents. *Ann Thorac Surg* 1996; **62**: 963–7.

54. Conio M, Caroli-Bosc F, Maes B *et al*. Early migration of a covered self-expanding metal stent corrected by implantation of a second stent. *Am J Gastroenterol* 1996; **91**: 2212–4.

55. Loizou LA, Rampton D & Bown SG. Treatment of malignant strictures of the cervical esophagus by endoscopic intubation using modified endoprostheses. *Gastrointest Endosc* 1992; **38**: 158–64.

56. Segalin A, Granelli P, Bonavina L, Siardi C, Mazzoleni L & Peracchia A. Self-expanding esophageal prosthesis. Effective palliation for inoperable carcinoma of the cervical esophagus. *Surg Endosc* 1994; **8**: 1343–5.

57. Wishingrad M, Kim M & Triadafilopoulos G. Early dysphagia after placement of a self-expanding esophageal stent: severe esophagitis mimicking luminal occlusion. *Am J Gastroenterol* 1995; **90**: 1525–6.

58. Maunoury V, Brunetaud JM, Cochelard D *et al*. Endoscopic palliation for inoperable malignant dysphagia: long term follow up. *Gut* 1992; **33**: 1602–7.

59. De Palma GD, Galloro G, Sivero L *et al*. Self-expanding metal stents for palliation of inoperable carcinoma of the esophagus and gastresophageal junction. *Am J Gastroenterol* 1995; **90**: 2140–2.

60. Simsek H, Oksuzoglu G & Akhan O. Endoscopic Nd:YAG laser therapy for esophageal wallstent occlusion due to tumor ingrowth. *Endoscopy* 1996; **28**: 400.

61. Schoefl R, Winkelbauer F, Haefner M, Poetzi R, Gangl A & Lammer J. Two cases of fractured esophageal nitinol stents. *Endoscopy* 1996; **28**: 518–20.

62. Hendra KP & Saukkonen JJ. Erosion of the right mainstem bronchus by an esophageal stent. *Chest* 1996; **110**: 857–8.

63. May A, Selmaier M, Hochberger J *et al*. Memory metal stents for palliation of malignant obstruction of the oesophagus and cardia. *Gut* 1995; **37**: 309–13.

64. Mason R. Palliation of malignant dysphagia: an alternative to surgery. *Ann R Coll Surg Engl* 1996; **78**: 457–62.

65. May A, Hahn EG & Ell C. Self-expanding metal stents for palliation of malignant obstruction in the upper gastrointestinal tract. Comparative assessment of three stent types implemented in 96 implantations. *J Clin Gastroenterol* 1996; **22**: 261–6.

66. Oliver SE, Robertson CS, Logan RFA *et al*. What does radiotherapy or chemothreapy add to survival over endoscopic palliation alone in inoperable squamous cell oesophageal cancer. *Gut* 1990; **31**: 750–2.

67. Reed CE, Marsh WH, Carlson LS *et al*. Prospective, randomised palliative treatment for unresectable cancer of the esophagus. *Ann Thorac Surg* 1991; **51**: 552–6.

68. Schmid EU, Alberts AS, Greeff F *et al*. The value of radiotherapy or chemotherapy after intubation for advanced esophageal carcinoma – a prospective randomized trial. *Radiother Oncol* 1993; **28**: 27–30.

69. Swain CP, Bown SG, Edwards DA, Kirkham JS, Salmon PR & Clark CG. Laser recanalization of obstructing foregut cancer. *Br J Surg* 1984; **71**: 112–15.

70. Krasner N, Barr H, Skidmore C & Morris AI. Palliative laser therapy for malignant dysphagia. *Gut* 1987; **28**: 792–8.

71. Fleischer D, Kessler F & Haye O. Endoscopic Nd: YAG laser therapy for carcinoma of the esophagus: a new palliative approach. *Am J Surg* 1982; **143**: 280–3.

72. Fleischer D & Kessler F. Endoscopic Nd:YAG laser therapy for carcinoma of the esophagus: a new form of palliative treatment. *Gastroenterology* 1983; **85**: 600–6.

73. Goldberg SJ & King KH. Endoscopic Nd:YAG laser coagulation as palliative therapy for obstructing esophageal carcinoma. *Am J Gastroenterol* 1986; **81**: 629–33.

74. Karlin DA, Fisher RS & Krevsky B. Prolonged survival and effective palliation in patients with squamous cell carcinoma of the esophagus following endoscopic laser therapy. *Cancer* 1987; **59**: 1969–72.

75. Radford CM, Ahlquist DA, Gostout CJ, Viggiano TR, Balm RK & Zinsmeister AR. Prospective comparison of contact with noncontact Nd:Yag laser therapy for palliation of esophageal carcinoma. *Gastrointest Endosc* 1989; **35**: 394–7.

76. Mason RC, Briht N & McColl I. Palliation of malignant dysphagia with laser therapy : predictability of results. *Br J Surg* 1991; **78**: 1346–7.

77. Murray FE, Bowers GJ, Birkett DH & Cave DR. Palliative laser therapy of advanced esophageal carcinoma: an alternative perspective. *Am J Gastroenterol* 1988; **83**: 816–19.

78. Naunheim KS, Petruska PJ, Roy TS, Schlueter JM, Kim H & Baue AE. Multimodality therapy

for adenocarcinoma of the esophagus. *Ann Thorac Surg* 1995; **59**: 1085–90.

79. Bader M, Dittler HJ, Ultsch B, Ries G & Siewert JR. Palliative treatment of malignant stenoses of the upper gastrointestinal tract using a combination of laser and afterloading therapy. *Endoscopy* 1986; **18** (Suppl): 27–31.

80. Sander R, Hagenmueller F, Sander C, Riess G & Classen M. Laser versus laser plus afterloading with iridium-192 in the palliative treatment of malignant stenosis of the esophagus: a prospective, randomized, and controlled study. *Gastrointest Endosc* 1991; **37**: 433–40.

81. Shmueli E, Srivastava E, Dawes PJ, Clague M, Matthewson K & Record CO. Combination of laser treatment and intraluminal radiotherapy for malignant dysphagia. *Gut* 1996; **38**: 803–5.

82. Spencer GM, Thorpe SM, Sargeant IR *et al*. Laser and brachytherapy in the palliation of adenocarcinoma of the oesophagus and cardia. *Gut* 1996; **39**: 726–31.

83. Bown SG. Palliation of malignant dysphagia: surgery, radiotherapy, laser, intubation alone or in combination? *Gut* 1991; **32**: 841–4.

84. Adam A, Ellul J, Watkinson AF *et al*. Palliation of inoperable esophageal carcinoma: a prospective randomized trial of laser therapy and stent placement. *Radiology* 1997; **202**: 344–8.

85. Loizou LA, Grigg D, Atkinson M, Robertson C & Brown SG. A prospective comparison of laser therapy and intubation in endoscopic palliation for malignant dysphagia. *Gastroenterology* 1991; **100**: 1303–10.

86. Alderson D & Wright PD. Laser recanalization versus endoscopic intubation in the palliation of malignant dysphagia. *Br J Surg* 1990; **77**: 1151–3.

87. Carter R, Smith JS & Anderson JR. Laser recanalization versus endoscopic intubation in the palliation of malignant dysphagia: a randomized prospective study. *Br J Surg* 1992; **79**: 1167–70.

88. Atkinson M. Esophageal intubation (Meeting abstract). *International Congress on Cancer of the Esophagus: Recent Advances in Biology, Prevention, Diagnosis and Treatment.* June 7–10, 1992, Genoa, Italy, 1992.

89. Sculpher MJ, Sargeant IR, Loizou LA, Thorpe SM, Spencer GM & Bown SG. A cost analysis of Nd:YAG laser ablation versus endoscopic intubation for the palliation of malignant dysphagia. *Eur J Cancer* 1995; **31A**: 1640–6.

90. Grund KE, Storek D, Zindel C & Becker HD. Highly flexible self-expanding metal mesh stents: a new kind of palliative therapy of malig-

nant dysphagia. *Z Gastroenterol* 1995; **33**: 392–8.

91. Barr H, Krasner N, Raouf A & Walker RJ. Prospective randomised trial of laser therapy only and laser therapy followed by endoscopic intubation for the palliation of malignant dysphagia. *Gut* 1990; **31**: 252–8.

92. Lindberg CG, Cwikiel W, Ivancev K, Lundstedt C, Stridbeck H & Tranberg KG. Laser therapy and insertion of Wallstents for palliative treatment of oesophageal carcinoma. *Acta Radiol* 1991; **32**: 345–8.

93. Sargeant IR, Loizou LA , Tulloch M, Thorpe S & Brown SG. Recanalization of tube overgrowth: a useful new indication for laser in palliation of malignant dysphagia. *Gastrointest Endosc* 1992; **38**: 165–9.

94. Tranberg KG, Stael von Holstein C, Ivancev K, Cwikiel W & Lunderquist A. The YAG laser and Wallstent endoprosthesis for palliation of cancer in the esophagus or gastric cardia. *Hepatogastroenterology* 1995; **42**: 139–44.

95. Sibille A, Lambert R, Souquet JC, Sabben G & Descos F. Long term survival after photodynamic therapy for esophageal cancer. *Gastroenterology* 1995; **108**: 337–44.

96. Regula J, MacRobert AJ, Gorchein A *et al*. Photosensitisation and photodynamic therapy of oesophageal, duodenal and colorectal tumors using 5-aminolaevulinic acid induced proptoporphryin IX – a pilot study. *Gut* 1995; **36**: 67–75.

97. Heier SK, Rothman KA, Heier LM & Rosenthal WS. Photodynamic therapy for obstructing esophageal cancer: light dosimetry and randomized comparison with Nd:YAG laser therapy. *Gastroenterology* 1995; **109**: 63–72.

98. Lightdale CJ, Heier SK, Marcon NE *et al*. Photodynamic therapy with porfimer sodium versus thermal ablation therapy with Nd:YAG laser for palliation of esophageal cancer: a multicenter randomized trial. *Gastrointest Endosc* 1995; **42**: 507–12.

99. Wang KK & Geller A. Photodynamic therapy for early esophageal cancers : light versus surgical might. *Gastroenterology* 1995; **108**: 593–607.

100. Hayata Y, Kato H, Konaka C *et al*. Photoradiation therapy in early stage cancer cases of the lung, esophagus and stomach. In: Andreoni A & Cubeddu R (eds) *Porphryins in Tumor Phototherapy.* New York: Plenum Press 1984: 405–12.

101. Okuda S, Mimura S, Otani T, Ichii M & Tatsuta M. Experimental and clinical studies on HPD-photoradiation therapy for upper gastrointest-

inal cancer. In: Andreoni A & Cubeddu R (eds) *Porphryins in Tumor Phototherapy*. New York: Plenum Press 1984: 413–7.

102. Okunaka T, Kato H, Conaka C, Yamamoto H, Bonaminio A & Eckhauser ML Photodynamic therapy of esophageal carcinoma. *Surg Endosc* 1990; **4**: 150–3.

103. McCaughan JS, Nims TA, Guy IT *et al.* Photodynamic therapy for oesophageal tumors. *Arch Surg* 1989; **124**: 74–80.

104. Marcon NE, Haber G, Kortan P & Kandel G. Photodynamic therapy (PDT) in the treatment of carcinoma of the esophagus and cardia (meeting abstract). Third Biennial Meeting of the International Photodynamic Association. July 17–21, Buffalo, NY, 1990: 31.

105. Marcon NE. Photodynamic therapy and cancer of the esophagus. *Semin Oncol* 1994; **21**: 20–3.

106. Patrice T, Foultier MT, Yactayo S *et al.* Endoscopic photodynamic therapy with hematoporphyrin derivative for primary treatment of gastrointestinal neoplasms in inoperable patients. *Dig Dis Sci* 1990; **35**: 545–52.

107. Messmann H, Holstege A, Szeimies RM, Lock G, Bown SG & Scholmerich J. Photodynamic therapy: a safe and effective treatment for tumor overgrowth in patients with oesophageal cancer and metal stents. *Endoscopy* 1995; **27**: 629.

108. Overholt BF & Panjehpour M. Photodynamic therapy in Barrett's esophagus: reduction of specialized mucosa, ablation of dysplasia, and treatment of superficial esophageal cancer. *Semin Surg Oncol* 1995; **11**: 372–6.

109. Angelini G, Pasini AF, Ederle A, Castagnini A, Talamini G & Bulighin G. Nd:YAG laser versus polidocanol injection for palliation of esophageal malignancy: a prospective, randomized study. *Gastrointest Endosc* 1991; **37**: 607–10.

110. Payne-James JJ, Spiller RC, Misiewicz JJ & Siolk DBA. Use of ethanol induced tumour necrosis to palliate dysphagia in patients with oesopha-gogastric cancer. *Gastrointest Endosc* 1990; **36**: 43–6.

111. Khansur T, Allred C & Tavassoli M. 5-Fluorouracil, adriamycin, and mitomycin C in adenocarcinoma of the esophagus or gastresophageal junction tumors. *Am J Clin Oncol* 1994; **17**: 506–8.

112. Ajani JA, Ilson DH, Daugherty K, Pazdur R, Lynch PM & Kelsen DP. Activity of taxol in patients with squamous cell carcinoma and adenocarcinoma of the esophagus. *J Natl Cancer Inst* 1994; **86**: 1086–91.

113. Javed T, Reed C , Walle T, Stuart RK, Ibrado AM & Bhalla K. A regimen of paclitaxel (P), cisplatin (CP) and 5-fluorouracil (FU) followed by G-CSF is highly active against epidermoid and adenocarcinoma of esophagus (Meeting abstract). *Proc Annu Meet Am Soc Clin Oncol* 1995; **14**: A456.

114. Wadler S, Fell S, Haynes H, Katz HJ, Rozenblit A, Kaleya R & Wiernik PH. Treatment of carcinoma of the esophagus with 5-fluorouracil and recombinant alfa-2a-interferon. *Cancer* 1993; **71**: 1726–30.

115. Wadler S, Haynes H, Beitler JJ *et al.* Phase II clinical trial with 5-fluorouracil, recombinant interferon- alpha-2b, and cisplatin for patients with metastatic or regionally advanced carcinoma of the esophagus. *Cancer* 1996; **78**: 30–4.

116. Walsh TN, Noonan N, Hollywood D, Kelly A, Keeling N & Hennessy TP. A comparison of multimodal therapy and surgery for esophageal adenocarcinoma. *N Engl J Med* 1996; **335**: 462–7.

117. Takiyama W, Fujii M & Moriwaki S. Small cell carcinoma of the esophagus: report of a case treated with chemotherapy. *Jpn J Surg* 1988; **18**: 330–5.

118. Clark T, Lee MJ & Munk PL. Primary small-cell carcinoma of the oesophagus with spontaneous oesophageal perforation following chemotherapy. *Australas Radiol* 1996; **40**: 250–3.

INDEX

Note: Page numbers in **bold type** indicate major discussions